Advanced Biomaterials for Dental Applications

Advanced Biomaterials for Dental Applications

Guest Editor
Ines Despotović

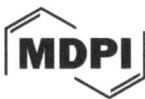

Basel • Beijing • Wuhan • Barcelona • Belgrade • Novi Sad • Cluj • Manchester

Guest Editor
Ines Despotović
Division of Physical Chemistry
Ruđer Bošković Institute
Zagreb
Croatia

Editorial Office
MDPI AG
Grosspeteranlage 5
4052 Basel, Switzerland

This is a reprint of the Special Issue, published open access by the journal *Materials* (ISSN 1996-1944), freely accessible at: https://www.mdpi.com/journal/materials/special_issues/C83L5K3Z14.

For citation purposes, cite each article independently as indicated on the article page online and as indicated below:

Lastname, A.A.; Lastname, B.B. Article Title. *Journal Name* **Year**, *Volume Number*, Page Range.

ISBN 978-3-7258-4001-4 (Hbk)
ISBN 978-3-7258-4002-1 (PDF)
https://doi.org/10.3390/books978-3-7258-4002-1

© 2025 by the authors. Articles in this book are Open Access and distributed under the Creative Commons Attribution (CC BY) license. The book as a whole is distributed by MDPI under the terms and conditions of the Creative Commons Attribution-NonCommercial-NoDerivs (CC BY-NC-ND) license (https://creativecommons.org/licenses/by-nc-nd/4.0/).

Contents

About the Editor vii

Joanna Wysokińska-Miszczuk, Katarzyna Piotrowska, Michał Paulo and Monika Madej
Composite Materials Used for Dental Fillings
Reprinted from: *Materials* 2024, 17, 4936, https://doi.org/10.3390/ma17194936 1

Jolanta Szymańska, Monika Krzywicka, Zbigniew Kobus, Anna Malm and Agnieszka Grzegorczyk
The Influence of Selected Titanium Alloy Micro-Texture Parameters on Bacterial Adhesion
Reprinted from: *Materials* 2024, 17, 4765, https://doi.org/10.3390/ma17194765 16

Moritz Waldecker, Stefan Rues, Peter Rammelsberg and Wolfgang Bömicke
Dimensional Accuracy of Novel Vinyl Polysiloxane Compared with Polyether Impression Materials: An In Vitro Study
Reprinted from: *Materials* 2024, 17, 4221, https://doi.org/10.3390/ma17174221 27

Matilde Ruiz-Linares, Vsevolod Fedoseev, Carmen Solana, Cecilia Muñoz-Sandoval and Carmen María Ferrer-Luque
Antibiofilm Efficacy of Calcium Silicate-Based Endodontic Sealers
Reprinted from: *Materials* 2024, 17, 3937, https://doi.org/10.3390/ma17163937 39

Nicolás Gutiérrez Robledo, Miquel Punset Fuste, Alejandra Rodríguez-Contreras, Fernando García Marro, José María Manero Planella, Oscar Figueras-Álvarez and Miguel Roig Cayón
In Vitro Assessment of a New Block Design for Implant Crowns with Functional Gradient Fabricated with Resin Composite and Zirconia Insert
Reprinted from: *Materials* 2024, 17, 3815, https://doi.org/10.3390/ma17153815 49

Ines Despotović, Željka Petrović, Jozefina Katić and Dajana Mikić
Alendronate as Bioactive Coating on Titanium Surfaces: An Investigation of CaP–Alendronate Interactions
Reprinted from: *Materials* 2024, 17, 2703, https://doi.org/10.3390/ma17112703 71

Isabela da Rocha Silva, Aline Tavares da Silva Barreto, Renata Santos Seixas, Paula Nunes Guimarães Paes, Juliana do Nascimento Lunz, Rossana Mara da Silva Moreira Thiré and Paula Mendes Jardim
Novel Strategy for Surface Modification of Titanium Implants towards the Improvement of Osseointegration Property and Antibiotic Local Delivery
Reprinted from: *Materials* 2023, 16, 2755, https://doi.org/10.3390/ma16072755 86

Michał Ciszyński, Bartosz Chwaliszewski, Wojciech Simka, Marzena Dominiak, Tomasz Gedrange and Jakub Hadzik
Zirconia Dental Implant Designs and Surface Modifications: A Narrative Review
Reprinted from: *Materials* 2024, 17, 4202, https://doi.org/10.3390/ma17174202 104

Ko Nakanishi, Tsukasa Akasaka, Hiroshi Hayashi, Kumiko Yoshihara, Teppei Nakamura, Mariko Nakamura, et al.
From Tooth Adhesion to Bioadhesion: Development of Bioabsorbable Putty-like Artificial Bone with Adhesive to Bone Based on the New Material "Phosphorylated Pullulan"
Reprinted from: *Materials* 2024, 17, 3671, https://doi.org/10.3390/ma17153671 118

Andrea Galve-Huertas, Louis Decadt, Susana García-González, Federico Hernández-Alfaro and Samir Aboul-Hosn Centenero
Immediate Implant Placement with Soft Tissue Augmentation Using Acellular Dermal Matrix Versus Connective Tissue Graft: A Systematic Review and Meta-Analysis
Reprinted from: *Materials* **2024**, *17*, 5285, https://doi.org/10.3390/ma17215285 . . . . **134**

About the Editor

Ines Despotović

Dr. Ines Despotović is a senior research associate at the Ruđer Bošković Institute in Zagreb, Croatia. She received her BSc (1993), MSc (1996) and PhD (2002) degrees in Computational Organic Chemistry from the University of Zagreb, Croatia. She is a Guest Editor for a Special Issue of MDPI's *Materials*. Her main research interests relate to the following topics: multifunctional dental materials, bone tissue engineering, mechanical behavior of dental materials, surface modification and surface characterization methods.

Composite Materials Used for Dental Fillings

Joanna Wysokińska-Miszczuk [1], Katarzyna Piotrowska [2,*], Michał Paulo [1] and Monika Madej [2]

[1] Faculty of Medical Dentistry, Medical University of Lublin, ul. Chodźki 6 Ave, 20-093 Lublin, Poland; joanna.wysokinska-miszczuk@umlub.pl (J.W.-M.); michal.paulo@umlub.pl (M.P.)
[2] Faculty of Mechatronics and Mechanical Engineering, Kielce University of Technology, al. Tysiąclecia Państwa Polskiego 7, 25-314 Kielce, Poland; mmadej@tu.kielce.pl
* Correspondence: kpawelec@tu.kielce.pl

Abstract: This article explores the properties of composite materials employed in dental fillings. A traditional nano-hybrid composite containing nanofiller particles exceeding 82% by weight served as a benchmark. The remaining samples were fabricated from ormocer resin, maintaining an identical nanofiller content of 84%. In all specimens, the nanoparticles were dispersed randomly within the matrix. This study presents findings from investigations into surface geometry, hardness, wettability, and tribological behavior. The microscopic observations revealed that ormocer-based samples exhibited greater surface roughness than those composed of the traditional composite. Hardness testing indicated that both ceramic addition and sample preparation significantly influenced mechanical properties. Ceramic-enhanced samples demonstrated superior hardness, surpassing the reference composite by 30% and 43%, respectively. Contact angle measurements revealed hydrophilic characteristics in the classic composite, contrasting with the hydrophobic nature of ceramic-containing samples. Tribological evaluations revealed the superiority of the classic composite in terms of friction coefficients and volumetric wear compared to ormocer-based materials.

Keywords: dental composites; ormocer resin; surface texture; hardness; wettability; friction; wear

1. Introduction

Modern dentistry offers a range of advanced materials capable of restoring both the function and esthetics of teeth, such as the shape and color of damaged tissues. These solutions are tailored to the individual needs and expectations of patients, and dental services not only provide therapeutic benefits but also enhance the quality of life [1]. Materials used for dental fillings must possess suitable mechanical, tribological, and physicochemical properties while maintaining biocompatibility with natural tooth tissues.

When designing new dental composites, it is crucial to achieve composites with a low coefficient of friction and minimal wear while exerting minimal influence on the wear of opposing tooth tissues. To reduce wear and the coefficient of friction of dental materials, the composition of the fillers used is intensively modified [2]. The latest literature indicates a significant impact of nanoparticles on the structure and performance properties of composites. Compared to commonly used macro- and microparticles, nanoparticles are characterized by uniform dispersion in the resin on a nanoscale. As a result, nanocomposites exhibit greater hardness and wear resistance. Additionally, the presence of nanoparticles contributes to a reduction in polymerization shrinkage, a decrease in water absorption, and an increase in the likelihood of achieving a smoother surface due to polishing [3,4].

A key aspect of designing new dental composites is achieving materials with low friction coefficients and wear resistance, ensuring longer service life and minimal impact on the wear of opposing tooth tissues. Dental composites should exhibit a synergistic interaction with natural tooth tissues. To improve these properties, the composition of the fillers used is continuously modified, with the use of nanoparticles playing an increasingly important role. Nanoparticles, due to their uniform distribution in the resin matrix, significantly improve the hardness, wear resistance, and esthetic properties of composites. This distribution, on a nanoscale, allows for the creation of a more homogeneous structure, which reduces stress concentration and improves the strength of the material. The large specific surface area of nanoparticles enables better bonding with the matrix, increasing adhesion between the components of the composite. The use of nanoparticles also improves the esthetic properties of dental composites, as they have the ability to scatter light in a manner closer to that of natural tooth tissue. When reconstructing teeth in visible areas, using nanocomposites allows for better color matching and translucency. Additionally, the use of nanocomposites increases durability and reduces the risk of material degradation, as they exhibit higher resistance to chemical agents present in the oral cavity, such as acids and enzymes. All these aspects are crucial for the long-term success of dental treatment. Modifying dental composite fillers by introducing nanoparticles into the polymer matrix represents a modern approach to improving the quality and effectiveness of materials used in dentistry [4–6].

The literature features extensive research on nanofiller-reinforced dental composites [7–11], yet the diversity of components complicates direct comparisons of their performance characteristics.

The researchers in [12] examined how adding silica nanoparticles to ceramic–polymer composites affected their mechanical and wear-and-tear properties. They focused on how the type, amount, and size of the filler particles influenced the overall performance of the composite. The researchers primarily used silica powder with particles $5 \div 10$ μm in diameter and a density of 2.38 g/cm^3. They incorporated a nanofiller, silanized silica R709, with particles measuring 40 nm and a density of 2.20 g/cm^3. The organic component consisted of methacrylate monomers: Bis-GMA and TEGMA. The filler constituted 55–60% of the composite's volume. The prepared samples were solidified using a light-activated polymerization process.

Vickers microhardness testing revealed that adding nanofillers enhanced the composite's hardness. Samples composed entirely of micro-silica powder, with 60.7% filler, exhibited a hardness of 58.8 kPa. However, when 15% of the filler was replaced with nanopowder, the hardness increased to 65.5 kPa, exceeding the original hardness by over 10%. Wear-and-tear evaluations demonstrated that samples containing both micro- and nano-silica powders, with a total filler content of 60% and 10% nanopowder, exhibited the lowest wear. Furthermore, the friction coefficients were lowest when 10% of the filler consisted of nanopowder. According to these authors, the addition of SiO nanopowder has a positive impact on microhardness and tribological properties, with the best results obtained at 10–15% volume of the composite.

In [13], the authors also investigated the tribological properties of ceramic–polymer composites. The composites had an organic matrix comprising a mixture of Bis-GMA, TEGDMA, and DEA-EMA resins, and a system of photoinitiators and stabilizers. The authors introduced powdered fillers such as fluoride, nanosilica (n-SiO_2), and a friction modifier—polyethylene (PE)—into the organic matrix. The fillers underwent a silanization process in a silane solution. This process involved depositing active silane groups onto the surface of the filler particles in a vacuum evaporator. After homogenization, the composites were cured in PTFE molds for 40 s. Friction tests were conducted on a specially designed dental friction simulator—a pneumatically controlled pin-on-disc tribological tester operating in reciprocating motion under lubrication with a pH 6.8 solution, corresponding to the pH of human saliva. The counter sample was human enamel embedded in an aluminum frame. The results showed that both the strontium fluoride-based composite and the ytterbium fluoride-added composite exhibited similar friction coefficient values, with slightly lower values recorded for the composite with added ytterbium fluoride. Simultaneously, greater linear and volumetric wear was recorded for this material. During the study, the authors observed that the wear of ceramic–polymer composites intended for permanent dental fillings depended on the type of powdered filler and was lower for a composite with strontium fluoride.

Studies [14–21] indicate that the tribological properties of dental resin-based composites are significantly influenced by the morphology, homogeneity, and concentration of inorganic fillers. The authors of [16] investigated the effect of hydroxyapatite (HA) particles on the tribological behavior of resin-based composites. They found that a composite containing 0.4% by volume of filler particles exhibited optimal hardness, reduced wear, and a lower coefficient of friction. In addition to HA particles, [17] explored the effect of reinforcing the polymer matrix with two distinct types of ceramic particles, alumina and silica. The authors concluded that incorporating alumina into the polymer matrix enhances wear resistance. In turn, [18] observed that composites with organic fillers demonstrated the lowest coefficient of friction and wear.

Recent studies have dealt with the application of nanomaterials to different medicine areas, which has led to a new discipline known as nanomedicine. Nanotechnology has the potential to revolutionize the field of healthcare diagnostics by improving the accuracy, sensitivity, and speed of medical tests. Polymer nanocomposites offer new opportunities for modern medicine to generate products for antibacterial treatment [22], tissue engineering [23], cancer therapy [24], medical imaging [25], dental applications [26], drug delivery, etc. [27]. There are also potential uses in designing medical tools and processes for the new generation of medical scientists.

This study comprehensively characterized the surface layer and mechanical/physicochemical properties of materials used for dental fillings. A key aspect was evaluating their tribological behavior when lubricated with artificial saliva. The innovative approach involved applying materials in single or multiple layers and conducting tests at 37 °C to mimic oral conditions.

2. Materials and Methods

The NHO-1 and NHO-4 test materials were made of ormocer resin. These materials have indications for single-layer restorations up to 4 mm. They consisted of nanoscale particles and did not differ in filler content, with the filler particles being randomly dispersed in the matrix (in all tested composites). The NH sample, on the other hand, served as a reference material with a nano-hybrid structure containing nanoparticle fillers. Samples were prepared according to the manufacturer's recommendations. The characteristics of the composite resins used are presented in Table 1.

Table 1. Test materials were prepared according to the description below.

Parameters	Materials		
	NH	NHO-1	NHO-4
Sample	Classic composite	Bulk fill one layer	Bulk fill four layers
Type	Nano-hybrid	Nano-hybrid ormocer	Nano-hybrid ormocer
Matrix and filler	Based on silicone dioxide	Based on silicone dioxide	Based on silicone dioxide
Filler content (%by weight)	>82	84	84

For NHO-1 and NHO-4 (VOCO, Cuxhaven, Germany), each 0.5 mm thick layer was applied directly from the package and then condensed using dental instruments (a flat plastic tool) for 60 s. A flat plastic tool is a basic dental instrument used for applying and modeling fillings. It has two tips: a spatula and a ball. The spatula is suitable for applying the material, modeling the cusps, and giving the filling its final shape. The ball end (a ball burnisher) works perfectly when condensing the material. The first layer was applied directly to the surface of the metal piston, and then, using an LED Translux Wave lamp (KULZER, Hanau, Germany) with a power of >1200 mW/cm^2 and a wavelength of 440–480 nm, the first 0.5 mm thick layer was irradiated for 60 s. Subsequent portions of the composite were applied to the already polymerized layers and irradiated again. For each irradiation, the SoftStart function was used (this involves starting the polymerization with a relatively low-intensity light, which gradually increases during the device's operating cycle). Before each use of the lamp, its power was checked using the measuring device installed in the lamp base. Samples were produced using the composite at room temperature. The NH material (Megadenta, Radeberg, Germany) was prepared as a single 3 mm thick layer. It was applied in a single portion directly to the device piston and then condensed using dental instruments for 120 s (a flat dental condenser and a ball condenser). The thickness of a single layer was permissible by the manufacturer according to the instructions (a layer up to 4 mm thick). Then, using an LED Translux Wave lamp with a power of >1200 mW/cm^2 and a wavelength of 440–480 nm, the entire 3 mm thick layer was irradiated for 60 s.

The samples were prepared using a device (Figure 1) designed for creating individual color guides for composite or porcelain materials. This tool enabled the production of discs with a diameter of 12 mm and a thickness of 3 mm. Thanks to the design of this tool and the embedded scale, it was possible to precisely measure the thickness of each individual layer applied to create the final sample in the form of a disc.

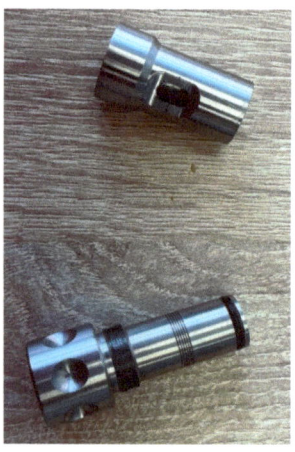
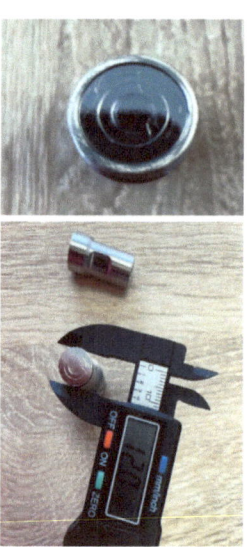

Figure 1. A device for creating custom composite samples.

A single operator prepared the test materials and avoided using additional dental equipment for polishing (Smile Line USA Inc., Wheat Ridge, CO, USA) after polymerization. The final layer was condensed and smoothed with a dental flat plastic tool to achieve smooth surfaces. The geometric structure of the surfaces before the tribological tests was observed using a DCM8 confocal microscope (Leica, Geneva, Switzerland). Surface topography analysis was performed based on 3D axonometric images, surface profiles, material composition curves, and selected amplitude parameters (Sq, Sv, Sp, Ssk, and Sku). The surface area under analysis was 0.157 mm^2. The results of the experiments are presented in Section 3.1.

To determine the mechanical properties, an ultra-nanoindentation hardness tester (UNHT) (Anton Paar, Baden, Switzerland) and a Berkovich indenter were employed in the instrumental indentation method. Hardness, Young's modulus, plastic work, and elastic work were calculated from the load–displacement curve. A constant loading and unloading rate of 100 mN/min, a maximum load of 50 mN, and a 5 s hold were used. The results of these tests are presented in Section 3.2.

Wettability was assessed using an Attention Theta (Biolin Scientific, Tietäjäntie, Finland) optical tensiometer and the sessile drop method. A 4 µL droplet of demineralized water and artificial saliva solution was placed on the sample surface, and the contact angle was immediately measured. Average angle values were determined from five sets of measurements. The tests were conducted at a temperature of $23 \pm 1\ °C$ and $55 \pm 5\%$ humidity. The results are presented in Section 3.3.

Tribological tests were performed using an TRB3 tribometer (Anton Paar, Baden, Switzerland). The tests were conducted in reciprocating motion under simulated saliva lubrication at 37 °C. The test parameters included a load of 1 N, frequency of 1 Hz, stroke length of 3 mm, angle of 60°, and 10,000 cycles of friction. A schematic of the friction junction is presented in Figure 2. The results are presented in Section 3.4.

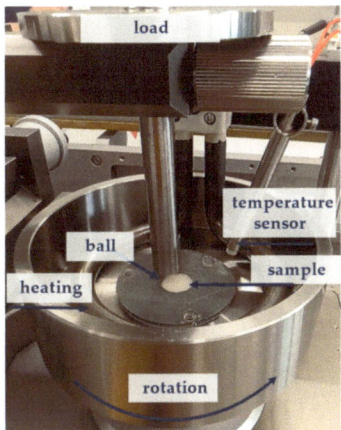

Figure 2. Friction pair.

The counter sample in the tested friction junctions was a 6 mm diameter ZrO_2 ball (Table 2).

Table 2. Mechanical and physicochemical properties of ZrO_2 [28].

			Resistance To		
Vickers Hardness, GPa	Bending Strength, MPa	Thermal Shock, °C	Chemical Exposure	Thermal Expansion Coefficient, $\times 10^{-6}/°C$	Thermal Conductivity, W/(m × K)
13	1000	280	good	7.7	3

The chemical composition of the lubricant is presented in Table 3.

Table 3. Chemical composition of the lubricant—artificial saliva [29].

			Artifical Saliva, g/dm³		
NaCl	KCl	$CaCl_2 \times 2H_2O$	$NaH_2PO_4 \times 2H_2O$	$Na_2S \times 9H_2O$	Urea
0.4	0.4	0.795	0.780	0.005	1.0

Following tribological testing, the samples were subjected to microscopic observations. The measurement area for each sample was 800 by 1000 µm. The study determined the volumetric wear of the wear tracks. To complement the study, amplitude parameters within the wear tracks were determined. The parameters were analyzed on areas of 150 by 200 µm and compared to values outside the wear track. The results are presented in Section 3.5.

3. Results

3.1. Confocal Microscopy Results

Figures 3–5 present 3D isometric views (a), material ratio curves (b), and mean primary profiles (c). Additionally, core roughness parameters were determined based on the material ratio curves: Sk—core roughness depth, Spk—mean peak height above the core roughness level, and Svk—mean valley depth below the core roughness profile (Figure 6).

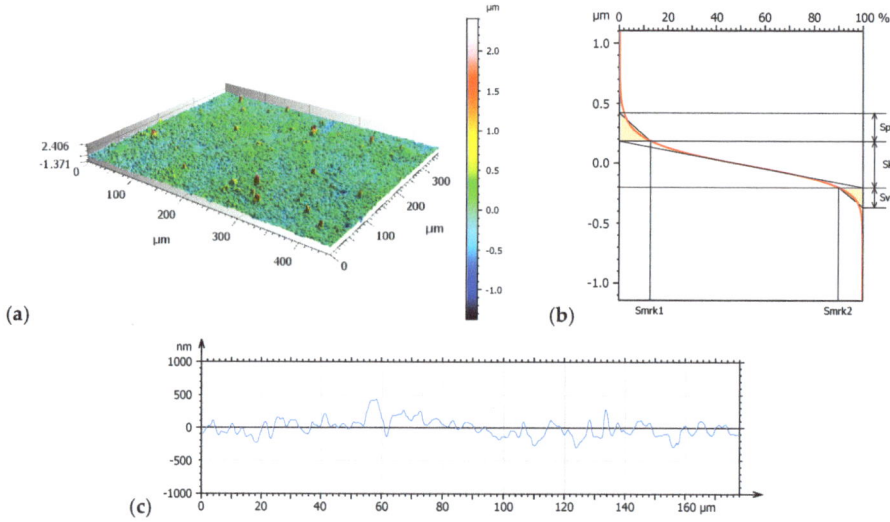

Figure 3. NH—axonometric image 3D (**a**), material ratio curve (**b**), primary surface profile (**c**).

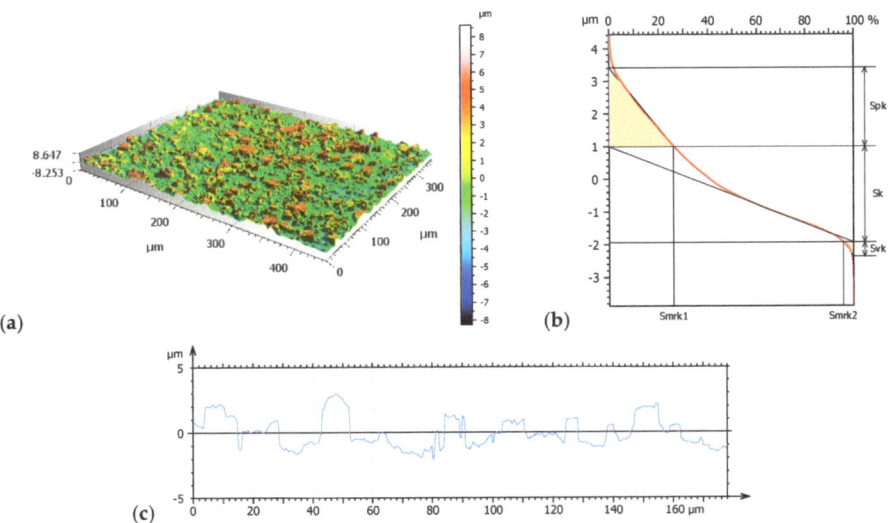

Figure 4. NHO-1—axonometric image 3D (**a**), material ratio curve (**b**), primary surface profile (**c**).

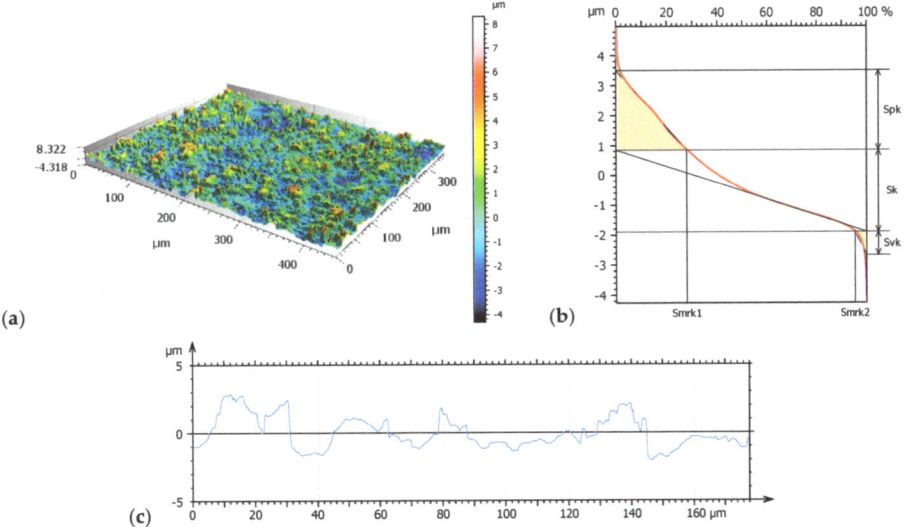

Figure 5. NHO-4—axonometric image 3D (**a**), material ratio curve (**b**), primary surface profile (**c**).

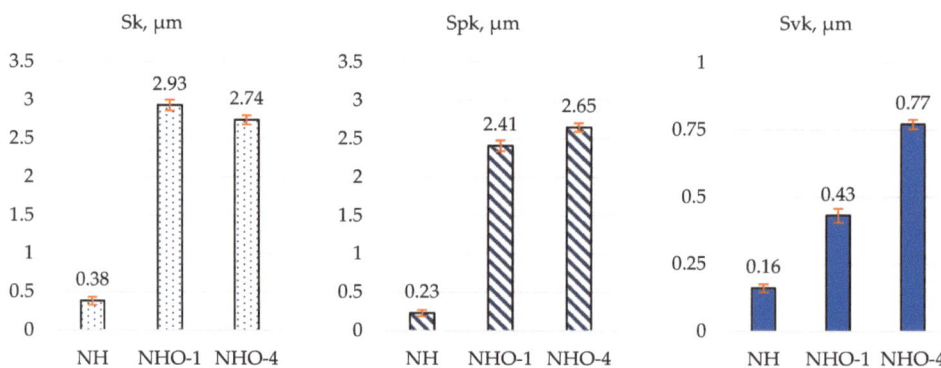

Figure 6. Core roughness parameters.

Amplitude parameters of the mean profile were determined to supplement the study. The results are shown in Table 4.

Table 4. The parameters of surface texture.

Parameter	NH		NHO-1		NHO-4	
	Mean	Stand. Dev.	Mean	Stand. Dev.	Mean	Stand. Dev.
Sq [μm]	0.21	0.02	1.58	0.15	1.53	0.15
Sv [μm]	1.66	0.16	4.58	0.45	3.84	0.45
Sp [μm]	1.81	0.19	4.91	0.23	4.45	0.23
Ssk	−0.05	0.27	0.69	0.25	0.68	0.25
Sku	4.27	0.45	2.49	0.34	2.44	0.34

Geometric surface texture analysis revealed that samples NHO-1 and NHO-4 exhibited the most pronounced surface topography. This is evidenced by the values of the amplitude parameters: Sq, Sv, and Sp. The positive values of the skewness parameter (Ssk) for all tested samples indicate the presence of steep peaks with sharp crests, most notably in samples NHO-1 and NHO-4. The kurtosis value (Sku), a measure of the peakedness of the height distribution, is also sensitive to isolated peaks or valleys. A value close to 3 indicates a normal height distribution—an even distribution of peaks and valleys on the surface. Samples NHO-1 and NHO-4 exhibit such a distribution.

Analysis of the material ratio curves (Figure 6) suggests that samples NHO-1 and NHO-4 will exhibit both the longest running-in period and the best lubrication due to the highest values of the Svk and Spk parameters compared to the classical composite. The values of these parameters were more than 10 times higher than the classical composite. Additionally, for both samples, a higher friction force is expected in the initial phase of the tribological test.

3.2. Hardness

Figure 7 shows the average values of the mechanical parameters, instrumental hardness (HIT) and Young's modulus (EIT), calculated from 10 measurement series.

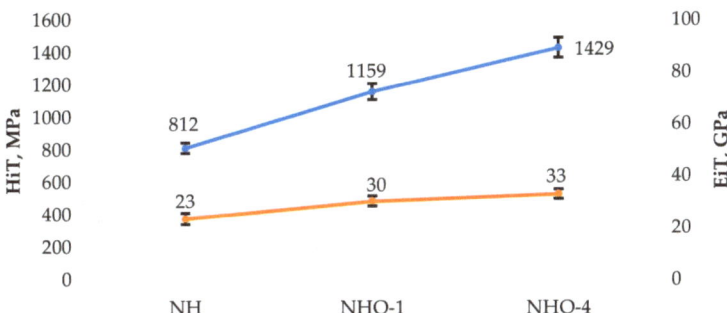

Figure 7. Results of mechanical tests: instrumental hardness (HIT), Young's modulus (EIT).

The hardness testing results indicated that the reference sample (NH) exhibited the lowest instrumental hardness of 812 MPa and a Young's modulus of 23 GPa. These parameters were approximately 47% and 30% lower, respectively, compared to the values obtained for sample number 3.

Sample NH was a nano-hybrid material (possessing typical micro-hybrid properties with the advantages of nanotechnology) with a filler content >82% by weight. As a classic composite material without ceramic additives, it exhibited the poorest performance. Additionally, its polymerization shrinkage coefficient was <1.9%, while for samples NHO-1 and NHO-4 it was <1.25%. Samples NHO-1 and NHO-4 were ceramic-based materials, with both the filler and the composite matrix made of silicon dioxide. The filler volume fraction was 84%. These properties were responsible for achieving better results. The difference between samples NHO-1 and NHO-4 is related to the sample preparation method. Disk NHO-4 was made of six layers, each 0.5 mm thick. In contrast, disk NHO-1 was made from a single 3 mm thick layer that was then polymerized as a whole, unlike sample NHO-4, where each layer was polymerized separately. Preparing the disk from multiple layers of material reduced polymerization shrinkage and improved the material's strength properties [30,31].

3.3. Contact Angle

The contact angle plays a significant role in the performance of tribological systems. Figures 8 and 9 show example images of demineralized water droplets deposited on the surfaces of the analyzed materials, while Figure 10 presents the average values of the recorded contact angles.

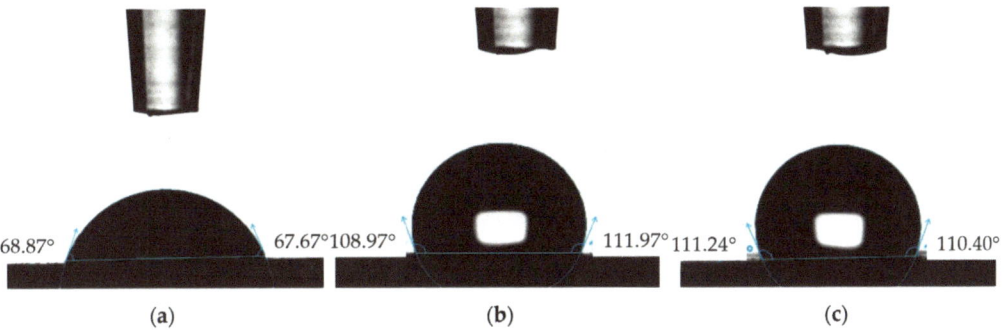

Figure 8. Examples of demineralized water droplets: (**a**) NH, (**b**) NHO-1, (**c**) NHO-4.

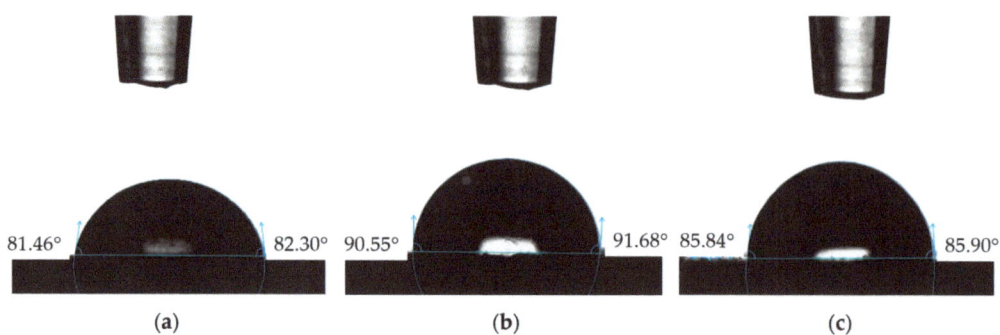

Figure 9. Examples of artificial saliva droplets: (**a**) NH, (**b**) NHO-1, (**c**) NHO-4.

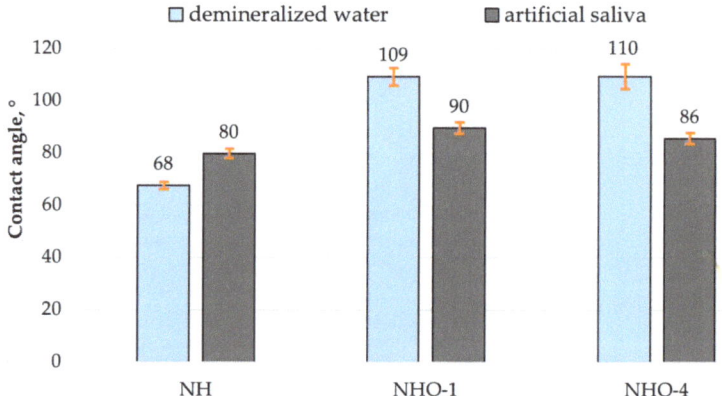

Figure 10. Average contact angle.

The results presented in Figure 10 indicate that the nature of the surface topography influences the contact angle values. The lowest contact angle values for demineralized water and artificial saliva were recorded for the reference sample NH, which had the least developed surface, while the highest values were for sample NHO-1, which had the highest roughness. Sample NH was characterized by good wettability and exhibited hydrophilic properties. In the case of samples NHO-1 and NHO-4, the contact angles with demineralized water were 110° and 109°, respectively, indicating their hydrophobic properties.

In a clinical context, dental fillings should exhibit hydrophobic properties [32]. Within the oral cavity, every tooth surface, as well as dental fillings used to restore tooth shape and function, comes into contact with saliva. Dental caries is an infectious disease, and bacteria migrate and settle on the surfaces of teeth and dental restorations. Increased hydrophilicity of dental materials can accelerate the degradation of bonds, thereby increasing the likelihood of microleakage between the patient's tissues and the composite filling. This is particularly dangerous in areas that are poorly cleaned by the patient, such as class II and V restorations. In such cases, the risk of secondary caries is significantly increased. With increasing hydrophilicity of composite materials, there is an increased risk of discoloration at the interface between the materials and the patient's tissues, as well as on the fillings themselves, which directly translates into a deterioration of the esthetic effect and increased patient dissatisfaction with treatment [33–38].

3.4. Tribological Tests

The purpose of the tribological tests was to determine the friction coefficients of the friction pairs tested. Figure 11 shows graphs of average friction coefficients recorded during friction with lubrication by the artificial saliva solution.

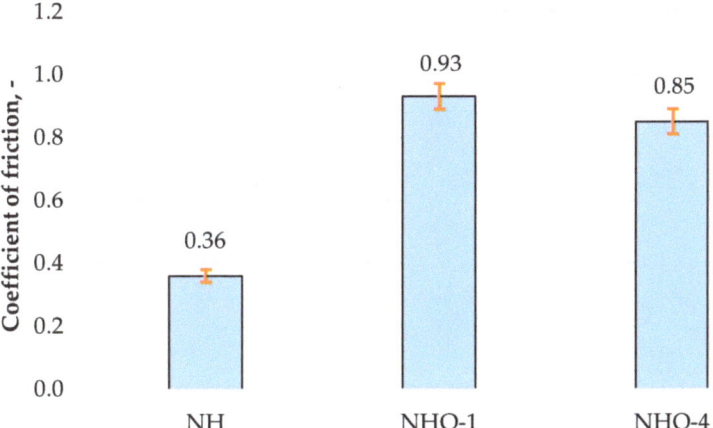

Figure 11. Friction coefficient.

Based on the results of tribological tests, it was determined that the stereometric parameters of the surface layer have a significant impact on tribological properties. The sample with the least developed surface, NH, exhibited the lowest friction coefficients, while the highest values were recorded for NHO-1. These were approximately 60% higher compared to the reference material. In the case of sample NHO-4, the recorded coefficients of friction were approximately 10% lower compared to NHO-1. This is most likely due to the better lubricating properties of this surface, related to the parameter Svk—i.e., the average depth of valleys below the core profile. The interaction of two elements moving relative to each other results in tribological wear, which largely depends on the stereometric properties of the triboelement surfaces.

3.5. Assessment of Surface Geometric Structure of Samples

Figure 12 presents microstructural images (a) and profiles (b) of the wear tracks (red area), Figure 13 shows photographs of the wear tracks on the balls, and Figure 14 presents the average wear track volume determined based on five series of measurements.

The microscopic examination results indicated that the greatest wear traces were recorded for the sample with a ceramic additive—NHO-1—and the least for the classic composite material—NH. The volumetric wear of sample NHO-4 was approximately 30% less compared to NHO-1 and resulted from the sample preparation method. In the case of NHO-1, the 3 mm thick material was polymerized as a whole, while in the case of NHO-4, each of the six layers, 0.5 mm thick, was polymerized separately, which improved its hardness and wear resistance.

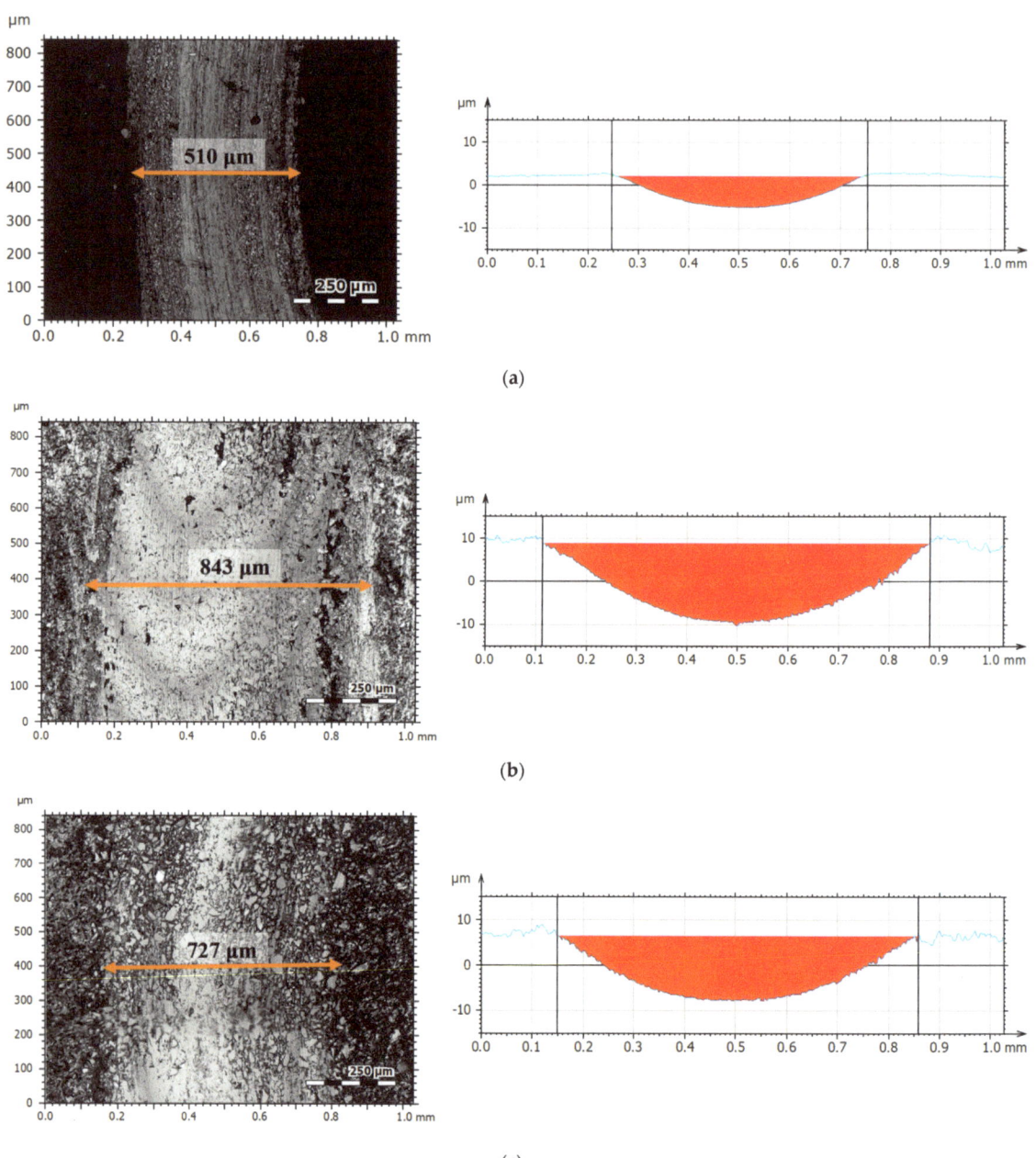

Figure 12. Wear microstructure and profiles: (**a**) NH, (**b**) NHO-1, (**c**) NHO-4.

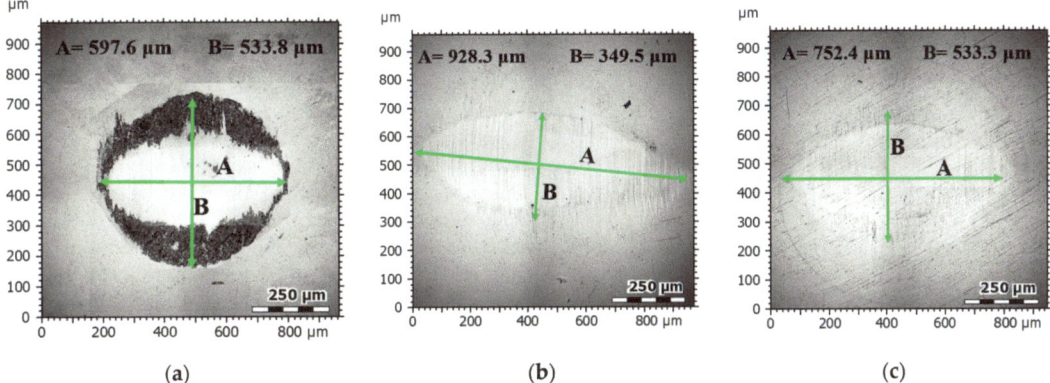

Figure 13. Ball wear track images: (a) NH, (b) NHO-1, (c) NHO-4.

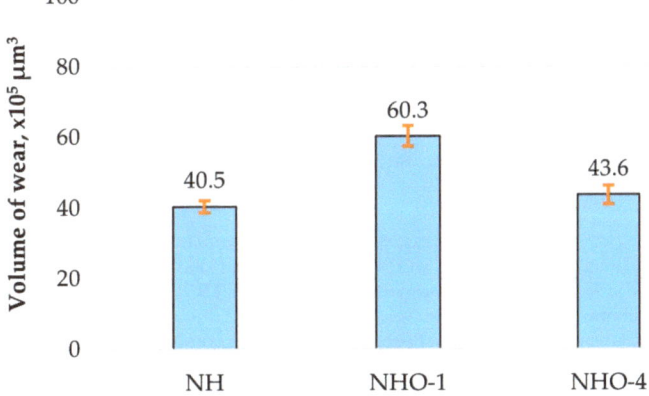

Figure 14. Volumetric wear of the samples.

4. Conclusions

The microscopic analysis showed that samples NHO-1 and NHO-4 had the most complex surface structures. Based on their material composition curves, these samples were predicted to exhibit the longest run-in time and best lubrication. The hardness tests confirmed that both the ceramic additive and the layer-by-layer polymerization method significantly improved the material's mechanical properties. Compared to the standard composite, NHO-1 and NHO-4 were 30% and 43% harder, respectively. Moreover, building up the material in 0.5 mm layers provided better results than curing it in a single 3 mm block.

The results of contact angle measurements indicated the hydrophilic properties of the classic composite, while the samples with ceramic additives were hydrophobic. From a clinical standpoint, poorly wettable materials are more desirable, as an increased hydrophilicity of dental materials can accelerate bond degradation, increase the likelihood of microleakage between the patient's tissues and the filling, and pose a potential risk of secondary caries development.

Based on the results of friction and wear tests, it was determined that the stereometric parameters of the surface layer have a significant impact on tribological properties. The classic composite exhibited the lowest friction coefficients, while the highest values were recorded for NHO-1. For the NHO-4 sample, the recorded values were approximately

10% lower compared to NHO-1, most likely due to the better lubricating properties of this surface.

The microscopic observations of the wear tracks after tribological tests showed that the classic composite—NH—exhibited the highest wear resistance. However, the material with ceramic additives—NHO-4—showed slightly worse results. The volumetric wear of this sample was only about 8% higher compared to NH.

The results suggest that further research is necessary to optimize polishing processes for improved surface quality. This includes determining optimal time and tools. Additionally, the influence of polishing pastes and composite wear under varying forces, temperatures, and coatings should be investigated to enhance the understanding of composite behavior in clinical settings, leading to the development of more durable and esthetically pleasing dental material.

Author Contributions: Conceptualization, J.W.-M. and M.M.; methodology, K.P., M.P. and M.M.; investigation, K.P. and M.P.; writing—original draft preparation, J.W.-M., K.P., M.P. and M.M.; writing—review and editing, J.W.-M., K.P., M.P. and M.M. All authors have read and agreed to the published version of the manuscript.

Funding: This research received no external funding.

Institutional Review Board Statement: Not applicable.

Informed Consent Statement: Not applicable.

Data Availability Statement: The original contributions presented in the study are included in the article, further inquiries can be directed to the corresponding author.

Conflicts of Interest: The authors declare no conflict of interest.

References

1. Nemeth, K.D.; Haluszka, D.; Seress, L.; Lovasz, B.V.; Szalma, J.; Lempel, E. Effect of Air-Polishing and Different Post-Polishing Methods on Surface Roughness of Nanofill and Microhybrid Resin Composite. *Polimers* **2022**, *14*, 1643. [CrossRef] [PubMed]
2. Siejka-Kulczyk, J.; Mystkowska, J.; Lewandowska, M.; Dąbrowski, J.R.; Kurzydłowski, K.J. The influence of nano-silica on the wear resistance of ceramic-polymer composites intended for dental fillings. *Solid State Phenom.* **2009**, *151*, 135–138. [CrossRef]
3. Mandikos, M.N.; McGivney, G.P.; Davis, E.; Bush, P.J.; Carter, M. A comparison of the wear resistance and hardness of indirect composite resins. *J. Prosthet. Dent.* **2001**, *85*, 386–395. [CrossRef] [PubMed]
4. Wilżak, A.; Nowak, J.; Szram, O.; Sokołowski, J.; Łukomska-Szymańska, M. Dental composites—The chemical structure and properties of components. Literature review. *Stomatol. Estet.* **2014**, 75–83.
5. Kleczewska, J.; Bielinski, D.; Ranganathan, N.; Sokołowski, J. Characterization of Light-Cured Dental Composites. In *Materials Characterization: Modern Methods and Applications*; Jenny Stanford Publishing: London, UK, 2015; pp. 117–148.
6. Mousavinasab, S.M. Effects of filler content on mechanical and optical properties of dental composite resin. In *Metal, Ceramic and Polymeric Composites for Various Uses*; Scitus Academics LLC.: Wilmington, DE, USA, 2011.
7. Khurshid, Z.; Zafar, M.; Qasim, S.; Shahab, S.; Naseem, M.; Abu Reqaiba, A. Advances in nanotechnology for restorative dentistry. *Materials* **2015**, *8*, 717–731. [CrossRef]
8. Zafar, M.S.; Khurshid, Z.; Najeeb, S.; Zohaib, S.; Rehman, I.U. Therapeutic applications of nanotechnology in dentistry. In *Nanostructures for Oral Medicine*; Elsevier: Amsterdam, The Netherlands, 2017; pp. 833–862.
9. Abuelenain, D.A.; Neel, E.A.A. Surface and mechanical properties of different dental composites. *Austin J. Dent.* **2015**, *2*, 1019.
10. Halvorson, R.H.; Erickson, R.L.; Davidson, C.L. The effect of filler and silane content on conversion of resin-based composite. *Dent. Mater.* **2003**, *19*, 327–333. [CrossRef]
11. Alqahtani, A.S.; Sulimany, A.M.; Alayad, A.S.; Abdulaziz, A.S.; Omar, A.B. Evaluation of the Shear Bond Strength of Four Bioceramic Materials with Different Restorative Materials and Timings. *Materials* **2022**, *15*, 4668. [CrossRef]
12. Szafran, M.; Bobryk, E.; Szczęsna, B.; Jałbrzykowski, M. Wpływ dodatku nanowypełniacza na właściwości mechaniczne i tribologiczne kompozytów ceramiczno-polimerowych do zastosowań stomatologicznych. *Kompozyty* **2006**, *6*, 83–87.
13. Mystkowska, J.; Dąbrowski, J.R. Tribological characteristics of the kinematics couple: Tooth—Composite material for permanent dental fillings. *Eksploat. I Niezawodn.* **2010**, *3*, 4–9.
14. Altaie, A.; Bubb, N.L.; Franklin, P.; Dowling, A.H.; Fleming, G.J.; Wood, D.J. An approach to understanding tribological behaviour of dental composites through volumetric wear loss and wear mechanism determination; beyond material ranking. *J. Dent.* **2017**, *59*, 41–47. [CrossRef] [PubMed]

15. Tricco, A.C.; Lillie, E.; Zarin, W.; O'Brien, K.K.; Colquhoun, H.; Levac, D.; Moher, D.; Peters, M.D.J.; Horsley, T.; Weeks, L.; et al. Research and reporting methods PRISMA Extension for Scoping Reviews (PRISMA-ScR): Checklist and explanation. *Ann. Intern. Med.* **2018**, *169*, 467–473. [CrossRef] [PubMed]
16. Akhtar, K.; Pervez, C.; Zubair, N.; Khalid, H. Calcium hydroxyapatite nanoparticles as a reinforcement filler in dental resin nanocomposite. *J. Mater. Sci. Mater. Med.* **2021**, *32*, 129. [CrossRef] [PubMed]
17. Vargas, S.; Estevez, M.; Hernandez, A.; Laiz, J.C.; Brostow, W.; Hagg Lobland, H.E.; Rodriguez, J.R. Hydroxyapatite based hybrid dental materials with controlled porosity and improved tribological and mechanical properties. *Mater. Res. Innov.* **2013**, *17*, 154–160. [CrossRef]
18. Mystkowska, J.; Dąbrowski, J.R. The influence of selected powder fillers on the tribological properties of composite materials for dental fillings. *SSP* **2009**, *144*, 33–38. [CrossRef]
19. Antunes, P.V.; Ramalho, A. Influence of pH values and aging time on the tribological behaviour of posterior restorative materials. *Wear* **2009**, *267*, 718–725. [CrossRef]
20. Suryawanshi, A.S.; Behera, N. Tribological behavior of dental restorative composites in chewable tobacco environment. *Proc. Inst. Mech. Eng. H.* **2020**, *234*, 1106–1112. [CrossRef]
21. Yadav, R.; Meena, A. Comparative investigation of tribological behavior of hybrid dental restorative composite materials. *Ceram. Int.* **2021**, *48*, 6698–6706. [CrossRef]
22. Ozdal, M.; Gurkok, S. Recent advances in nanoparticles as antibacterial agent. *Admet Dmpk* **2022**, *10*, 115–129. [CrossRef]
23. Hasan, A.; Morshed, M.; Memic, A.; Hassan, S.; Webster, T.J.; El-Sayed Marei, H. Nanoparticles in tissue engineering: Applications, challenges and prospects. *Int. J. Nanomed.* **2018**, *13*, 5637–5655. [CrossRef]
24. Cheng, Z.; Li, M.; Dey, R.; Chen, Y. Nanomaterials for cancer therapy: Current progress and perspectives. *J. Hematol. Oncol.* **2021**, *4*, 85. [CrossRef] [PubMed]
25. Han, X.; Xu, K.; Taratula, O.; Farsad, K. Applications of Nanoparticles in Biomedical Imaging. *Nanoscale* **2019**, *11*, 799–819. [CrossRef] [PubMed]
26. Sreenivasalu, P.K.P.; Dora, C.P.; Swami, R.; Jasthi, V.C.; Shiroorkar, P.N.; Nagaraja, S.; Asdaq, S.M.B.; Anwer, M.K. Nanomaterials in Dentistry: Current Applications and Future Scope. *Nanomaterials* **2022**, *12*, 1676. [CrossRef] [PubMed]
27. Singh, R.P.; Choi, J.W.; Tiwari, A.; Pandey, A.C. *Biomedical Materials and Diagnostic Devices*; Tiwari, A., Ramalingam, M., Kobayashi, H., Turner, A.P.F., Eds.; Scribener Publ.: Beverly, MA, USA; Wiley & Sons Inc.: Hoboken, NJ, USA, 2012; Volume 7, pp. 217–262.
28. TOPSEIKO. Available online: https://top-seiko.com/pl/works/material-cat/ceramics/zirconia/ (accessed on 20 September 2024).
29. PN-EN ISO 10993-15:2023-10; Biological Evaluation of Medical Devices—Part 15: Identification and Quantification of Degradation Products of Metals and Alloys. International Organization for Standardization: Geneva, Switzerland, 2023.
30. Bociong, K.; Szczesio, A.; Krasowski, M.; Sokolowski, J. The influence of filler amount on selected properties of new experimental-resin dental composite. *Open Chem.* **2018**, *16*, 905–911. [CrossRef]
31. Bucuta, S.; Ilie, N. Light transmittance and micro-mechanical properties of bulk fill vs. conventional resin based composites. *Clin. Oral. Investig.* **2014**, *18*, 1991–2000. [CrossRef]
32. Moussa, D.G.; Fok, A.; Aparicio, C. Hydrophobic and Antimicrobial Dentin: A Peptide-based 2-tier Protective System for Dental Resin Composite Restorations. *Acta Biomater.* **2019**, *88*, 251–265. [CrossRef]
33. Malacarne, J.; Carvalho, R.M.; de Goes, M.F.; Svizero, N.; Pashley, D.H.; Tay, F.R.; Yiu, C.K.; de Oliveira Carrilho, M.R. Water sorption/solubility of dental adhesive resins. *Dent. Mater.* **2006**, *22*, 973–980. [CrossRef]
34. Sideridou, I.D.; Karabela, M.M. Sorption of water, ethanol or ethanol/water solutions by light-cured dental dimethacrylate resins. *Dent. Mater.* **2011**, *27*, 1003–1010. [CrossRef]
35. Sideridou, I.; Tserki, V.; Papanastasiou, G. Study of water sorption, solubility and modulus of elasticity of light-cured dimethacrylate-based dental resins. *Biomaterials* **2003**, *24*, 655–665. [CrossRef]
36. Oysaed, H.; Ruyter, I.E. Water sorption and filler characteristics of composites for use in posterior teeth. *J. Dent. Res.* **1986**, *65*, 1315–1318. [CrossRef]
37. Teughles, W.; Van Assche, N.; Sliepen, I.; Quirynen, M. Effect of material characteristics and/or surface topography on biofilm develpoment. *Clin. Oral. Imp. Res.* **2006**, *17*, 68–81. [CrossRef] [PubMed]
38. Aykent, F.; Aykent, F.; Yondem, I.; Ozyesil, A.G.; Gunal, S.K.; Avunduk, M.C.; Ozkan, S. Effect of different finishing techniques for restorative materials on surface roughness and bacterial Adhesion. *J. Prosthet. Dent.* **2010**, *103*, 221–227. [CrossRef] [PubMed]

Disclaimer/Publisher's Note: The statements, opinions and data contained in all publications are solely those of the individual author(s) and contributor(s) and not of MDPI and/or the editor(s). MDPI and/or the editor(s) disclaim responsibility for any injury to people or property resulting from any ideas, methods, instructions or products referred to in the content.

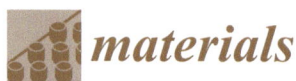

Article

The Influence of Selected Titanium Alloy Micro-Texture Parameters on Bacterial Adhesion

Jolanta Szymańska [1], Monika Krzywicka [2,*], Zbigniew Kobus [2], Anna Malm [3] and Agnieszka Grzegorczyk [3]

[1] Chair of Comprehensive Dentistry, Medical University of Lublin, 20-059 Lublin, Poland; jolanta.szymanska@umlub.pl
[2] Department of Technology Fundamentals, University of Life Sciences in Lublin, 20-950 Lublin, Poland; zbigniew.kobus@up.lublin.pl
[3] Chair and Department of Pharmaceutical Microbiology with Laboratory for Microbiological Diagnostics, Medical University of Lublin, 20-059 Lublin, Poland; anna.malm@umlub.pl (A.M.); agnieszka.grzegorczyk@umlub.pl (A.G.)
* Correspondence: monika.krzywicka@up.lublin.pl

Abstract: The colonization of microbes and the resulting formation of biofilms on dental implants are significant contributors to peri-implantitis and the failure of these implants. The aim of the research was to analyze the impact of density and depth of laser texturing of the Ti-6Al-7Nb alloy surface on the colonization of selected microorganisms and biofilm formation. Standard strains of Gram-negative and Gram-positive bacteria and yeasts from the American Type Culture Collection—ATCC—were used to demonstrate the ability to form single-species biofilms in vitro. The study evaluated three types of titanium samples with different texture density and depth. The colonization and biofilm formation abilities of the tested microorganisms were assessed. The obtained results were subjected to statistical analysis. Among the analyzed strains, *L. rhamnosus* showed the highest colonization of the tested surfaces. It was found that there is no relationship between the texture parameters and the number of colony-forming units (CFU/mL) for *C. albicans*, *S. mutans*, and *L. rhamnosus*. For the *F. nucleatum* strain, it was shown that the number of colony-forming bacteria is related to the texture density.

Keywords: laser surface texturing; titanium alloys; microorganism colonization; biofilm

Citation: Szymańska, J.; Krzywicka, M.; Kobus, Z.; Malm, A.; Grzegorczyk, A. The Influence of Selected Titanium Alloy Micro-Texture Parameters on Bacterial Adhesion. *Materials* **2024**, *17*, 4765. https://doi.org/10.3390/ma17194765

Academic Editor: Piotr Piszczek

Received: 3 September 2024
Revised: 25 September 2024
Accepted: 26 September 2024
Published: 28 September 2024

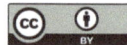

Copyright: © 2024 by the authors. Licensee MDPI, Basel, Switzerland. This article is an open access article distributed under the terms and conditions of the Creative Commons Attribution (CC BY) license (https://creativecommons.org/licenses/by/4.0/).

1. Introduction

The final stage of prosthetic treatment using implants of missing teeth involves the proper functioning of the stomatognathic system and an aesthetic appearance [1]. Biofilm—a multi-microbial formation that consists mainly of bacteria, as well as protozoa, viruses and fungi—is constantly present in the oral cavity. Biofilm contains up to 100 bacterial species [2]. It is found on hard and soft tissues of the oral cavity, as well as on surfaces like orthodontic bands, clear aligners or dentures [3,4]. The presence of supragingival and subgingival biofilm can be the cause of the evolution of periodontitis and peri-implantitis—polymicrobial inflammatory diseases that cause the destruction of the tissue supporting the tooth/implant; the inflammation of the mucous membrane around the implant (peri-implant mucositis); and/or the inflammation of the tissues involved in the osseointegration of the implant (peri-implantitis) [4].

Both the bone and the surrounding soft tissues (epithelium, gingival connective tissue) are involved in the process of implant osseointegration, and the presence of opportunistic pathogens in the biofilm on the mentioned tissues around the implants and on their surface, including microcracks in the implant surface, disturbs this process. The consequence of the inflammatory cascade caused by microorganisms in the biofilm is the destruction of supporting tissues [5–7].

A short adhesion time and intensive multiplication of microorganisms, including opportunistic pathogens, cause the formation of a biofilm, which is a favorable environment for the survival of microorganisms and the maintenance of infections [2]. Modern methods of microbiological identification have allowed for the detection of the presence of some common oral pathogens around the implants, such as *Tannerella forsythia*, *Porphyromonas gingivalis* (*P. gingivalis*), *Prevotella intermedia* (*P. intermedia*) and *Fusobacterium nucleatum* (*F. nucleatum*) [8,9].

The "early colonizers" are mainly considered to be Gram-positive aerobic bacteria—*Streptococcus* spp. and *Actinomyces* spp., which influence the local environment around the implant, making it suitable for "secondary colonizers" such as *F. nucleatum*. This bacterium acts as a "bridge species". Through coaggregation, it facilitates the adhesion of "late colonizers" and periopathogens, such as *P. gingivalis* [10]. Studies have shown that *P. gingivalis* and *P. intermedia* are mainly accountable for peri-implantitis among "late colonizers" [11]. Severe peri-implantitis may be followed by the loss of the implant at various times. In cases of both early and late implant loss, *F. nucleatum* and *P. gingivalis* were prevalent. Implants that were lost later exhibited greater bacterial diversity and had higher levels of *Treponema*, *Fretibacterium*, *Pseudoramibacter*, and *Desulfobulbus*. In contrast, the microbial communities associated with implants that experienced early loss were highly variable and did not display any significantly more abundant bacterial taxa [12].

The physicochemical properties of the surface of the implants like surface roughness, hydrophobicity, surface free energy, and surface electrochemistry, may influence the formation of the bacterial biofilm [13]. The surface roughness, a common feature of the implant, is one of the factors contributing to the greater colonization and formation of a multimicrobial biofilm [14].

The surface modification of titanium biomaterials plays an important role in the success of surgical procedures, including dental implants. The use of surface engineering methods allows us to obtain the desired functional properties and biological functions. In the past few years, there has been increased interest in laser processing, such as laser ablation, laser-induced periodic surface structures—LIPSS, laser melting, direct laser interference patterning—DLIP, and matrix-assisted pulsed evaporation—MAPLE [15]. Laser technology is also used for surface texturing. Laser surface texturing has numerous advantages, such as high efficiency, ease of operation, environmental friendliness, and the ability to produce controlled and repeatable geometries [16–18]. Laser surface texturing has a significant impact on the moisturizing properties and adhesion of bacteria, which is crucial for biomedical applications [19,20]. An important research problem is the selection of appropriate texture parameters, such as the shape and size of the produced dimples and density [21].

Based on the literature review, it was determined that no detailed analysis of the correlation between texture parameters, such as the density and depth of individual texture elements and the adhesion of *Candida albicans* (*C. albicans*), *Streptococcus mutans* (*S. mutans*), *Lactobacillus rhamnosus* (*L. rhamnosus*), *Fusobacterium nucleatum* (*F. nucleatum*) has been performed. Therefore, the novelty of our research is the analysis of the relationship between texture parameters and the adhesion of selected bacteria. The aim of this article is to analyze the effect of selected parameters (density, depth) of the texture of the surface of the Ti-6Al-7Nb alloy on the number of adhering microorganisms.

2. Materials and Methods

2.1. Laser Surface Texture Preparation

The samples made of Ti-6Al-7Nb titanium alloy (ChM sp. z o.o., Juchnowiec Kościelny, Poland) were the subject of the research. The chemical composition of the alloy complied with ISO 5832-11. Table 1 shows the chemical composition of the alloy.

Table 1. The chemical composition of Ti-6Al-7Nb.

Fe	O	N	C	H	Al	Nb	Ta	Ti
max. 0.25%	max. 0.2%	max. 0.05%	max. 0.08%	max. 0.009%	5.5–6.5%	6.5–7.5%	max. 0.5%	rest

The surface roughness (Ra) of the samples was 0.06 μm. The laser surface texturing process was carried out as described in the work by Krzywicka et al. [19]. Laser surface texturing was performed in argon shield at 100% power, and the surface scanning was carried out with a laser beam, with a speed of 50 mm/s. After scanning the surface twice with a laser beam with the frequency of 80 kHz, individual textured elements with the depth of approx. 5 μm were obtained. Depths of about 78 μm were obtained using a frequency of 100 kHz, and the surface was scanned 35 times.

In order to determine the number of adhering microorganisms (CFU/mL), dimples with the following density and depth were produced:
–50%, 5 μm,
–10%, 5 μm,
–10%, 78 μm.

The diameter of the dimples was approximately 200 μm. The microgeometric characteristics of the texture were examined utilizing the HIROX KH-8700 digital microscope (Hirox, Tokyo, Japan). Following the laser texturing process, the samples were immersed in distilled water at a temperature of 55 °C within an ultrasonic cleaner (Ultron, Dywity, Poland) for 10 min.

2.2. Fungal and Bacterial Cell Culture and Assessment of Different Species of Oral Microbiota Colonization and Biofilm Formation

The following American Type Culture Collection (ATTC) strains were used in the study: *C. albicans* ATCC 10231—yeast-like fungi, *S. mutans* ATCC 25175—Gram-positive bacteria, *L. rhamnosus* GG ATCC 53103—Gram-positive bacteria, and *F. nucleatum* ATCC 25586—Gram-negative bacteria, which may affect biofilm formation on the surface of dental plaque. The microorganisms were used to show the capacity to form in vitro single-species biofilms composed of all the reference strains.

The study was conducted using sterile 6-well polystyrene titration plates (NUNC) and the following reagents: crystal violet, 1% solution (BioMerieux, Warsaw, Poland), ethyl alcohol 96% pure p. a., sterile phosphate-buffered saline (PBS) with calcium and magnesium ions, pH 7.4 ± 0.2, osmolarity 270–290 mOsmol/L (BioMaxima, Lublin, Poland).

Preparation of Microorganisms for Analysis

An assessment of the number of adhering microorganisms was carried out (CFU/mL). The prepared bacterial and fungal inocula were transferred into the wells on the 6-well plates containing the appropriate media; the starting densities obtained were 1.5×10^7 CFU/mL (for bacteria) and 5×10^5 CFU/mL fungi. At the same time, the titanium alloy samples were coated with mucin—1% solution (Sigma, Lublin, Poland)—and subsequently placed on the media with a given microorganism suspension, each in a separate well.

The samples were incubated at 35 °C for an hour (adhesion period) under aerobic or anaerobic conditions, depending on the microorganism. After that time, the samples were thoroughly rinsed with 5 mL PBS, placed in fresh sterile media, and incubated at 35 °C under atmospheric conditions suited to each of the microorganisms for 24 h (biofilm formation period) and another 24 h (biofilm maturation). After each 24 h period, the samples were rinsed with 5 mL sterile PBS and the biomaterials were placed in fresh media.

After 48 h incubation, the samples were rinsed once more, placed in test tubes with 3 mL PBS, and shaken at 1000 rpm for 30 min. Next, 10^{-1} to 10^{-10} dilutions were made, plated in the appropriate media, and incubated at 35 °C for 48 h. After incubation, the colonies were counted (Counter Colony Scan 1200; Interscience, Fisher Scientific, Porto Salvo, Portugal) and converted into CFU/mL. At the same time, substrate control and microbial viability control were carried out.

2.3. Statistical Analysis

Using Dell Statistica v. 13.1 (Dell Inc., Cracow, Poland, 2016), an examination was carried out to analyze the relationships between variables. Initially, the presence of a correlation between independent variables (density, depth) and dependent variables (CFU/mL) was investigated. Once a correlation was confirmed, a regression function was derived to quantify the relationships. The next step involved verifying the model by checking the assumptions such as the significance of linear regression, the significance of partial regression coefficients, the absence of collinearity between independent variables, homoscedasticity, the absence of autocorrelation of residuals, the normal distribution of residuals, and the expected value of the random component being 0. The data were considered statistically significant at $p < 0.1$.

3. Results and Discussion

3.1. The Microbial Reference Strains Representing Oral Microbiota Colonization and Biofilm Formation

The reference sample was not subjected to the laser surface texturing (Ra = 0.06 μm). Figures 1 and 2 show the profiles of the individual texture elements.

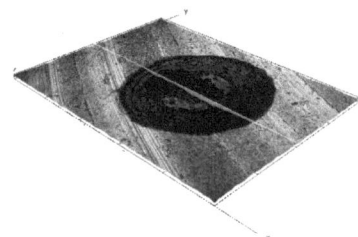

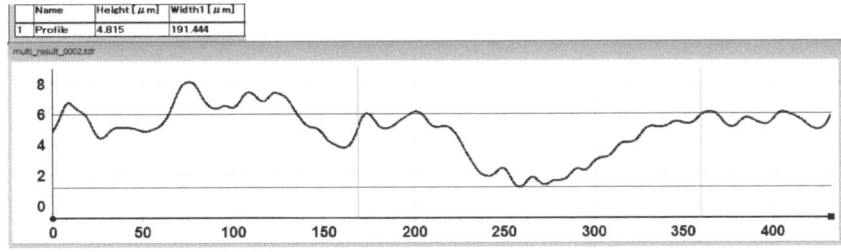

Figure 1. The profile of a single texture element in the form of a dimple with a diameter of 191.44 μm and a depth of 4.82 μm.

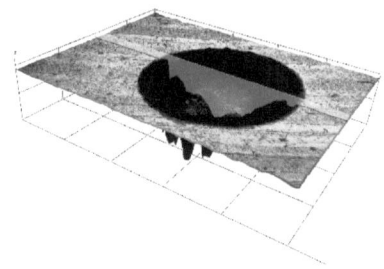

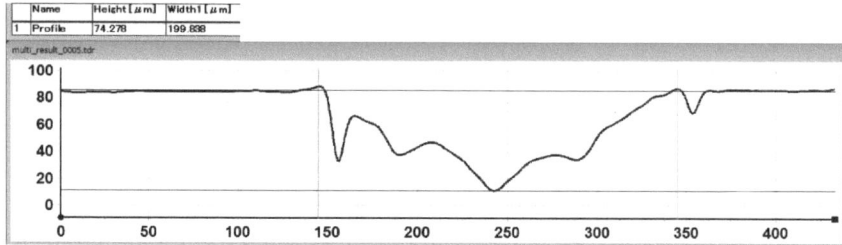

Figure 2. The profile of a single texture element in the form of a dimple with a diameter of 199.84 μm and a depth of 74.28 μm.

Table 2 shows the number of CFU/mL of the microbial references strains representing oral microbiota forming a biofilm on the titanium alloy samples.

Table 2. The number of CFU/mL of the microbial references strains representing oral microbiota forming a biofilm on the titanium alloy samples.

Microbial Species	Sample	Biofilm Size	
		CFU/mL	log CFU/mL
C. albicans ATCC 10231	Model	$0.75 \times 10^4 \pm 0.13 \times 10^4$	3.88 ± 3.11
	10%, 5 μm	$0.8 \times 10^4 \pm 0.15 \times 10^4$	3.90 ± 3.17
	10%, 78 μm	$2.0 \times 10^4 \pm 0.36 \times 10^4$	4.30 ± 3.55
	50%, 5 μm	$1.7 \times 10^4 \pm 0.53 \times 10^4$	4.23 ± 3.72
S. mutans ATCC 25175	Model	$0.61 \times 10^4 \pm 0.23 \times 10^4$	3.78 ± 3.36
	10%, 5 μm	$2.50 \times 10^4 \pm 0.36 \times 10^4$	4.39 ± 3.55
	10%, 78 μm	$4.36 \times 10^4 \pm 1.7 \times 10^4$	4.63 ± 4.23
	50%, 5 μm	$3.05 \times 10^4 \pm 1.9 \times 10^4$	4.48 ± 4.28
L. rhamnosus ATCC 53103	Model	$2.13 \times 10^7 \pm 1.09 \times 10^7$	7.32 ± 7.03
	10%, 5 μm	$4.47 \times 10^7 \pm 2.4 \times 10^7$	7.65 ± 7.38
	10%, 78 μm	$3.36 \times 10^7 \pm 1.25 \times 10^7$	7.53 ± 7.10
	50%, 5 μm	$2.77 \times 10^7 \pm 1.5 \times 10^7$	7.44 ± 7.17
F. nucleatum ATCC 25586	Model	$0.27 \times 10^6 \pm 0.10 \times 10^6$	5.43 ± 5.00
	10%, 5 μm	$0.48 \times 10^6 \pm 0.19 \times 10^6$	5.68 ± 5.28
	10%, 78 μm	$0.56 \times 10^6 \pm 0.19 \times 10^6$	5.74 ± 5.28
	50%, 5 μm	$2.96 \times 10^6 \pm 0.94 \times 10^6$	6.47 ± 5.97

All analyzed strains showed the lowest adhesion to the non-textured surface. The lowest adhesion to the Ti-6Al-7Nb surface among all analyzed strains was demonstrated by *S. mutans*, and the highest was demonstrated by *L. rhamnosus*.

C. albicans ATCC 10231 showed the lowest biofilm formation on the textured surface, on which dimples of the lowest depth were created. The CFU/mL value for the sample on the surface of which textures with a depth of 5 μm and density of 10% were created is 6.67% higher than the untextured sample. Comparing the biofilm formation on the surface on which dimples of the same depth and different densities were created, it can be seen that a significantly lower CFU/mL value was recorded for the lower density.

S. mutans ATCC 25175 showed the lowest biofilm formation on the textured surface on which dimples of the lowest depth were created. The CFU/mL value for the sample on the surface of which textures with a depth of 5 μm and density of 10% were created is 309.8% higher than the untextured sample. Compared to the surface on which dimples of the same depth and different densities were created, it can be seen that a significantly lower CFU/mL value was recorded for the lower density.

L. rhamnosus GG ATCC 53103 showed the lowest adhesion to the textured surface on which dimples with a depth of 5 μm and a density of 50% were created. The CFU/mL value for the sample on the surface of which textures with a depth of 5 μm and density of 50% were created is 30% higher compared to the untextured sample. Comparing the colonization and biofilm formation on the surface on which dimples of the same density were created, it can be seen that a lower CFU/mL value was recorded for the higher depth of the dimples.

F. nucleatum ATCC 25586 showed the lowest biofilm formation on the textured surface on which dimples with a depth of 5 μm and a density of 10% were created. The CFU/mL value for the sample on the surface of which textures with a depth of 5 μm and density of 10% were created is 77.8% higher than the untextured sample. Comparing the biofilm formation on the surface on which dimples of the same density were created, it can be seen that a lower CFU/mL value was recorded for the lower depth of the dimples.

3.2. The Dependence of the Number of Adhering Microorganisms on Texture Geometry

It was found that there is no correlation between the texture parameters and CFU/mL for *C. albicans* ATCC 10231, *S. mutans* ATCC 25175 and *L. rhamnosus* GG ATCC 53103, and therefore no regression function can be found.

For the *F. nucleatum* ATCC 25586 strain, it was shown that the independent variable density is correlated ($p < 0.1$) with the dependent variable CFU/mL. There is a correlation between the studied characteristics. The standard error of the estimate for the intercept about its value is relatively large. The coefficient of determination is 0.9; hence, the model explains 99.9% of the variability in CFU/mL. The linear correlation coefficient R is equal to 0.999; thus, there is an almost completely linear relationship between the dependent variable and the independent variables. Linearity is checked with the F-test. The *p*-value for this test is 0.020, which means that the regression equation is significant. The standard error of the estimation is 56,569, which means that the predicted values of the CFU/mL variable differ from the empirical values by an average of 56,569. The residual distribution is assumed to be normal. The value of the d statistic is 2.5, which implies that there is autocorrelation of the residuals. This may be due to a small number of data (3) or other factors affecting the CFU/mL value. The random component εi has an expected value of 0. The average value of the residuals is equal to 0. The analyses carried out show that sample no. 3, on the surface of which dimples with a depth of 5 μm and a density of 50% were created, has a significantly large impact on the load of the regression equation. This could be the cause of the high standard error value.

The regression equation is:

$$\text{CFU/mL} = -90{,}000 + 6{,}100{,}000 \times \text{Density} \pm 51{,}962 \qquad (1)$$

This means that if the density increases by 1%, the CFU/mL value increases by 6.1×10^6.

The model verification showed that the assumptions of unbiased residuals, random deviations and the lack of autocorrelation of residuals are not met. This could be attributed to a limited data set (3) or other factors affecting the CFU/mL value.

4. Discussion

The CFU/mL values were significantly different for individual bacterial strains. The lowest adhesion to the control sample was shown by *S. mutans*. The studies showed increased bacterial adhesion to the textured surface. The highest CFU/mL value for *C. albicans* and *S. mutans* was recorded for the sample on the surface of which textures with a depth of 78 μm and density of 10% were produced, which is 166.7% and 614.8% higher in comparison to the non-textured sample, respectively. The highest CFU/mL value for *L. rhamnosus* was recorded on the surface where the dimples with the lowest density and depth were created, and this value was 109.9% higher than for the control sample. The highest CFU/mL value for *F. nucleatum* was recorded on the surface where the dimples with the lowest depth and highest density were created, and this value was 996.3% higher than for the control sample. The lowest percentage increase in adhesion compared to the control sample was shown by *L. rhamnosus*, which also showed the highest adhesion to the Ti-6Al-7Nb alloy. The lowest CFU/mL value for *C. albicans*, *S. mutans*, *F. nucleatum* was shown for the lowest depth of a single textural element and the lowest density. The lowest CFU/mL value was recorded for the highest density for *L. rhamnosus* alone. The mechanism of bacterial adhesion is complex. Undoubtedly, laser micromachining causes increased roughness, and thus increases the contact surface. The diameters of all analyzed bacteria were smaller than the distance between the dimples as well as the diameter, and the depth of the generated textures, so it can be assumed that the generated textures promoted bacterial migration, penetration into dimples, and biofilm formation. The most similar results were obtained for *S. mutans* and *C. albicans*, despite these being pathogens from different groups—a Gram-positive bacterium and a fungus, respectively. The sizes of these pathogens also differed significantly, with *C. albicans* measuring 2–4 μm in diameter and *S. mutans* approximately 0.5–0.75 μm in diameter [22]. The most similar sizes were found in *L. rhamnosus* (from 0.8 to 1.0 μm in width) [23] and *S. mutans*, and both strains belong to Gram-positive bacteria. Despite these similarities, extremely different CFU/mL values were obtained.

The available literature reports present divergent results on the effects of laser surface texturing on microorganism adhesion. Similar results to ours were obtained by Singh et al. [24], Esfahanizadeh et al. [25], and Uhlmann et al. [26]. Singh et al. [24] produced fish-scale, octagonal, and hexagonal features with varying densities of 43.4%, 55%, 74.7%, heights of 97 μm, 102 μm, 127 μm, and a diameter/edge of pillar of 135 × 95 μm, 53 μm, 1.06 μm on the surface of the Ti-6Al-4V alloy. An average bacterial area coverage of *Staphylococcus aureus* (*S. aureus*) could be approximated to 35% for untextured and to 60% for textured. Singh et al. [24] also indicate that the size of the textures has an influence on bacterial adhesion. Esfahanizadeh et al. [25] report that a higher pathogen count was found on the surface of the treated titanium (with similar microgrooves at 8 μm intervals) compared to the untreated sample. The mean count of *Aggregatibacter actinomycetemcomitans* was 11.3163 and 9.6941 log CFUs/mL, with 11.3437 and 10.0831 log CFUs/mL for *P. intermedia*, and 12.1176 and 10.1213 log CFUs/mL for *P. gingivalis* in the laser and titanium groups, respectively. Uhlmann et al. [26] produced textures of various parameters on the surface of the Ti-6Al-4V alloy and showed that the adhesion of *S. mutans* to the surface on which the LIPSS was made, with a height of 300 nm, a microcavity width of 15 μm, a length of 30 μm, a height of 5 μm, and a microcavity length of 15 μm (rest unchanged), showed similar results for bacterial attachment, and these values are significantly higher than for the control sample subjected to chemical polishing. Based on the conducted research and the results of the above-mentioned authors [24–26], the production of textures with the size of single micrometers will promote the adhesion of various bacterial strains.

Grössner-Schreiber et al. [27] performed a Ti Grade 2 laser treatment and found no difference in the adhesion of *S. mutans* and *Streptococcus sanguis* between polished Ti and Ti laser. Hauser-Gerspach et al. [28] treated the surface of commercially pure titanium using different laser energy densities (12.74 J/cm^2 and 63.69 J/cm^2). They showed no differences in the adhesion of *Streptococcus sanguinis* and *P. gingivalis* bacteria between laser-processed and polished samples. Du et al. [29] produced the LIPSS on the Ti Grade 4 surface, which showed no statistically significant difference in OD (optical density) between the polished surface (*Escherichia coli* (*E. coli*): 0.973; *S. aureus*: 0.971) and the LIPSS surface (*E. coli*: 0.969; *S. aureus*: 0.955). It is worth emphasizing that Grössner-Schreiber et al. [27], Hauser-Gerspach et al. [28], and Du et al. [29] do not provide the sizes of the textures produced, so it is impossible to compare them with the results of our research and the size of the analyzed bacteria. Many authors obtained different results and showed that laser surface texturing reduces bacterial adhesion [30–36]. Parmar et al. [30] produced micro-pits of various diameters (24–35 μm) and depths (4.58–78 μm) on the surface of the Ti-6Al-4V alloy. In our studies, a depth of 78 μm was also analyzed, but with a much larger diameter of 200 and other pathogens and alloys. The studies carried out showed a 75% decrease in the adhesion of *S. aureus* compared to the untreated sample. Additionally, in the case of the textured sample, a reduction in CFU/mL by 80% was demonstrated after 72 h, compared to a 20% reduction for the non-textured sample. Shiju et al. [31] performed laser texturing of the Ti-6Al-4V alloy surface and produced dimples with a depth of 2.5 μm and a diameter of 10 μm. The textures produced are significantly smaller in size than those produced in our studies, but are still larger than the size of the bacteria when using confocal microscopy; it was shown that *S. aureus* adhesion was lower on the surface of treated samples than on untreated samples [31]. Doll et al. [32] carried out the laser processing of titanium, on the surface of which three different types of Sharklet™-like textures were produced (grooves with a width of 2 μm, a depth of ≥2 μm, and various lengths from 4 μm to 16 μm, arranged in a periodic diamond-like pattern at fixed intervals 2 μm between elements), with linear grooves (2 μm wide, ≥2 μm deep and a fixed interval of 2 μm) and grid structures (an orthogonal overlap of two structural grooves with the same dimensions as above). The analysis showed the reduced adhesion of *S. aureus* on all tested microstructures compared to smooth titanium surfaces. Based on the studies conducted by Doll et al. [32], who also produced micrometer-sized textures, larger than the diameter of *S. aureus*, it can be concluded that not only the size but also the shape of the produced textures plays an important role in limiting bacterial adhesion. Eghbali et al. [33] proved that the surface modification of the Ti-6Al-4V alloy at depths ranging from 0.5 to 50 μm inhibits *E. coli* adhesion when using a higher laser frequency of 160 kHz. However, increasing the groove distances to over 50 μm and using a lower laser frequency of 20 kHz decreases laser pulse overlaps, leading to enhanced cell adhesion. Chik et al. [34] produced LIPSS (pulse duration 380 fs, power 0.11 W, wavelength 515 μm, frequency 200 kHz) on the surface of Ti Grade 5. Laser-treated surfaces were characterized by lower bacterial adhesion compared to polished surfaces (by >80% in the case of *E. coli* and >20% in the case of *S. aureus*). Our experiments, as well as the studies by Chik et al. [34], showed that individual bacterial strains adhere to a given surface to a varying extent. Zwahr et al. [35] produced crater-like structures on the Ti Grade 4 surface (separation distance of 50 μm), then, directly on this texture, a hole-like pattern with a 5 μm spatial period was generated. The adhesion of *E. coli* bacteria was reduced by 30% compared to the control sample. Research conducted by Zwahr et al. [35] indicated that the appropriately selected shapes of textures, even micrometer-sized, can limit the adhesion of bacteria. Yao et al. [36] subjected Ti to laser processing and produced a circular pattern on the surface of the samples. The laser-treated samples exhibited lower roughness than the control disks subjected to autoclaving treatments and were characterized by slightly less *P. gingivalis* adhesion and less *P. gingivalis* colonization than the control samples. Yao et al. [36] did not provide texture sizes; hence, it is impossible to compare them with our research results.

The authors [37–40] who produced textures with sizes below 1 micrometer, including nanotextures, showed reduced bacterial adhesion. Orazi et al. [37], on the surface of the Ti-6Al-4V alloy, using different laser operating parameters (the first treatment—the pulse energy of 16 μJ and an overall dose of 27 J/cm^2, the second treatment—the pulse energy of 32 μJ and an overall dose of 270 J/cm^2), created an LIPSS with dimensions of 100–200 nm. Based on the conducted research, it was shown that laser-treated surfaces exhibit lower

S. aureus adhesion (2 log$_{10}$ CFU) compared to the untreated surface (5 log$_{10}$ CFU). Meinshausen et al. [38] created wavy textures on the surface of Ti Grade 4 with a spacing of 0.7 to 5 μm and a height of 100 to 800 nm, and demonstrated that laser-treated surfaces show a lower adhesion of *S. aureus* bacteria compared to the control sample. Luo et al. [39] conducted laser treatment on 99.7% pure titanium and created three types of nano-ripples on the surface of the samples: LIPSS (400 nm), columns with overlapped LIPSS, and similar periods with LIPSS, but with nano-ripples interrupted by shallow sinuous grooves (1 μm pitch) vertically. It was shown that the tested textures could prevent bacterial colonization and biofilm formation, and their antibacterial effectiveness against *E. coli* ranged from 43% to 56%. Donaghy et al. [40] produced a spiky surface and decreasing peak-to-peak distance between ripples (0.63 to 0.315 μm) on the Ti-35Nb-7Zr-6Ta surface, and showed a significant reduction in *S. aureus* adhesion on the treated surface compared to the control sample.

The presented research results indicate that the laser texturing of the surface of titanium alloys requires further optimization. In particular, it is necessary to take into account the species of bacteria that form biofilms and which, as proved by the research results, show varying adhesion to the surfaces of alloys used for implants.

5. Conclusions

Laser surface texturing has an impact on microorganism colonization and biofilm formation. Drawing from the research carried out, it can be concluded that different species of oral microbiota react in varying degrees to the produced textures. *C. albicans, S. mutans, F. nucleatum* showed the lowest colonization and biofilm formation to the lowest depth textures, while *L. rhamnosus* demonstrated the lowest depth but with different densities—50% for *L. rhamnosus*. Among the analyzed strains, *L. rhamnosus* showed the highest adhesion to the tested surfaces. It was found that there is no relationship between texture parameters and the CFU/mL value for *C. albicans, S. mutans* and *L. rhamnosus*. For the *F. nucleatum* strain, it was shown that the number of colony-forming bacteria is related to the texture density.

There is a need to continue research on micro- and nanotextures of titanium surfaces for dental implants, which minimize colonization by microorganisms and thus limit the development of inflammatory processes around implants, promoting the proper course of osteointegration.

Author Contributions: Conceptualization, M.K. and J.S.; methodology, M.K., J.S., A.M. and A.G.; formal analysis, M.K. and A.M; investigation, M.K. and A.G.; data curation, M.K. and A.G.; writing—original draft preparation, M.K. and J.S.; writing—review and editing, M.K. and J.S.; visualization, M.K.; supervision, M.K. and Z.K.; project administration, M.K.; funding acquisition, J.S. All authors have read and agreed to the published version of the manuscript.

Funding: This research was funded as part of the statutory activity of the Medical University of Lublin, Poland, grant number DS 290.

Institutional Review Board Statement: Not applicable.

Informed Consent Statement: Not applicable.

Data Availability Statement: The original contributions presented in the study are included in the article, further inquiries can be directed to the corresponding author.

Conflicts of Interest: The authors declare no conflicts of interest.

References

1. Szpak, P.; Szymańska, J. The survival of dental implants with different implant-abutment connection systems. *Curr. Issues Pharm. Med. Sci.* **2016**, *29*, 11–13. [CrossRef]
2. Larsen, T.; Fiehn, N.E. Dental biofilm infections-an Update. *APMIS* **2017**, *125*, 376–384. [CrossRef] [PubMed]
3. Meto, A.; Colombari, B.; Castagnoli, A.; Sarti, M.; Denti, L.; Blasi, E. Efficacy of a Copper–Calcium–Hydroxide Solution in Reducing Microbial Plaque on Orthodontic Clear Aligners: A Case Report. *Eur. J. Dent.* **2019**, *13*, 478–484. [CrossRef]

4. Lasserre, J.F.; Brecx, M.C.; Toma, S. Oral microbes, biofilms and their role in periodontal and peri-implant diseases. *Materials* **2018**, *11*, 1802. [CrossRef]
5. Shrivastava, D.; Srivastava, K.C.; Ganji, K.K.; Alam, M.K.; Al Zoubi, I.; Sghairee, M.G. Quantitative assessment of gingival inflammation in patients undergoing nonsurgical periodontal therapy using photometric CIELab Analysis. *BioMed. Res. Int.* **2021**, *30*, 6615603. [CrossRef]
6. Shrivastava, D.; Srivastava, K.C.; Dayakara, J.K.; Sghaireen, M.G.; Gudipaneni, R.K.; Al-Johani, K.; Baig, M.N.; Khurshid, Z. Bactericidal Activity of Crevicular Polymorphonuclear Neutrophils in Chronic Periodontitis Patients and Healthy Subjects under the Influence of Areca Nut Extract: An In Vitro Study. *Appl. Sci.* **2020**, *10*, 5008. [CrossRef]
7. Dhir, S. Biofilm and dental implant: The microbial link. *J. Indian Soc. Periodontol.* **2013**, *17*, 5–11. [CrossRef] [PubMed]
8. Charalampakis, G.; Belibasakis, G.N. Microbiome of peri-implant infections: Lessons from conventional, molecular and metagenomic analyses. *Virulence* **2015**, *6*, 183–187. [CrossRef]
9. Sahrmann, P.; Gilli, F.; Wiedemeier, D.B.; Attin, T.; Schmidlin, P.R.; Karygianni, L. The microbiome of peri-implantitis: A systematic review and meta-analysis. *Microorganisms* **2020**, *8*, 661. [CrossRef]
10. Siddiqui, D.A.; Fidai, A.B.; Natarajan, S.G.; Rodrigues, D.C. Succession of oral bacterial colonizers on dental implant materials: An in vitro biofilm model. *Dent. Mater.* **2022**, *38*, 384–396. [CrossRef]
11. Mombelli, A.; Lang, N.P. Microbial aspects of implant dentistry. *Periodontol. 2000* **1994**, *4*, 74–80. [CrossRef] [PubMed]
12. Korsch, M.; Marten, S.M.; Stoll, D.; Prechtl, C.; Dötsch, A. Microbiological findings in early and late implant loss: An observational clinical case-controlled study. *BMC Oral Health* **2021**, *21*, 112. [CrossRef] [PubMed]
13. Yuan, C.; Wang, X.; Gao, X.; Chen, F.; Liang, X.; Li, D. Effects of surface properties of polymer-based restorative materials on early adhesion of Streptococcus mutans in vitro. *J. Dent.* **2016**, *54*, 33–40. [CrossRef]
14. Nakanishi, E.Y.; Palacios, J.H.; Godbout, S.; Fournel, S. Interaction between Biofilm Formation, Surface Material and Cleanability Considering Different Materials Used in Pig Facilities—An Overview. *Sustainability* **2021**, *13*, 5836. [CrossRef]
15. Ferraris, S.; Cochis, S.A.; Scalia, A.C.; Tori, A.; Rimondini, L.; Spriano, S. Laser surface texturing of Ti-cp and Ti6Al4V alloy for the improvement of fibroblast adhesion and alignment and the reduction of bacterial adhesion. *J. Mater. Res. Technol.* **2024**, *29*, 5464–5472. [CrossRef]
16. Wang, S.; Wang, W.; Xu, Y.; Zhang, X.; Chen, C.; Geng, P.; Ma, N. Effect of nanosecond pulsed laser parameters on texturing formation of metallic surface: Experiment and modelling. *J. Mater. Res. Technol.* **2023**, *26*, 7775–7788. [CrossRef]
17. Costa, R.C.; Nagay, B.E.; Bertolini, M.; Costa-Oliveira, B.E.; Sampaio, A.A.; Retamal-Valdes, B.; Shibli, J.A.; Feres, M.; Barão, V.A.R.; Souza, J.G.S. Fitting pieces into the puzzle: The impact of titanium-based dental implant surface modifications on bacterial accumulation and polymicrobial infections. *Adv. Colloid Interface Sci.* **2021**, *298*, 102551. [CrossRef]
18. Souza, J.C.M.; Sordi, M.B.; Kanazawa, M.; Ravindran, S.; Henriques, B.; Silva, F.S.; Aparicio, C.; Cooper, L.F. Nano-scale modification of titanium implant surfaces to enhance osseointegration. *Acta Biomater.* **2019**, *94*, 112–131. [CrossRef] [PubMed]
19. Krzywicka, M.; Szymańska, J.; Tofil, S.; Malm, A.; Grzegorczyk, A. Surface Properties of Ti6Al7Nb Alloy: Surface Free Energy and Bacteria Adhesion. *J. Funct. Biomater.* **2022**, *13*, 26. [CrossRef]
20. Corsaro, C.; Orlando, G.; Costa, G.; Latino, M.; Barreca, F.; Mezzasalma, A.M.; Neri, F.; Fazio, E. Wetting Behavior Driven by Surface Morphology Changes Induced by Picosecond Laser Texturing. *Materials* **2024**, *17*, 1719. [CrossRef]
21. Voisey, K.T.; Scotchford, C.A.; Martin, L.; Gill, H.S. Effect of Q-switched Laser Surface Texturing of Titanium on Osteoblast Cell Response. *Phys. Procedia* **2014**, *56*, 1126–1135. [CrossRef]
22. Microbe Notes. Available online: https://microbenotes.com (accessed on 24 September 2024).
23. Wood, B.J.B.; Holzapfel, W.H. *Genera of Lactic Acid Bacteria*; Blackie Academic and Professional: London, UK, 1995; p. 420. ISBN 075140215X.
24. Singh, S.M.; George, A.; Tiwari, J.; Ramkumar, K. Balani Influence of laser surface texturing on the wettability and antibacterial properties of metallic, ceramic, and polymeric surfaces. *J. Mater. Res.* **2021**, *36*, 398–3999. [CrossRef]
25. Esfahanizadeh, N.; Mirmalek, N.; Bahador, A.; Daneshparvar, H.; Akhoundi, N.; Pourhajibagher, M. Formation of biofilm on various implant abutment materials. *Gen. Dent.* **2018**, *65*, 39–44.
26. Uhlmann, E.; Schweitzer, L.; Kieburg, H.; Spielvogel, A.; Huth-Herms, K. The effects of laser microtexturing of biomedical Grade 5 Ti-6Al-4V dental implants (Abutment) on biofilm formation. *Procedia CIRP* **2018**, *68*, 184–189. [CrossRef]
27. Grössner-Schreiber, B.; Griepentrog, M.; Haustein, I.; Müller, W.-D.; Briedigkeit, H.; Göbel, U.B.; Lange, K.-P. Plaque formation on surface modified dental implants. *Clin. Oral Implant. Res.* **2001**, *12*, 543–551. [CrossRef]
28. Hauser-Gerspach, I.; Mauth, C.; Waltimo, T.; Meyer, J.; Stübinger, S. Effects of Er:YAG laser on bacteria associated with titanium surfaces and cellular response in vitro. *Laser Med. Sci.* **2014**, *29*, 1329–1337. [CrossRef]
29. Du, C.; Wang, C.; Zhang, T.; Zheng, L. Antibacterial performance of Zr-BMG, stainless steel, and titanium alloy with laser-induced periodic surface structures ACS. *Appl. Bio. Mater.* **2022**, *5*, 272–284. [CrossRef]
30. Parmar, V.; Kumar, A.; Mani Sankar, M.; Datta, S.; Vijaya Prakash, G.; Mohanty, S.; Kalyanasundaram, D. Oxidation facilitated antimicrobial ability of laser micro-textured titanium alloy against gram-positive *Staphylococcus aureus* for biomedical applications. *J. Laser Appl.* **2018**, *30*, 032001. [CrossRef]
31. Shiju, V.P.; Abhijith, N.V.; Sudeep, U. Experimental study on the influence of hydrophilicity on bacterial adhesion in bioimplants. *J. Phys: Conf. Ser.* **2019**, *1355*, 012028. [CrossRef]

32. Doll, K.; Fadeeva, E.; Stumpp, N.S.; Grade, S.; Chichkov, B.N.; Stiesch, M. Reduced bacterial adhesion on titanium surfaces micro-structured by ultra-short pulsed laser ablation. *BioNanoMaterials* 2016, *17*, 53–57. [CrossRef]
33. Eghbali, N.; Naffakh-Moosavy, H.; Sadeghi Mohammadi, S.; Naderi-Manesh, H. The influence of laser frequency and groove distance on cell adhesion, cell viability, and antibacterial characteristics of Ti-6Al-4V dental implants treated by modern fiber engraving laser. *Dent. Mater.* 2021, *37*, 547–558. [CrossRef] [PubMed]
34. Chik, N.; Wan, W.S.; Zain, M.d.; Mohamad, A.J.; Sidek, M.Z.; Wan, W.H.; Reif, A.; Rakebrandt, J.H.; Pfleging, W.; Liu, X. Bacterial Adhesion on the Titanium and Stainless-Steel Surfaces Undergone Two Different Treatment Methods: Polishing and Ultrafast Laser Treatment. *IOP Conf. Ser. Mater. Sci. Eng.* 2018, *358*, 012034. [CrossRef]
35. Zwahr, C.; Helbig, R.; Werner, C.; Lasagni, A.F. Fabrication of multifunctional titanium surfaces by producing hierarchical surface patterns using laser based ablation methods. *Sci. Rep.* 2019, *9*, 6721. [CrossRef]
36. Yao, W.L.; Lin, J.C.Y.; Salamanca, E.; Pan, Y.-H.; Tsai, P.-Y.; Leu, S.-J.; Yang, K.-C.; Huang, H.-M.; Huang, H.-Y.; Chang, W.-J. Er,Cr:YSGG Laser Performance Improves Biological Response on Titanium Surfaces. *Materials* 2020, *13*, 756. [CrossRef] [PubMed]
37. Orazi, L.; Pogorielov, M.; Deineka, V.; Husak, V.; Korniienko, O.; Mishchenko, O.; Reggiani, B. Osteoblast cell response to LIPSS-modified Ti-implants. *Key Eng. Mater.* 2019, *813*, 322–327. [CrossRef]
38. Meinshausen, A.K.; Herbster, M.; Zwahr, C.; Soldera, M.; Müller, A.; Halle, T.; Lasagni, A.F.; Bertrand, J. Aspect ratio of nano/microstructures determines *Staphylococcus aureus* adhesion on PET and titanium surfaces. *J. Appl. Microbiol.* 2021, *131*, 1498–1514. [CrossRef] [PubMed]
39. Luo, X.; Yao, S.; Zhang, H.; Cai, M.; Liu, W.; Pan, R.; Chen, C.; Wang, X.; Wang, L.; Zhong, M. Biocompatible nano-ripples structured surfaces induced by femtosecond laser to rebel bacterial colonization and biofilm formation. *Opt. Laser Technol.* 2020, *124*, 105973. [CrossRef]
40. Donaghy, C.L.; McFadden, R.; Smith, G.C.; Kelaini, S.; Carson, L.; Malinov, S.; Margariti, A.; Chan, C.-W. Fibre Laser Treatment of Beta TNZT Titanium Alloys for Load-Bearing Implant Applications: Effects of Surface Physical and Chemical Features on Mesenchymal Stem Cell Response and *Staphylococcus aureus* Bacterial Attachment. *Coatings* 2019, *9*, 186. [CrossRef]

Disclaimer/Publisher's Note: The statements, opinions and data contained in all publications are solely those of the individual author(s) and contributor(s) and not of MDPI and/or the editor(s). MDPI and/or the editor(s) disclaim responsibility for any injury to people or property resulting from any ideas, methods, instructions or products referred to in the content.

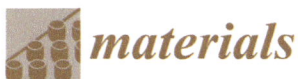 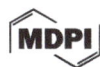

Article

Dimensional Accuracy of Novel Vinyl Polysiloxane Compared with Polyether Impression Materials: An In Vitro Study

Moritz Waldecker, Stefan Rues, Peter Rammelsberg and Wolfgang Bömicke *

Department of Prosthetic Dentistry, University Hospital Heidelberg, University of Heidelberg, 69120 Heidelberg, Germany; moritz.waldecker@med.uni-heidelberg.de (M.W.); stefan.rues@med.uni-heidelberg.de (S.R.); peter.rammelsberg@med.uni-heidelberg.de (P.R.)
* Correspondence: wolfgang.boemicke@med.uni-heidelberg.de; Tel.: +49-6221-56-6052

Abstract: Transferring the intraoral situation accurately to the dental laboratory is crucial for fabricating precise restorations. This study aimed to compare the dimensional accuracy of a new hydrophilic quadrofunctional vinyl polysiloxane (VPS) and polyether (PE), in combination with different impression techniques (mono-phase single step or dual-phase single step). The reference model simulated a partially edentulous mandible. Stainless-steel precision balls were welded to specific teeth and were used to detect dimensional deviations. Fifteen impressions were made for each of the following four test groups: (1) VPS mono-phase, (2) PE mono-phase, (3) VPS dual-phase, and (4) PE dual-phase. Global accuracy was measured by deviations from the reference model, while local accuracy focused on the trueness and precision of abutment tooth surfaces. Statistical analysis was conducted using ANOVA ($\alpha = 0.05$). All distances were underestimated, with the highest global inaccuracies for the cross-arch distance, ranging from -82 µm to -109 µm. The abutment tooth surfaces showed excellent local accuracy for all the materials and techniques, with crown surface trueness < 10 µm and precision < 12 µm. Inlay surfaces had higher inaccuracies (trueness < 15 µm, precision < 26 µm). Within the limitations of this study, all impression materials and techniques can be used to produce models with clinically acceptable accuracy.

Keywords: accuracy; impression technique; vinyl polysiloxane; polyether

Citation: Waldecker, M.; Rues, S.; Rammelsberg, P.; Bömicke, W. Dimensional Accuracy of Novel Vinyl Polysiloxane Compared with Polyether Impression Materials: An In Vitro Study. *Materials* **2024**, *17*, 4221. https://doi.org/10.3390/ma17174221

Academic Editor: Ines Despotović

Received: 15 July 2024
Revised: 9 August 2024
Accepted: 23 August 2024
Published: 27 August 2024

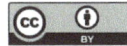

Copyright: © 2024 by the authors. Licensee MDPI, Basel, Switzerland. This article is an open access article distributed under the terms and conditions of the Creative Commons Attribution (CC BY) license (https://creativecommons.org/licenses/by/4.0/).

1. Introduction

The accuracy of fit of tooth-supported restorations depends on many factors during the fabrication process, of which the accuracy of the impression and the resulting cast are probably the most important. The basic prerequisite for accurately fitting dental restorations is an almost error-free transfer of the intraoral situation to the dental laboratory. Today, dentists have two basic approaches to making an impression—the conventional approach using plastic impression materials and the digital approach using an intraoral scan.

Digital impressions are currently the focus of much scientific attention and are being used more and more in everyday practice. Compared with conventional impressions, digital impressions save time [1,2], increase patient comfort [1,2] and, depending on the indication, improve accuracy. However, despite these clinical and economic benefits, there are limitations. One limitation is that subgingival preparation margins, poorly visible proximal contact areas, insufficient mouth opening, or anatomical features in the retromolar space can make digital impressions difficult or even impossible. Another limitation is that intraoral scanners are only feasible for certain indications. While superior fit has been reported for single crowns and three-unit fixed partial dentures fabricated using digital impressions [3], scan volumes larger than half a jaw are considered unsuitable for the fabrication of fixed partial dentures [4–7]. Finally, for technical or physical reasons, there is currently no straightforward way to fabricate removable partial or complete dentures based on digital impressions alone [8,9]. Therefore, conventional impressions still play an important role in everyday dental practice.

Two main materials are used to take conventional impressions of teeth or implants supporting fixed or removable dental prosthesis—polyether (PE) and vinyl polysiloxane (VPS) [10,11].

There is no ideal material for every situation [12,13], with each material having its own limitations. Therefore, the dental industry continues to develop improved or even novel materials for conventional impressions. However, the suitability of these new materials must be scientifically tested.

The aim of this study was to compare the dimensional accuracy of a novel VPS material with improved hydrophilicity (hydrophilic quadrofunctional vinyl polysiloxane) with that of established PE materials in combination with different impression techniques (monophase single step or dual-phase single step) over short and long distances as well as their accuracy (trueness and precision) and angular changes at the abutment tooth level. The null hypotheses were that accuracy would not be influenced by material class, impression technique, or impression material.

2. Materials and Methods

An edentulous mandibular arch was fabricated from steel and fitted with cobalt–chromium teeth (Figure 1). The partially edentulous arch model simulated the conditions for a fixed partial denture with complete crown preparations on the left first premolar (LP) and first molar (LM) and a trihydral inlay preparation on the right second premolar (RP). Stainless-steel precision balls (diameter = 3.175 mm; G3; shape deviation $\leq$ 0.08 µm; mean roughness value Ra $\leq$ 0.01 µm; variation of ball diameter $\leq$ 0.13 µm) were welded onto the right second molar (B_1 with center P_1), onto the left first molar (B_2 with center P_2), and between the central incisors (B_3 with center P_3). The model was covered with polymethyl methacrylate resin to simulate the attached gingiva.

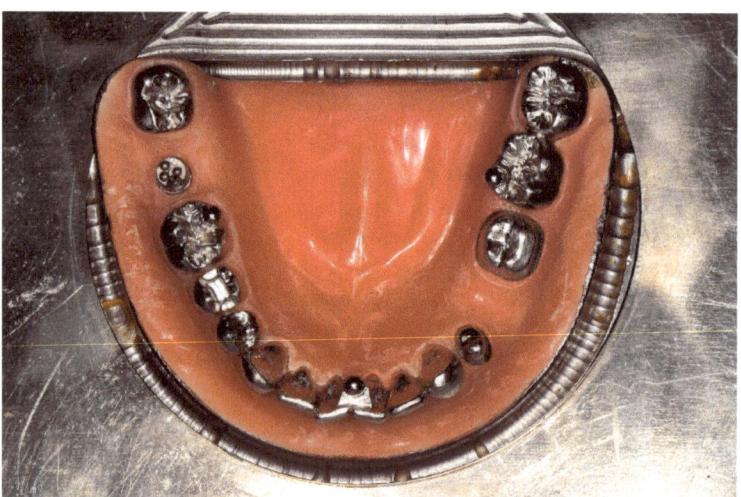

Figure 1. Occlusal view of the reference model.

Before being welded to the model base, all prepared teeth were measured with high precision to create a digital reference dataset on the tooth level (µscan with CF4 sensor, NanoFocus AG (Oberhausen, Germany); surface grid = 50 µm; accuracy < 1 µm). To determine the spatial positioning of the precision balls and the prepared teeth after being welded to the steel base, measurements were made using a coordinate measuring machine (Mar-Vision 222, Hexagon Metrology (Wetzlar, Germany); accuracy < 1–2 µm).

A global coordinate system was defined by the centers of the precision balls (P_1, P_2, and P_3) as follows (Figure 2): P_1 as the origin, x-axis in the direction P_1P_2, and the xy-plane defined by all three center points, with the y-axis oriented in the anterior direction. A local coordinate system with axes parallel to those of the global coordinate system was added at the respective center of the margin of each prepared tooth, resulting in angles of 0° between the corresponding tooth axes in the reference model. The reference distances between the center points of the precision balls and of the margins are shown in Table 1.

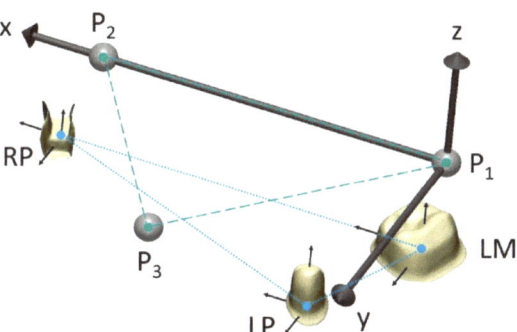

Figure 2. Defined distances between center of each precision ball (turquoise dashed) and between center points on margin level of prepared teeth (blue dotted). LM, left first molar; LP, left first premolar; RP, right first premolar; P_1, center point of precision ball 1; P_2, center point of precision ball 2; P_3, center point of precision ball 3.

Table 1. Reference distances between center points of precision balls and margins (margin level) as well as between intersection points of vertical axis of local coordinate systems (z-axis) with respective tooth surface (surface level).

Distances between Precision Balls			Distances between Prepared Teeth					
[mm]								
P_1P_2	P_1P_3	P_2P_3	LPLM		LMRP		LPRP	
			Margin level	Surface level	Margin level	Surface level	Margin level	Surface level
40.338	35.916	31.927	15.400	15.359	41.515	41.500	36.578	36.498

A total of 15 impressions per test group were made from the reference model (Table 2). All impressions were removed from the model after 12 min, which is twice the clinical setting time of the PE material and 2.4 times the setting time of the VPS material. The extended setting time at room temperature for VPS was chosen because shrinkage effects could still be detected 10 min (which would be twice the setting time of the material) after mixing. Metallic rim-lock trays were used, individualized with an incisal stop and a dorsal dam, to guarantee a minimum distance between the tray and the metallic reference model and positional stability during setting as well as to support a seamless flow of the impression material to the tooth row. All impressions were disinfected for 5 min (PrintoSept-ID, Alpro Medical GmbH (St. Georgen, Germany)) and then poured with type IV gypsum (esthetic-base gold, dentona AG (Dortmund, Germany)) no earlier than 1 h after removal from the model. The saw-cut models were scanned using a laboratory scanner (D2000, 3shape A/S (Kopenhagen, Denmark)) with a quality control software to generate a digital dataset in the STL file format.

First, the position of the ball centers (given diameter d = 3.175 mm) was determined by optimization (method of least squares; squared deviations at the triangle corner points were weighted with proportionate surface area using MATLAB version R2020a, MathWorks (Natick, MA, USA), and the deviations for distances defined by the ball centers, ΔP_1P_2, ΔP_1P_3, and ΔP_2P_3, were calculated in relation to the respective reference distances. For the prepared teeth, each reference tooth surface, together with its local coordinate system, was aligned separately to the scan data by means of a best-fit algorithm (Geomagic Design X;

3D Systems (Rock Hill, SC, USA). Distance deviations (ΔLMLP, ΔLMRP, and ΔLPRP) were then assessed between the origins of the coordinate systems (margin level), located at the center of the margin line, and between the intersection points of the vertical axes (z-axes) of the local coordinate systems with the respective occlusal tooth surface (surface level). In addition, angular deviations between the x-axes (Δα), the y-axes (Δβ), and the z-axes (Δγ) after individual tooth alignment were assessed.

Table 2. Test groups differing in impression material/material combination, material class, and impression technique.

Test Group	Impression Material/Material Combinations	Material Class	Impression Technique
VPS-MP	Aquasil Ultra+ Medium	Vinyl polysiloxane	Mono-phase
PE-MP	Impregum Penta Soft	Polyether	Mono-phase
VPS-DP	Aquasil Ultra+ Heavy/XLV	Vinyl polysiloxane	Dual-phase
PE-DP	Impregum Penta H Duo Soft/Garant L Duo Soft	Polyether	Dual-phase

Distance deviations were analyzed using both signed and unsigned values. The accuracy of the individual surfaces of the prepared teeth within the margin line was analyzed in terms of trueness (mean mesh deviation between reference and scan) and precision (standard deviation of the mesh deviations along the surface). To evaluate trueness and precision, unsigned (absolute) values were used.

All results were displayed as boxplot diagrams for descriptive analysis. In boxplots, circles/asterixes mark mild/extreme outliers deviating more than 1.5/3.0 times the interquartile range from the respective quartile value. Significant ($\alpha = 0.05$) factors were quantified using ANOVA and Tukey's post hoc tests (SPSS 24 (Armonk, NY, USA)).

3. Results

In general, distances were underestimated independent of the test group. Mean distance deviations between the precision ball centers were highest for the cross-arch distance (P_1P_2) and ranged between -82 μm for the PE-DP group and -109 μm for the VPS-MP group (Table 3, Figure 3). Distances between the abutment teeth (Table 3, Figure 4) were reproduced more accurately. Mean distance deviations were not larger than -63 μm (measured for VPS-DP) at the margin line level and -84 μm (measured for VPS-MP) at the surface level for long distances (LMRP and LPRP). All the gypsum models showed high accuracy independent of the impression material for the frequent clinical application of three-unit fixed partial dentures. The mean deviations for the distance between the respective abutment teeth (LMLP) never exceeded -18 μm (measured for PE-MP) at the margin line level and -16 μm (measured for VPS-MP, PE-MP, and VPS-DP) at the surface level.

Gypsum casts fabricated from PE impressions showed slightly less deviation from the reference model than those fabricated from the VPS impression materials. The accuracy between the VPS and the PE did not differ more than 15 μm for the mono-phase impressions and 27 μm for the dual-phase impressions. No statistically significant influence of material class was found for distances defined by the precision ball centers ($p = 0.131$), whereas distances between the abutment teeth did have a significant effect ($p = 0.001$).

For the impression technique (mono-phase/dual-phase), a significant effect was found for both distances defined by the precision ball centers and for distances between the abutment teeth at the surface level ($p \leq 0.036$) but not for distances between the abutment teeth at the margin line level ($p = 0.169$).

Concerning the distances defined by the precision ball center points, multiple comparisons revealed no significant differences between the two mono-phase impression materials, VPS-MP and PE-MP ($p = 0.989$), and the two dual-phase impression materials, VPS-DP and PE-DP ($p = 0.265$). For distances between the abutment teeth at the margin line and surface level, a significant difference was observed between the dual-phase impression materials ($p < 0.001$) but not for the mono-phase impression materials ($p \geq 0.145$).

Table 3. Deviations in distances between center points of precision balls and of margins (margin level) as well as between intersection points of vertical axis of local coordinate systems (z-axis) with respective tooth surface (surface level).

Test group	Distance	Level	Distance Deviations [μm]				
			Mean Value	Standard Deviation	Minimum	Median	Maximum
VPS-MP	P_1P_2	-	−109	24	−154	−109	−60
	P_1P_3	-	−83	14	−106	−87	−64
	P_2P_3	-	−66	15	−92	−67	−39
	LMLP	Margin	−13	11	−32	−13	4
		Surface	−16	13	39	−16	5
	LMRP	Margin	−58	21	−109	−53	−28
		Surface	−84	17	−123	−82	−59
	LPRP	Margin	−58	23	−109	−53	−23
		Surface	−84	17	−114	−80	−47
PE-MP	P_1P_2	-	−94	20	−131	−89	−65
	P_1P_3	-	−93	25	−141	−91	−50
	P_2P_3	-	−66	26	−132	−56	−42
	LMLP	Margin	−18	14	−36	−23	6
		Surface	−16	16	−38	−23	17
	LMRP	Margin	−49	12	−69	−45	−33
		Surface	−69	15	−96	−72	−48
	LPRP	Margin	−48	19	−80	−42	−23
		Surface	−69	20	−96	−66	−37
VPS-DP	P_1P_2	-	−91	25	−120	−97	−15
	P_1P_3	-	−80	27	−134	−82	−38
	P_2P_3	-	−56	18	−78	−58	−8
	LMLP	Margin	−13	11	−37	−13	7
		Surface	−16	14	−46	−13	4
	LMRP	Margin	−63	28	−107	−61	−10
		Surface	−83	28	−125	−89	−19
	LPRP	Margin	−59	27	−104	−58	−21
		Surface	−79	26	−127	−76	−45
PE-DP	P_1P_2	-	−82	40	−161	−77	20
	P_1P_3	-	−68	36	−140	−66	19
	P_2P_3	-	−47	32	−114	−47	8
	LMLP	Margin	−12	16	−43	−10	18
		Surface	−9	19	−42	−10	36
	LMRP	Margin	−36	31	−88	−43	35
		Surface	−53	37	−111	−63	34
	LPRP	Margin	−34	29	−74	−40	20
		Surface	−56	29	−101	−60	−5

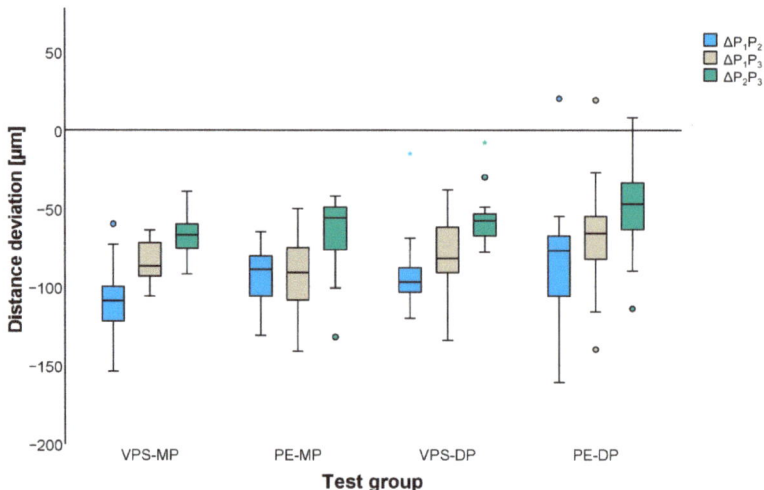

Figure 3. Distance deviations displayed for distances between precision ball center points P_1, P_2, and P_3.

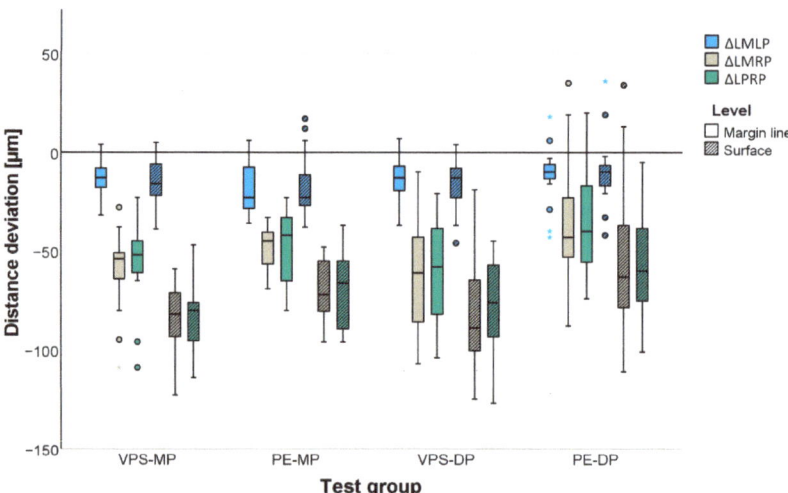

Figure 4. Distance deviations displayed for distances between abutment teeth measured at margin level and at surface level.

The mean angular deviations between the tooth axes (given by the attached local coordinate systems) ranged between 0.8° and 1.2° for all three axes and all test groups. Maximum angular changes never exceeded 2°. For the most important case, angular changes between the vertical tooth axes (z-axes), the results are given in Table 4. Once again, excellent accuracy was observed for the three-unit fixed partial denture, with mean angular changes of about 0.2° independent of the impression material. For longer distances, the upper limit was 0.8°.

Table 4. Vertical angular deviations for prepared teeth.

Angular Deviation	Test Group	Mean Value	Standard Deviation	Minimum	Median	Maximum
				[°]		
Δα	VPS-MP	1.0	0.1	0.8	1.0	1.3
	PE-MP	1.0	0.2	0.7	1.0	1.8
	VPS-DP	1.0	0.1	0.7	1.0	1.2
	PE-DP	1.1	0.3	0.8	1.1	1.9
Δβ	VPS-MP	1.1	0.1	0.9	1.1	1.2
	PE-MP	1.1	0.2	1.0	1.1	1.7
	VPS-DP	1.0	0.1	0.9	1.0	1.2
	PE-DP	1.2	0.2	1.0	1.2	2.0
Δγ	VPS-MP	0.8	0.1	0.6	0.9	1.0
	PE-MP	0.8	0.1	0.7	0.8	1.1
	VPS-DP	0.8	0.1	0.7	0.8	0.9
	PE-DP	0.9	0.1	0.7	0.8	1.1

The local accuracy of the gypsum master casts was comparable in all test groups ($p = 0.089$, Table 5 and Figure 5). Excellent accuracy was obtained for the abutment teeth with full crown preparations (trueness < 10 μm, precision < 12 μm), whereas inlay preparations were more challenging and showed significantly lower accuracy ($p < 0.001$; trueness < 15 μm, precision < 26 μm).

Table 5. Trueness (precision) for individual prepared teeth.

Tooth	Test Group	Mean Value	Standard Deviation	Minimum	Median	Maximum
				[μm]		
LP	VPS-MP	8 (7)	2 (2)	6 (5)	7 (6)	13 (10)
	PE-MP	8 (7)	1 (2)	6 (5)	8 (7)	11 (12)
	VPS-DP	9 (10)	2 (2)	7 (6)	8 (7)	14 (39)
	PE-DP	7 (6)	1 (1)	6 (5)	8 (6)	9 (7)
LM	VPS-MP	10 (9)	3 (3)	5 (6)	10 (8)	17 (16)
	PE-MP	9 (11)	4 (6)	5 (5)	8 (9)	16 (27)
	VPS-DP	10 (9)	5 (5)	5 (5)	9 (8)	21 (26)
	PE-DP	8 (9)	2 (4)	6 (5)	8 (7)	13 (20)
RP	VPS-MP	13 (23)	3 (14)	10 (13)	12 (18)	22 (56)
	PE-MP	13 (24)	2 (9)	10 (13)	13 (19)	15 (40)
	VPS-DP	14 (26)	2 (14)	11 (13)	14 (22)	20 (70)
	PE-DP	13 (25)	2 (11)	10 (14)	13 (22)	17 (48)

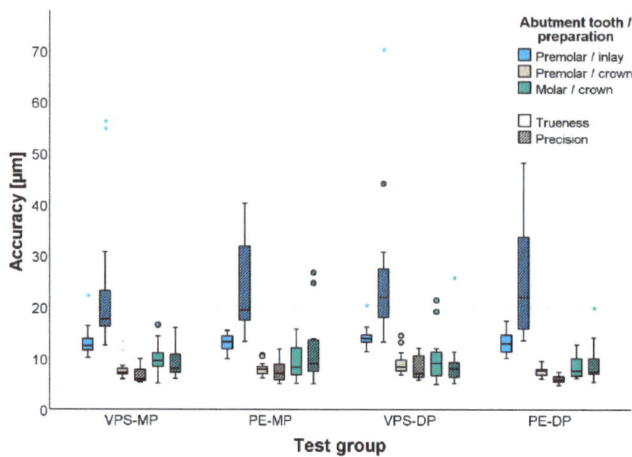

Figure 5. Accuracy (trueness and precision) of prepared teeth.

4. Discussion

The null hypothesis that accuracy would not be influenced by material class, impression technique, or impression material had to be partially rejected. The local accuracy of the plaster master casts was not different between the groups but did differ between the preparation designs. With respect to global accuracy, the results suggest that the deviations in the plaster master casts generated on the basis of VPS and PE materials were, in general, small but partially significant different.

This study involved every stage of the workflow, including disinfection of the impression. Disinfection has been shown to influence the impression material's dimensional accuracy and the surface detail reproduction [14,15]. There is no standard method for disinfecting dental impressions. Various alternative methods can be found in the literature, including the following: ethylene oxide [16], autoclave [16], microwave [17], ultraviolet radiation [18,19], immediate pour and disinfection of the cast [20,21], and chemical disinfection, by the spray or immersion method [22,23]. Chemical disinfection by immersion is considered the most effective method for reducing most microorganisms. As different impression materials have different chemical and physical properties, the manufacturer's recommendations for disinfection of the respective impression material in terms of duration and method should be strictly adhered to [24–26]. Accordingly, this study used a disinfectant in the manner intended by the manufacturer for the impression materials used. Dimensional accuracy and stability of impression materials are crucial factors for successive production of dental restorations. According to Walker et al., regardless of the disinfection protocol (not disinfected or disinfected with two different disinfectant solutions, in combination, with two different time intervals), no significant difference was found for VPS in terms of dimensional accuracy [14]. For PE, a significant difference was found between the disinfected and non-disinfected impressions. This is due to the expansion of PE caused by the absorption of water from the disinfectant solution [14]. In addition to the global accuracy, the local accuracy of an impression is also important. While the surfaces of the VPS impressions showed no changes after disinfection, NaOCL (0.5%) had a significant effect on the surface quality of PE impression, resulting in a mottled or matte/sticky surface. If an impression is not poured directly, the long-term stability of the impression materials is also important. VPS and PE were reported to show a significant difference in their dimensional stability over time. This effect was observed for the non-disinfected and disinfected impressions. However, it is important to emphasize at this point that any changes in accuracy caused by different disinfection methods or registered by measurements at different times have no clinically relevant influence [14,15,22,27,28].

Nevertheless, it seemed reasonable and important to consider disinfection as an integral step in the clinical process of model fabrication, as well as to reflect any potential impact on model accuracy in the results of this study.

Irrespective of the impression material and impression technique, all plaster casts were scaled down overall, and all molded structures experienced a certain degree of lingual tilt. This further shortened the distances at the occlusal surface level compared with distance deviations at the margin level. The direction of scale remains controversial in the literature. Some studies have reported an enlarged scale [29], while others have reported both enlarged and scaled-down measurements [7,30,31]. The reference situation in the present study might have been underestimated because a plaster with less than 0.1% expansion was used, which may not have compensated for the shrinkage of the impression material. Since all distances were too short, a higher expansion of the plaster cast would have improved the accuracy. To compensate the -80 μm to -100 μm deviation on the 40 mm cross-arch distance, a plaster with 0.20% to 0.25% more expansion than the one used in our study would have been necessary. This problem cannot be completely solved in such a simplistic manner since there will be shape deviations that cannot be compensated for by a scaling process, but a higher expansion would have been beneficial in our study since all the distances were underestimated.

Additionally, the results show that impression accuracy depends on the impression technique, with lower deviations when using the dual-phase technique. This is in contrast to the findings of previous studies. Johnson et al. reported better accuracy with the mono-phase technique than with the dual-phase technique [32], and an earlier study on the same reference model showed that regular-setting polyether impressions performed better with the mono-phase technique than those with the dual-phase technique [33]. Nevertheless, the results are in line with the expectation that the dual-phase technique has greater dimensional stability. Dimensional deviations should be lower with the dual-phase technique because the filler content is higher in the highly viscous phase.

With regard to local accuracy of the impressions/plaster casts, both trueness and precision were excellent, independent of the material class, impression technique, and impression material. However, the full-crown preparations deviated significantly less than the inlay-preparations, indicating that accurate impressions/plaster casts of inlay preparations are more challenging than those for full-crown-preparations. This might be because of the accessibility of an inlay cavity during the scanning process is much worse than that of a full-crown preparation when digitizing the plaster cast or the more challenging situation during impression-making and pouring of the plaster-casts. However, in general, the observed accuracy of the tested impression materials/techniques is in the range of that which has been demonstrated in previous studies [31,33].

Both impression material class and impression technique are suitable for taking highly accurate impressions of single crowns, fixed partial dentures, inlays, or a complete dental arch. Accuracy differs only slightly between impression materials, so it is reasonable to assume that other factors determine which impression material should be used in a daily routine. This decision may be influenced by economic factors (price, shelf life, storability), patient-related factors (taste, demolding force), physical properties (tear strength, compatibility with astringents or disinfectants, tolerance towards moisture), biological properties (toxicity), and handling differences. Seen in this way, the almost five times higher tear strength of the VPS-DP compared to the PE-DP, in combination with the two to three times easier removal of a VPS impression compared to a PE impression due to less adhesion to the tooth hard substances, might represent a noticeable advantage [13,14]. Impression materials with clinical approval were used in this study. The probability of the impression materials used triggering an allergic or toxic reaction is therefore low. Nevertheless, the literature attributes a certain cytotoxic potential to impression materials [34]. Roberta et al. were able to show that PE drastically reduces cell proliferation in comparison with VPS. At the same time, however, no difference was found between the two materials in terms of their cytotoxicity [35]. A cytotoxic effect was found even after a short exposure time of 10 min of the human gingival fibroblast cells to various impression materials. Dentists should therefore select an impression material with low cytotoxicity and the shortest possible setting time and ensure that all impression residues are removed from the oral cavity [36].

As digital impressions cannot currently be used for all indications, it seems reasonable to continue the development of new impression materials and the further development and enhancement of existing impression materials [4–9,37]. The focus should be on conventional impression materials that set quickly or whose setting behavior can be controlled by the clinician.

There are some limitations to this study. This was an in vitro study looking at one partially edentulous situation with prepared and unprepared metal teeth, so the results may not apply to other dental situations. Future studies should be conducted on additional models of different partially edentulous situations.

That being said, metal teeth do not have uncharacteristically higher demolding forces compared with natural teeth [38]. It can be stated that the material properties of the metal reference teeth in relation to the demolding forces are comparable to the properties of natural teeth.

Another limitation is that the workflow in this study represents a best-case scenario. The impression tray was fixed and completely immobile during the setting of the impression material, so the clinically relevant influences of patient movements or changes in the position of the impression tray on accuracy were not observed. In addition, the effects of moisture or saliva, sulcus fluid, and blood could not be investigated in vitro.

Moreover, the number of samples is limited. However, 15 samples seem to be a sufficient sample size. In a previous study using an identical model and an identical evaluation strategy, significant differences were found with an even smaller (n = 10) or a similar number of samples (n = 16) [33,38].

5. Conclusions

Within the limitations of this study, the following conclusions were drawn:
1. VPS and PE impression materials have adequate accuracy for all clinical applications.
2. The dual-phase impression technique may give a more accurate impression.
3. Short distances are displayed more accurately than long distances regardless of the impression material.
4. Inlay preparations are less accurate than full crown preparations, regardless of the impression material used.
5. The choice of impression material and impression technique lies with the treating clinician and is not only dependent on the accuracy of the impression material.

Author Contributions: Conceptualization, M.W., S.R., P.R. and W.B.; methodology, M.W., S.R. and W.B.; formal analysis, M.W., S.R. and W.B.; writing—original draft preparation, M.W.; writing—review and editing, S.R., P.R. and W.B.; visualization, M.W.; project administration, M.W., S.R. and W.B. All authors have read and agreed to the published version of the manuscript.

Funding: Moritz Waldecker is funded by the Physician-Scientist Program of University of Heidelberg, Faculty of Medicine. The study was financially supported by Dentsply Sirona.

Institutional Review Board Statement: Not applicable.

Informed Consent Statement: Not applicable.

Data Availability Statement: The original contributions presented in the study are included in the article, further inquiries can be directed to the corresponding author.

Acknowledgments: The authors would like to thank Dorothee Ruckes for conducting the tests.

Conflicts of Interest: The authors declare no conflicts of interest.

References

1. Yuzbasioglu, E.; Kurt, H.; Turunc, R.; Bilir, H. Comparison of digital and conventional impression techniques: Evaluation of patients' perception, treatment comfort, effectiveness and clinical outcomes. *BMC Oral Health* **2014**, *14*, 10. [CrossRef]
2. Schepke, U.; Meijer, H.J.; Kerdijk, W.; Cune, M.S. Digital versus analog complete-arch impressions for single-unit premolar implant crowns: Operating time and patient preference. *J. Prosthet. Dent.* **2015**, *114*, 403–406.e1. [CrossRef]
3. Chochlidakis, K.M.; Papaspyridakos, P.; Geminiani, A.; Chen, C.J.; Feng, I.J.; Ercoli, C. Digital versus conventional impressions for fixed prosthodontics: A systematic review and meta-analysis. *J. Prosthet. Dent.* **2016**, *116*, 184–190.e12. [CrossRef] [PubMed]
4. Waldecker, M.; Rues, S.; Behnisch, R.; Rammelsberg, P.; Bomicke, W. Effect of scan-path length on the scanning accuracy of completely dentate and partially edentulous maxillae. *J. Prosthet. Dent.* **2024**, *131*, 146–154. [CrossRef]
5. Waldecker, M.; Bömicke, W.; Behnisch, R.; Rammelsberg, P.; Rues, S. In-vitro accuracy of complete arch scans of the fully dentate and the partially edentulous maxilla. *J. Prosthodont. Res.* **2021**, *66*, 538–545. [CrossRef] [PubMed]
6. Waldecker, M.; Rues, S.; Rammelsberg, P.; Bömicke, W. Accuracy of complete-arch intraoral scans based on confocal microscopy versus optical triangulation: A comparative in vitro study. *J. Prosthet. Dent.* **2020**, *126*, 414–420. [CrossRef] [PubMed]
7. Waldecker, M.; Rues, S.; Awounvo Awounvo, J.S.; Rammelsberg, P.; Bömicke, W. In vitro accuracy of digital and conventional impressions in the partially edentulous maxilla. *Clin. Oral Investig.* **2022**, *26*, 6491–6502. [CrossRef] [PubMed]
8. Cameron, A.B.; Evans, J.L.; Robb, N.D. A technical and clinical digital approach to the altered cast technique with an intraoral scanner and polyvinyl siloxane impression material. *J. Prosthet. Dent.* **2022**, *132*, 315–319. [CrossRef]
9. Chebib, N.; Imamura, Y.; El Osta, N.; Srinivasan, M.; Muller, F.; Maniewicz, S. Fit and retention of complete denture bases: Part II—Conventional impressions versus digital scans: A clinical controlled crossover study. *J. Prosthet. Dent.* **2022**, *131*, 618–625. [CrossRef]
10. Hamalian, T.A.; Nasr, E.; Chidiac, J.J. Impression materials in fixed prosthodontics: Influence of choice on clinical procedure. *J. Prosthodont.* **2011**, *20*, 153–160. [CrossRef]
11. Jayaraman, S.; Singh, B.P.; Ramanathan, B.; Pazhaniappan Pillai, M.; MacDonald, L.; Kirubakaran, R. Final-impression techniques and materials for making complete and removable partial dentures. *Cochrane Database Syst. Rev.* **2018**, *4*, CD012256. [CrossRef] [PubMed]
12. Guo, Y.Q.; Ma, Y.; Cai, S.N.; Yu, H. Optimal impression materials for implant-supported fixed complete dentures: A systematic review and meta-analysis. *J. Prosthet. Dent.* **2023**, in press. [CrossRef] [PubMed]
13. Hüttig, F.; Klink, A.; Kohler, A.; Mutschler, M.; Rupp, F. Flowability, Tear Strength, and Hydrophilicity of Current Elastomers for Dental Impressions. *Materials* **2021**, *14*, 2994. [CrossRef] [PubMed]
14. Walker, M.P.; Rondeau, M.; Petrie, C.; Tasca, A.; Williams, K. Surface quality and long-term dimensional stability of current elastomeric impression materials after disinfection. *J. Prosthodont.* **2007**, *16*, 343–351. [CrossRef]
15. Kotsiomiti, E.; Tzialla, A.; Hatjivasiliou, K. Accuracy and stability of impression materials subjected to chemical disinfection—A literature review. *J. Oral Rehabil.* **2008**, *35*, 291–299. [CrossRef]
16. Holtan, J.R.; Olin, P.S.; Rudney, J.D. Dimensional stability of a polyvinylsiloxane impression material following ethylene oxide and steam autoclave sterilization. *J. Prosthet. Dent.* **1991**, *65*, 519–525. [CrossRef]
17. Abdelaziz, K.M.; Hassan, A.M.; Hodges, J.S. Reproducibility of sterilized rubber impressions. *Braz. Dent. J.* **2004**, *15*, 209–213. [CrossRef]
18. Ishida, H.; Nahara, Y.; Tamamoto, M.; Hamada, T. The fungicidal effect of ultraviolet light on impression materials. *J. Prosthet. Dent.* **1991**, *65*, 532–535. [CrossRef]
19. Larsen, T.; Fiehn, N.E.; Peutzfeldt, A.; Owall, B. Disinfection of dental impressions and occlusal records by ultraviolet radiation. *Eur. J. Prosthodont. Restor. Dent.* **2000**, *8*, 71–74.
20. Ivanovski, S.; Savage, N.W.; Brockhurst, P.J.; Bird, P.S. Disinfection of dental stone casts: Antimicrobial effects and physical property alterations. *Dent. Mater.* **1995**, *11*, 19–23. [CrossRef]
21. Stern, M.A.; Johnson, G.H.; Toolson, L.B. An evaluation of dental stones after repeated exposure to spray disinfectants. Part I: Abrasion and compressive strength. *J. Prosthet. Dent.* **1991**, *65*, 713–718. [CrossRef] [PubMed]
22. Ahuja, B.M.; Pawashe, K.G.; Sanyal, P.K.; Al-Qarni, M.A.; Alqahtani, N.M.; Alqahtani, S.M.; Ahmed, A.R.; Abdul Khader, M.; Elmahdi, A.E.; Chaturvedi, S. Assessment of dimensional stability of novel VPES impression material at different time intervals with standard disinfectants. *BMC Oral Health* **2024**, *24*, 579. [CrossRef] [PubMed]
23. Hardan, L.; Bourgi, R.; Cuevas-Suarez, C.E.; Lukomska-Szymanska, M.; Cornejo-Rios, E.; Tosco, V.; Monterubbianesi, R.; Mancino, S.; Eid, A.; Mancino, D.; et al. Disinfection Procedures and Their Effect on the Microorganism Colonization of Dental Impression Materials: A Systematic Review and Meta-Analysis of In Vitro Studies. *Bioengineering* **2022**, *9*, 123. [CrossRef] [PubMed]
24. Chidambaram, S.R.; George, A.M.; Muralidharan, N.P.; Prasanna Arvind, T.R.; Subramanian, A.; Rahaman, F. Current overview for chemical disinfection of dental impressions and models based on its criteria of usage: A microbiological study. *Indian J. Dent. Res.* **2022**, *33*, 30–36.
25. Vrbova, R.; Bradna, P.; Bartos, M.; Roubickova, A. The effect of disinfectants on the accuracy, quality and surface structure of impression materials and gypsum casts: A comparative study using light microscopy, scanning electron microscopy and micro computed tomography. *Dent. Mater. J.* **2020**, *39*, 500–508. [CrossRef]
26. Lepe, X.; Johnson, G.H. Accuracy of polyether and addition silicone after long-term immersion disinfection. *J. Prosthet. Dent.* **1997**, *78*, 245–249. [CrossRef]

27. Awod Bin Hassan, S.; Ali, F.A.A.; Ibrahim, N.A.L.; Heboyan, A.; Ravinder, S.S. Effect of chemical disinfection on the dimensional stability of polyvinyl ether siloxane impression material: A systemic review and meta-analysis. *BMC Oral Health* **2023**, *23*, 471. [CrossRef]
28. Soganci, G.; Cinar, D.; Caglar, A.; Yagiz, A. 3D evaluation of the effect of disinfectants on dimensional accuracy and stability of two elastomeric impression materials. *Dent. Mater. J.* **2018**, *37*, 675–684. [CrossRef]
29. Caputi, S.; Varvara, G. Dimensional accuracy of resultant casts made by a monophase, one-step and two-step, and a novel two-step putty/light-body impression technique: An in vitro study. *J. Prosthet. Dent.* **2008**, *99*, 274–281. [CrossRef]
30. Hoods-Moonsammy, V.J.; Owen, P.; Howes, D.G. A comparison of the accuracy of polyether, polyvinyl siloxane, and plaster impressions for long-span implant-supported prostheses. *Int. J. Prosthodont.* **2014**, *27*, 433–438. [CrossRef]
31. Stober, T.; Johnson, G.H.; Schmitter, M. Accuracy of the newly formulated vinyl siloxanether elastomeric impression material. *J. Prosthet. Dent.* **2010**, *103*, 228–239. [CrossRef] [PubMed]
32. Johnson, G.H.; Lepe, X.; Aw, T.C. The effect of surface moisture on detail reproduction of elastomeric impressions. *J. Prosthet. Dent.* **2003**, *90*, 354–364. [CrossRef] [PubMed]
33. Zenthöfer, A.; Rues, S.; Rammelsberg, P.; Ruckes, D.; Stober, T. Accuracy of a New Fast-Setting Polyether Impression Material. *Int. J. Prosthodont.* **2020**, *33*, 410–417. [CrossRef]
34. Sydiskis, R.J.; Gerhardt, D.E. Cytotoxicity of impression materials. *J. Prosthet. Dent.* **1993**, *69*, 431–435. [CrossRef]
35. Roberta, T.; Federico, M.; Federica, B.; Antonietta, C.M.; Sergio, B.; Ugo, C. Study of the potential cytotoxicity of dental impression materials. *Toxicol. Vitro.* **2003**, *17*, 657–662. [CrossRef]
36. Chen, S.Y.; Chen, C.C.; Kuo, H.W. Cytotoxicity of dental impression materials. *Bull. Environ. Contam. Toxicol.* **2002**, *69*, 350–355. [CrossRef] [PubMed]
37. Boehm, S.; Rues, S.; Balzer, A.; Rammelsberg, P.; Waldecker, M. Effect of a calibration aid and the intraoral scanner on the registration of a partially edentulous maxilla: An in vitro study. *J. Prosthet. Dent.* **2024**, *in press*. [CrossRef]
38. Rues, S.; Stober, T.; Bargum, T.; Rammelsberg, P.; Zenthöfer, A. Disposable plastic trays and their effect on polyether and vinyl polysiloxane impression accuracy-an in vitro study. *Clin. Oral Investig.* **2021**, *25*, 1475–1484. [CrossRef]

Disclaimer/Publisher's Note: The statements, opinions and data contained in all publications are solely those of the individual author(s) and contributor(s) and not of MDPI and/or the editor(s). MDPI and/or the editor(s) disclaim responsibility for any injury to people or property resulting from any ideas, methods, instructions or products referred to in the content.

Antibiofilm Efficacy of Calcium Silicate-Based Endodontic Sealers

Matilde Ruiz-Linares [1,2,*], Vsevolod Fedoseev [1], Carmen Solana [1,2], Cecilia Muñoz-Sandoval [3] and Carmen María Ferrer-Luque [1,2,*]

1. Department of Stomatology, University of Granada, 18071 Granada, Spain; drfedoseev@correo.ugr.es (V.F.)
2. Instituto de Investigación Biosanitaria, 18012 Granada, Spain
3. Cariology Unit, Department of oral Rehabilitation, Faculty of Dentistry, University of Talca, Talca 3344158, Chile; cemunoz@efom.cl
* Correspondence: matr@ugr.es (M.R.-L.); cferrer@ugr.es (C.M.F.-L.)

Abstract: Background: Using endodontic sealers with long-term antimicrobial properties can increase the success of endodontic treatment. This study aimed to assess the antimicrobial activity over time of two calcium silicate (CS)-based sealers, AH Plus Bioceramic and BioRoot RCS, and to compare them with an epoxy resin-based sealer, AH Plus Jet, against mature polymicrobial biofilms grown on human radicular dentin. Methods: The antimicrobial activity of the sealers was tested using a direct contact test after 1 and 6 weeks of contact with the biofilms. Cell viability was determined by the adenosine triphosphate (ATP) method and flow cytometry (FC). The results of the ATP test were analyzed using an ANOVA with Welch's correction, followed by the Games–Howell test. The number of cells with damaged membranes obtained by FC in each period was compared by means of an ANOVA and Duncan's test. For the comparison between times, a Student's t-test was used. Results: Globally, after a week of contact, the epoxy resin-based sealer obtained the best results. However, at 6 weeks, the two CSs showed the highest antimicrobial efficacy, with a significant increase in this activity over time. Conclusions: Calcium silicate-based sealers exert long-term antimicrobial activity against endodontic biofilms.

Keywords: AH Plus Jet; AH Plus Bioceramic; biofilms; BioRoot RCS; long-term antimicrobial activity

1. Introduction

The aim of endodontic treatment is the prevention and healing of apical periodontitis [1,2]. Using biocompatible filling materials that additionally have antimicrobial properties may be beneficial for endodontic treatment. A bioactive endodontic sealer that hermetically fills the root canal and potentially inhibits the growth of any residual bacteria is desirable [3].

AH Plus® Jet [AH, Dentsply Sirona, Ballaigues, Switzerland] is an epoxy resin-based endodontic sealer that is widely used due to its good physicochemical characteristics, long-term dimensional stability, good adhesion to dentin, fluidity, and biocompatibility [4]. However, its bioactivity and osteogenic potential are limited [5]. Although it has demonstrated some antimicrobial properties, the antiseptic capacity is limited after setting [6]. In addition, mutagenicity, cytotoxicity, inflammatory responses, and hydrophobicity have been reported [7].

Calcium silicate (CS)-based sealers have been gaining popularity, given their bioactivity and biocompatibility [8]. The main components of these materials are calcium silicate, monocalcium phosphate, calcium hydroxide, zirconium oxide, fillers, and thickeners [3,7]. Calcium silicate sealers are hydraulic, and their setting is conditioned by the presence of humidity [9]. Antimicrobial and biomineralization properties are exerted during the setting process through an increasing pH and a release of ions from the material [3,9]. However, these properties can vary greatly depending on the additives in each formulation [8], potentially influencing its indications and clinical application. The first to be marketed were powder–liquid formulations that required manual mixing. More recently, premixed ready-to-use CS formulations have a setting reaction that depends on the moisture existing in the dentinal tubules [9]. Some are still in the early stages of development, requiring more clinical and laboratory studies for their clinical recommendation [7].

BioRoot™ RCS [BR, Septodont, Saint-Maur-des-Fossés, France] is supplied in powder and liquid form. In addition to having good physical properties [10], it has demonstrated low cytotoxicity, inducing the secretion of osteogenic and angiogenic growth factors, and high immunomodulatory properties, which means that it can contribute to the in vivo healing and regeneration process of periapical lesions [11]. It has generally shown antimicrobial capacity in vitro against planktonic bacteria [3] and mono-species biofilms [4,12,13]. Few laboratory studies have evaluated its antimicrobial activity against multispecies biofilms [14,15].

Marketed in 2021, AH Plus® Bioceramic [AHBC, Dentsply Sirona, Ballaigues, Switzerland] is a premixed CS that contains tricalcium silicate, but in a lower percentage than existing ones [16]. The manufacturer claims that it features rapid setting, high wear resistance, and radiopacity; it is safe and biocompatible and does not discolor the tooth. Owing to its recent commercialization, its physical and biological properties are currently being compared with those of other CSs [17–19].

To date, one study has evaluated its antimicrobial activity against planktonic cultures of *E. faecalis* [18], with its antibiofilm activity remaining unknown. Therefore, the present experimental study aimed to evaluate and compare the antimicrobial efficacy over time of two endodontic CSs, AHBC and BR, and an epoxy resin-based sealer, AH, against polymicrobial biofilms formed on dentin.

2. Materials and Methods

The protocol of this in vitro study was approved by the Ethics Committee of the University of Granada, Spain (N° 1076 CEIH/2020). Informed consent was obtained from all patients prior to the collection of microbiological samples or extracted teeth.

The antimicrobial activity of the sealers over time (1 and 6 weeks) was evaluated using a modified direct contact test (DCT) [20] against polymicrobial biofilms on root dentin (n = 12/group/time). The viability of microorganisms after the DCT was quantified by means of the adenosine triphosphate (ATP) assay and flow cytometry (FC) (n = 10/group/time) [20]. Images obtained by confocal laser scanning microscopy (CLSM) served as an in situ visualization of the residual biofilm in dentin (n = 2/group/time).

The study groups were (1) AH Plus Jet (AH), (2) AH Plus Bioceramic (AHBC), (3) Bioroot RCS (BR), and (4) a positive control (without exposure to any material). Twelve material samples per group and evaluation period (1 and 6 weeks) were prepared. The chemical composition of the sealers and handling instructions, specified by the manufacturer, are summarized in Table 1.

2.1. Preparation of Dentin Samples

One hundred and twelve sterile specimens of human radicular dentin (4 × 4 × 0.7 mm) from the root coronal third of 56 single-rooted non-carious teeth, extracted for orthodontic reasons, were utilized as substrate for forming biofilms, as previously reported [21]. Briefly, the dentin samples were standardized by cutting with an Accuton-50 machine (Struers, Copenhagen, Denmark), and discarding the middle and apical thirds of the root and the dental crown to obtain a dentin cylinder of the root coronal third. Then, they were sectioned following the root canal lumen, each giving two halves. The root cement was removed by polishing to a flat surface, and the inner face was polished with 150, 220, 500, and 800-grit silicon carbide paper (Figure 1).

Table 1. Endodontic sealers.

Material (Lot Number)	Composition	Manipulation
AH Plus Jet (AH) (Dentsply Sirona, Ballaigues, Switzerland) (2304000347)	Paste A: bisphenol-A epoxy resin (25–50%), epoxy resin bisphenol-F (2.5–10%), calcium tungstate, zirconium oxide, silica, iron oxide pigments Paste B: N,N'-dibenzyl-5-oxanonandiamine-1,9 (10–25%), amantadine (2.5–10%), calcium tungstate, zirconium oxide, silica, silicone oil	Dual self-mixing syringe
AH Plus Bioceramic (AHBC) (Dentsply Sirona, Ballaigues, Switzerland) (KI221118)	Zirconium dioxide (50–75%), tricalcium silicate (5–15%), dimethyl sulfoxide (10–30%), lithium carbonate (<0.5%), thickening agent (<6%)	Pre-mixed single syringe
Bioroot RCS (BR) (Septodont, Saint-Maur-des-Fossés, France) (B29755)	Powder: tricalcium silicate (25–50%), zirconium oxide (25–50%), povidone Liquid: water, calcium chloride, water-soluble polymer	Powder–liquid: 1 tablespoon of powder and 5 drops of liquid mixed for 60 s

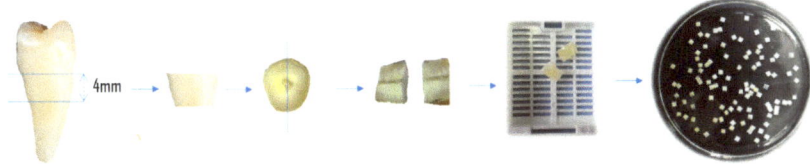

Figure 1. Root dentin sample preparation procedure.

To eliminate the smear layer formed during preparation, the samples were immersed in 17% ethylene diamine tetraacetic acid (EDTA, DIRECTA AB, Stockholm, Sweden) for 5 min and then washed with saline solution. Subsequently, each of the two halves obtained was randomly assigned to the different study groups. They were then autoclaved and incubated in Trypticase Soy Broth [TSB (Scharlau Chemie SA, Barcelona, Spain)] at 37 °C for 24 h to verify the absence of contamination.

2.2. Infection of Dentin Substrates

Microbiological samples were obtained clinically from root canals of necrotic teeth from three volunteer patients following a previous methodology [20] and served as inoculum for dentin infection and biofilm formation. The rubber dam and the tooth were disinfected with 3% H_2O_2 and 2.5% NaOCl, which was inactivated with 5% sodium thiosulfate. Pulp chamber access was gained using a sterile round bur, and the chamber was disinfected as previously described. The root canal was filled with sterile saline solution, taking care not to allow it to overflow; a sterile #15 K file (Dentsply Sirona, Ballaigues, Switzerland) was introduced 1 mm short of the apical foramen, and a gentle filing motion was carried out for 30 s before removal. Then, 3 sterile paper points were inserted into the root canal and left inside for 1 min to absorb the fluid. Both files and paper points were placed in microtubes with Tris-EDTA buffer and frozen at −20 °C until use.

For dentin infection, the samples were mixed in TSB and incubated for 24 h at 37 °C in anaerobiosis. Afterward, the cell density was adjusted in a spectrophotometer to a concentration of approximately 3.0×10^7 colony-forming units per milliliter in TSB. Dentin samples were infected in 24-well plates (Corning™, Fisher Scientific, Madrid, Spain) and inoculated with 200 µL of the microbial suspension described above and 1.8 mL of sterile TSB. Sterile dentin blocks were immersed in the inoculated wells and incubated at 37 °C in an anaerobic atmosphere for 3 weeks on a rocking table. The TSB medium was refreshed once a week to ensure the growth of the biofilms. Two dentin samples in each group were analyzed by CSLM to confirm biofilm growth. A negative control group (n = 4) was incubated only with TSB as a sterility control and processed the same way as the other groups.

2.3. Antimicrobial Activity Test (DCT)

To evaluate the antimicrobial activity of the materials (Figure 2), against polymicrobial biofilms, the dentin samples with the biofilms formed were put in direct contact with the materials. Under aseptic conditions, equal amounts of each sealer were dispensed in the bottom of the customized molds (1cm Ø × 3mm height). To standardize the volume of sealer in the mold, an area of 1 mm was delimited from its bottom, red dashed line in Figure 2a), and coated with each sealer. Sealers were handled following the manufacturer's instructions. The materials inside their molds were then introduced into the wells of a 24-well microtiter plate and stored for 24 h in an incubator at 100% humidity for setting. Next, they were sterilized with ultraviolet light, and 200 µL of sterile TSB was added to each mold.

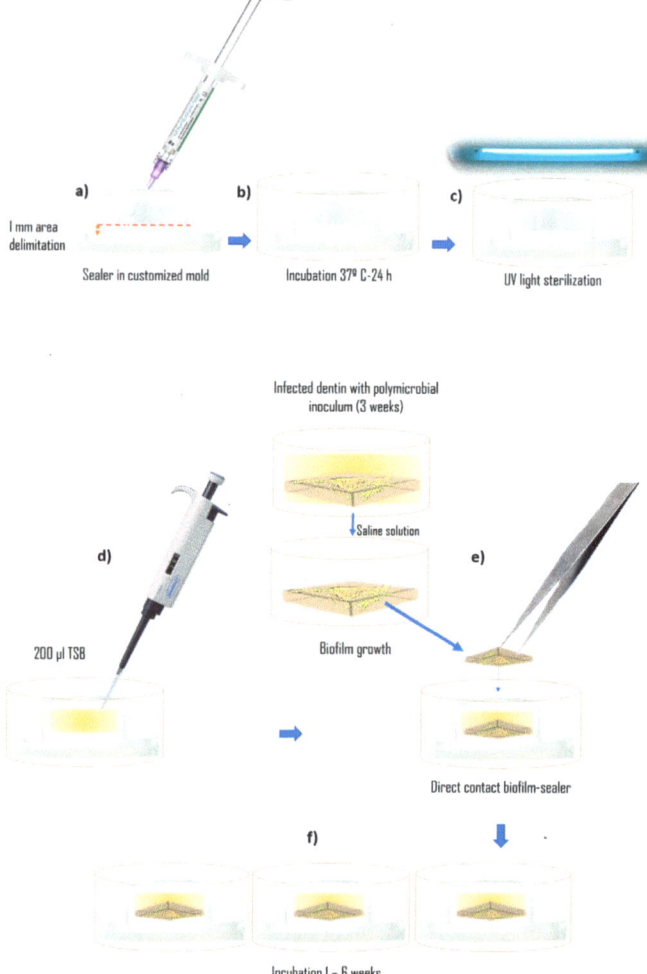

Figure 2. Antimicrobial activity test. Sealers were dispensed in customized mold (**a**), stored for 24 h/37 °C (**b**), and sterilized (**c**). Direct contact test (**d**–**f**).

Finally, the dentin blocks with the biofilm formed were placed in direct contact with the materials and incubated for 1 or 6 weeks at 37 °C under anaerobic conditions. Every three days, 100 µL of TSB was added to the molds to prevent desiccation.

After each contact time, 10 dentin blocks (group/time) were separated, placed in microtubes with 200 µL of TSB, stirred for 10 s, and then sonicated on a water-table sonicator (model 5510E-MT; Branson, Danbury, CT, USA) for 10 min to ensure recovery of biofilms. The remaining 2 dentin samples per group were observed under CSLM. For the control group, the same procedure was followed, except that there was no exposure to any material.

2.4. Microbial Viability

The cell viability of the recovered bacterial suspensions was evaluated by means of ATP and flow cytometry (FC) [22,23]. The ATP levels contained in the suspension of the recovered biofilms were evaluated with the BacTiter-Glo cell viability assay kit (BacTiter-Glo; Promega, Madison, WI, USA). For this end, 100 µL of the bacterial suspension was added to 100 µL of reagent in a 96-well opaque plate (Greiner, Monroe, NC, USA), followed by incubation at room temperature for 5 min. The luminescence produced was estimated using a luminometer (GloMax™ E6521, Promega, Madison, WI, USA) and expressed as an absolute value of relative light units (RLUs) in each group with respect to the control.

For FC, 100 µL of the microbial suspension was labeled using the LIVE/DEAD cell viability kit (BacLight™; Invitrogen, Eugene, OR, USA) to estimate the integrity of the cytoplasmic membrane. The kit includes two fluorescent nucleic acid dyes with different potentials to penetrate cells. SYTO 9 is a green dye that identifies microorganisms with intact and damaged membranes. Propidium iodide (IP) is a red stain that penetrates only cells with damaged membranes. After staining the microbial suspension with 100 µL of the fluorochromes, the tube was positioned in the FACS Canto II flow cytometer (BD Bioscience, San Jose, CA, USA), and the results were evaluated with the cytometer software (FACSDiva Version 6.1.3., Becton, Dickinson, San Jose, CA, USA). This provided a graph of two-dimensional dots showing the different cell populations within the microbiological sample, which had damaged membranes (considered dead) or undamaged ones (considered viable). Side and forward scatter gates were recognized to exclude debris. In all cases, 30,000 events were evaluated. The results were expressed as an absolute value of damaged/dead cells per milliliter.

For CSLM analysis, dentin specimens were stained with Syto 9/PI (LIVE/DEAD, BacLight; Invitrogen, Eugene, OR, USA) for 15 min [20], rinsed with saline solution, mounted on a 60 l-Dish (Ibidi, Martinsried, Germany) with mounting oil (BacLight™, Invitrogen), and then observed utilizing an inverted confocal laser scanning microscope (Leica TCS-SP5 II, Leica Microsystems, Mannheim, Germany). Microscopic confocal volumes (stacks) from random areas were acquired from each sample using the $40 \times$ oil lens, a 1 µm stepsize, and a format of 512×512 pixels.

2.5. Statistical Analysis

In previous statistical analyses, the normality of the data was estimated using the Shapiro–Wilk test, and the equality of variances was estimated with the Levene test. When the data followed a normal distribution and the variances were equal, an ANOVA test and a post hoc Duncan's test were used to show clusters. An ANOVA was performed with Welch's correction, followed by the Games–Howell test when the variances were not equal. In such cases, a Student's t-test was applied to compare times. Statistical analysis was conducted using SPSS v23.0 (IBM Corp, Armonk, NY, USA). In all instances, a p-value < 0.05 was considered significant.

3. Results

The results obtained with the ATP test are shown in Table 2. At one week, all sealers except AHBC significantly reduced RLUs with respect to the control ($p < 0.001$). The best results were obtained with AH, followed by BR. After 6 weeks of contact with the biofilms, all sealers obtained a significant decrease in RLUs compared to the control. The behavior of the SC-based sealers evaluated indicated a significant increase in antimicrobial activity over time. The antimicrobial activity of AH increased only slightly from 1 to 6 weeks. Similar findings using FC are shown in Table 3. The microscopic images obtained with CSLM are, moreover, consistent with the results obtained in the feasibility tests (Figure 3).

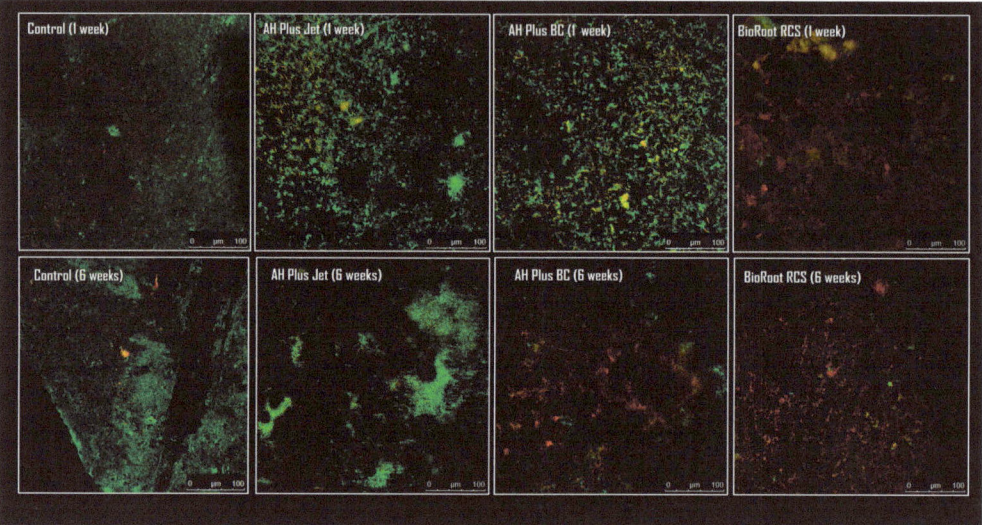

Figure 3. Representative CSLM microphotographs of 3-week biofilms after the direct contact test with the sealers of the different study groups/evaluation time. Syto-9 stained nucleic acid and emitted green fluorescence (considered as live cells), whereas damaged cells were stained by PI (red fluorescence for dead bacteria). The images were consistent with the results obtained in the microbial viability tests.

Table 2. Antimicrobial activity of endodontic sealers against polymicrobial biofilms determined by the ATP test. Mean (DE) (n = 10/group/time).

Group	ATP Test Relative Light Units (RLUs)		Comparison p-Value **
	1 Week	**6 Weeks**	
AH Plus Jet	42,931.2 (11,093.5) [a,1]	38,245.7 (11,429.3) [a,2]	0.023
AH Plus BC	201,947.8 (49,986.7) [b,d,1]	23,395.7 (7108.9) [b,2]	<0.001
BioRoot RCS	142,614.2 (49,986.1) [c,1]	20,216.5 (5455.3) [b,2]	<0.001
Control	228,075.5 (71,556.6) [d,1]	133,743.3 (21,459.7) [c,2]	
Comparison p-value *	<0.001	<0.001	

* Global comparison determined via an ANOVA with Welch's correction. Read vertically, the same letters in superscript show no significant differences determined by the Games–Howell test. ** A two-to-two comparison of 1- and 6-week RLUs. Read horizontally, the same numbers show no significant differences determined by the Student's t-test.

Table 3. Antimicrobial activity of endodontic sealers against polymicrobial biofilms determined by flow cytometry. Mean (SD) n = 10/group/time.

Group	Cells with Damaged Membrane/mL		Comparison p-Value **
	1 Week	6 Weeks	
AH Plus Jet	12,115 (4939) [a,1]	8557.6 (2950.3) [a,d,1]	0.066
AH Plus BC	4540.4 (1955.9) [b,d,1]	13,878.1 (3287.7) [b,2]	<0.001
BioRoot RCS	15,544.1 (1793) [c,1]	19,288.0 (903.3) [c,2]	<0.001
Control	6281 (2582.6) [d]	8266.5 (2416.1) [d]	
Comparison p-value *	<0.001	<0.001	

* Global comparison determined by an ANOVA. Read vertically, the same letters in superscript show no significant differences determined by Duncan's test. ** A two-to-two comparison of absolute values of cells with a damaged membrane at 1 and 6 weeks. Read horizontally, the same numbers show no significant differences determined by the Student's t-test.

4. Discussion

An ideal endodontic sealer should possess long-term antibacterial ability to reduce the residual bacterial load and prevent or limit microbial growth in the pulp space [3,6]. Because of its recent introduction, the antibiofilm properties of AHBC are still unknown. In turn, BR's efficacy against polymicrobial biofilms has been poorly evaluated [14,15]. AH was selected as a control.

To the best of our knowledge, this is the first study evaluating the long-term antimicrobial efficacy of AHBC and BR using a clinical endodontic polymicrobial biofilm growth model for 3 weeks [24] and human dentin. A follow-up of antimicrobial efficacy was performed for up to 6 weeks, whereas most research has focused on short-term evaluation [5,13].

To determine antimicrobial activity, a modified direct contact test was employed [20]. This approach is quantitative and reproducible and enables easy standardization; it simulates the contact between the microorganisms of the biofilm growing in the dentin and the applied materials [8]. Microbial viability was evaluated using two reproducible and quantitative approaches that have high sensitivity and specificity [23]. Since ATP is the primary energy molecule in all living cells, its quantification provides an estimate of the viable microbial population in a sample. The CF provides multiparametric information about individual cells within a heterogeneous population, permitting the discrimination of microbes having damaged versus unharmed membranes [23]. In addition, these techniques make it possible to discriminate the population of viable but non-cultivable cells that traditional cultures cannot detect [20]. CLSM also makes available a three-dimensional in situ image of the proportion of viable and non-viable bacteria without disturbing the cells attached to the substrate [24].

In the present study, after 7 days of contact with the biofilms, AH showed lower values of microbial viability according to the ATP test (Table 2), with a decrease in the values of RLUs at 6 weeks. Similar values were obtained with FC, showing only a 3.5% increase in dead cells over time (Table 3). The short-term efficacy of AH may be due to the bactericidal effect of formaldehyde released in small amounts during the setting process or to the toxicity of non-polymerized components [6]. These findings are consistent with those of previous investigations indicating that this sealer does not maintain its antimicrobial activity in the long term [3,6,25]. CSLM images confirmed these findings, with a predominance of cells stained with SYTO 9 in both time periods.

AHBC showed the opposite behavior. This sealer exerted very limited antimicrobial activity at one week, giving the same cell viability as the control group according to both evaluation methods. However, its efficacy over time increased significantly, with a reduction in RLUs of 82% and an increase in cells with damaged membranes (by FC) of around 68% compared to the control at 6 weeks of evaluation. Only one recent research study reports that this sealer could eradicate planktonic E. faecalis within 24 h [18], which are results that do not match those obtained in the present study, given the low activity of AHBC in the short term.

Overall, BR showed the best performance over time. After 7 days, a 37% decrease in RLUs was obtained, which increased to 85% in the last evaluation period, a significant difference between the two evaluated times. Likewise, FC indicated an increase in cells with damaged membranes of around 133% as the observation time increased, with significant differences from the rest of the groups (Table 3). This indicates that BR exerts short-term antimicrobial efficacy that is not lost in the long term. Images obtained by microscopy confirmed these findings. While there was a predominance of cells labeled by SYTO 9 at 7 days and by IP at 6 weeks for AHBC, a greater proportion of cells stained by IP was seen for BR in both time periods evaluated.

The results obtained with CS-based sealers could be related to increased alkalinizing conditions during hydration [13,26]. In the presence of water, calcium silicates form a hydrated calcium silicate gel (CSH, CaO SiO H_2O), which leads to the formation of calcium hydroxide ($Ca(OH)_2$) [8,9]. The dissociation of $Ca(OH)_2$ releases calcium (Ca^{2+}) and hydroxyl ions (OH^-), raising the pH. Nonetheless, although an alkaline pH in the microenvironment plays an important role in inhibiting bacterial viability, a significant correlation has been reported between the release of free Ca^{2+} and Si^{4+} ions and the antibacterial effect of SCs [27]. The released ions can cause bacterial membrane depolarization by binding Ca^{2+} and Si^{4+} ions to negatively charged bacterial membrane receptors, resulting in cell lysis [20,27].

The differences observed in this study between the two CSs evaluated over time may be due to their different compositions and the way they are dispensed, directly influencing their mode of hydration, hence the results obtained [8,13]. BR is a material that has a higher amount of CS in its composition than AHBC; and because it is mixed with water, hydration is always guaranteed regardless of the presence of fluids in the environment [13]. The sustained alkalinization of the medium over long periods and its capacity to release high concentrations of Ca^{2+} [4,10,15] leads to lower bacterial viability in the short [12,13] and long term [4], as demonstrated in the present study. On the other hand, it has been suggested that materials using the single-component presentation set in contact with ambient liquids are less antimicrobial than materials mixed with water [13]. AHBC is a ready-to-use sealer, and its setting reaction begins as soon as it obtains enough humidity; therefore, its hydration could have been delayed with respect to BR [11,16]. It also contained a lower percentage of SC in its composition (5–15%) and demonstrated a lower release of Ca^{2+} over time [19]. All these factors may contribute to a poor effect in the short term. The long-term effects of AHBC could be attributed to its composition. This includes dimethyl sulfoxide (DMSO) (10–30%), an organic solvent that has shown analgesic, anti-inflammatory, and antimicrobial properties [27]. Even at low concentrations, DMSO is not inert, and in some contexts, it shows antibacterial properties, generating changes in cellular processes [28], so its presence in the environment where the sealer is located could affect bacterial viability. Accordingly, the release of DMSO over time might contribute to its antibacterial efficacy. The fact that AHBC includes zirconium dioxide (ZrO_2) (50–75%) as a radiopacifier [19] also deserves mention. ZrO_2 nanoparticles have demonstrated antibacterial properties against oral [29] and other bacteria [30] by attracting the negatively charged cell wall against positively charged Zr ions. It has been reported recently that the AHBC sealer is highly soluble [16,18,19,31], which is attributed to the lower percentage of tricalcium silicate cement present in the sealer. This could strongly promote the release of DMSO and Zr from the sealer.

Still, the results cannot necessarily be extrapolated to the clinical situation, which is acknowledged as a limitation. Future studies, including ex vivo and in vivo research, should continue evaluating the antimicrobial and cytotoxic properties of bioceramics over time, as in vitro conditions do not fully represent the complexity or variability of a clinical situation.

5. Conclusions

Under the experimental conditions of this study, in the short term, AH Plus Jet and BioRoot RCS showed antimicrobial efficacy. BioRoot RCS and AH Plus BC obtained the best antibiofilm activity over time.

Author Contributions: Conceptualization, C.M.F.-L. and M.R.-L.; methodology, C.M.F.-L. and M.R.-L.; investigation and data collection, V.F. and C.S.; validation and formal analysis, C.M.-S.; writing—original draft preparation, C.M.F.-L., M.R.-L. and C.M.-S. All authors have read and agreed to the published version of the manuscript.

Funding: The research was funded by Research Group CTS-167 of Junta de Andalucía, Spain, and the Cátedra "Dentsply Sirona—UGR".

Institutional Review Board Statement: The procedures and study protocol described here were approved by the Ethics Committee of the University of Granada, Spain (no. 1076 CEIH/2020).

Informed Consent Statement: Informed consent was obtained from all subjects involved in the study.

Data Availability Statement: The data presented in this study are available upon reasonable request from the corresponding author due to privacy.

Acknowledgments: The authors thank Gertrudis Gómez Villaescusa, Ana Fernández Ibañez, Ana Santos Carro, and Gustavo Ortiz Ferrón for their technical assistance.

Conflicts of Interest: The authors declare no conflicts of interest.

References

1. Ng, Y.L.; Mann, V.; Rahbaran, S.; Lewsey, J.; Gulabivala, K. Outcome of primary root canal treatment: Systematic review of the literature—Part 2. Influence of clinical factors. *Int. Endod. J.* **2008**, *41*, 6–31. [CrossRef] [PubMed]
2. Waltimo, T.; Trope, M.; Haapasalo, M.; Orstavik, D. Clinical efficacy of treatment procedures in endodontic infection control and one year follow-up of periapical healing. *J. Endod.* **2005**, *31*, 863–866. [CrossRef] [PubMed]
3. Wang, Z.; Shen, Y.; Haapasalo, M. Antimicrobial and Antibiofilm Properties of Bioceramic Materials in Endodontics. *Materials* **2021**, *14*, 7594. [CrossRef] [PubMed]
4. Alsubait, S.; Albader, S.; Alajlan, N.; Alkhunaini, N.; Niazy, A.; Almahdy, A. Comparison of the antibacterial activity of calcium silicate- and epoxy resin-based endodontic sealers against Enterococcus faecalis biofilms: A confocal laser-scanning microscopy analysis. *Odontology* **2019**, *107*, 513–520. [CrossRef] [PubMed]
5. Long, J.; Kreft, J.U.; Camilleri, J. Antimicrobial and ultrastructural properties of root canal filling materials exposed to bacterial challenge. *J. Dent.* **2020**, *93*, 103283. [CrossRef] [PubMed]
6. AlShwaimi, E.; Bogari, D.; Ajaj, R.; Al-Shahrani, S.; Almas, K.; Majeed, A. In Vitro Antimicrobial Effectiveness of Root Canal Sealers against Enterococcus faecalis: A Systematic Review. *J. Endod.* **2016**, *42*, 1588–1597. [CrossRef]
7. Lim, M.; Jung, C.; Shin, D.H.; Cho, Y.B.; Song, M. Calcium silicate-based root canal sealers: A literature review. *Restor. Dent. Endod.* **2020**, *45*, e35. [CrossRef]
8. Camilleri, J.; Atmeh, A.; Li, X.; Meschi, N. Present status and future directions: Hydraulic materials for endodontic use. *Int. Endod. J.* **2022**, *55* (Suppl. S3), 710–777. [CrossRef]
9. Sfeir, G.; Zogheib, C.; Patel, S.; Giraud, T.; Nagendrababu, V.; Bukiet, F. Calcium Silicate-Based Root Canal Sealers: A Narrative Review and Clinical Perspectives. *Materials* **2021**, *14*, 3965. [CrossRef]
10. Siboni, F.; Taddei, P.; Zamparini, F.; Prati, C.; Gandolfi, M.G. Properties of BioRoot RCS, a tricalcium silicate endodontic sealer modified with povidone and polycarboxylate. *Int. Endod. J.* **2017**, *50* (Suppl. S2), e120–e136. [CrossRef]
11. Castro-Jara, S.; Antilef, B.; Osben, C.; Alcantara, R.; Fraga, M.; Nova-Lamperti, E.; Sánchez-Sanhueza, G. Bioactivity analysis of calcium silicate-based sealers and repair cements on the phenotype and cytokine secretion profile of CD14(+) monocytes: An ex vivo study. *Int. Endod. J.* **2023**, *56*, 80–91. [CrossRef] [PubMed]
12. Arias-Moliz, M.T.; Camilleri, J. The effect of the final irrigant on the antimicrobial activity of root canal sealers. *J. Dent.* **2016**, *52*, 30–36. [CrossRef] [PubMed]
13. Zancan, R.F.; Di Maio, A.; Tomson, P.L.; Duarte, M.A.H.; Camilleri, J. The presence of smear layer affects the antimicrobial action of root canal sealers. *Int. Endod. J.* **2021**, *54*, 1369–1382. [CrossRef] [PubMed]
14. Jerez-Olate, C.; Araya, N.; Alcántara, R.; Luengo, L.; Bello-Toledo, H.; González-Rocha, G.; Sánchez-Sanhueza, G. In vitro antibacterial activity of endodontic bioceramic materials against dual and multispecies aerobic-anaerobic biofilm models. *Aust. Endod. J.* **2022**, *48*, 465–472. [CrossRef] [PubMed]

15. Saavedra, F.M.; Pelepenko, L.E.; Boyle, W.S.; Zhang, A.; Staley, C.; Herzberg, M.C.; Marciano, M.A.; Lima, B.P. In vitro physicochemical characterization of five root canal sealers and their influence on an ex vivo oral multi-species biofilm community. *Int. Endod. J.* **2022**, *55*, 772–783. [CrossRef] [PubMed]
16. Donnermeyer, D.; Schemkamper, P.; Burklein, S.; Schafer, E. Short and Long-Term Solubility, Alkalizing Effect, and Thermal Persistence of Premixed Calcium Silicate-Based Sealers: AH Plus Bioceramic Sealer vs. Total Fill BC Sealer. *Materials* **2022**, *15*, 7320. [CrossRef] [PubMed]
17. Kwak, S.W.; Koo, J.; Song, M.; Jang, I.H.; Gambarini, G.; Kim, H.C. Physicochemical Properties and Biocompatibility of Various Bioceramic Root Canal Sealers: In Vitro Study. *J. Endod.* **2023**, *49*, 871–879. [CrossRef] [PubMed]
18. Souza, L.C.; Neves, G.S.T.; Kirkpatrick, T.; Letra, A.; Silva, R. Physicochemical and Biological Properties of AH Plus Bioceramic. *J. Endod.* **2023**, *49*, 69–76. [CrossRef] [PubMed]
19. Raman, V.; Camilleri, J. Characterization and Assessment of Physical Properties of 3 Single Syringe Hydraulic Cement-based Sealers. *J. Endod.* **2024**, *50*, 381–388. [CrossRef]
20. Ruiz-Linares, M.; Solana, C.; Baca, P.; Arias-Moliz, M.T.; Ferrer-Luque, C.M. Antibiofilm potential over time of a tricalcium silicate material and its association with sodium diclofenac. *Clin. Oral. Investig.* **2022**, *26*, 2661–2669. [CrossRef]
21. Ferrer-Luque, C.M.; Baca, P.; Solana, C.; Rodriguez-Archilla, A.; Arias-Moliz, M.T.; Ruiz-Linares, M. Antibiofilm Activity of Diclofenac and Antibiotic Solutions in Endodontic Therapy. *J. Endod.* **2021**, *47*, 1138–1143. [CrossRef] [PubMed]
22. Tan, K.S.; Yu, V.S.; Quah, S.Y.; Bergenholtz, G. Rapid method for the detection of root canal bacteria in endodontic therapy. *J. Endod.* **2015**, *41*, 447–450. [CrossRef] [PubMed]
23. Balouiri, M.; Sadiki, M.; Ibnsouda, S.K. Methods for in vitro evaluating antimicrobial activity: A review. *J. Pharm. Anal.* **2016**, *6*, 71–79. [CrossRef]
24. Shen, Y.; Stojicic, S.; Haapasalo, M. Antimicrobial efficacy of chlorhexidine against bacteria in biofilms at different stages of development. *J. Endod.* **2011**, *37*, 657–661. [CrossRef] [PubMed]
25. Ruiz-Linares, M.; Baca, P.; Arias-Moliz, M.T.; Ternero, F.J.; Rodriguez, J.; Ferrer-Luque, C.M. Antibacterial and antibiofilm activity over time of GuttaFlow Bioseal and AH Plus. *Dent. Mater. J.* **2019**, *38*, 701–706. [CrossRef]
26. Kapralos, V.; Sunde, P.T.; Camilleri, J.; Morisbak, E.; Koutroulis, A.; Ørstavik, D.; Valen, H. Effect of chlorhexidine digluconate on antimicrobial activity, cell viability and physicochemical properties of three endodontic sealers. *Dent. Mater.* **2022**, *38*, 1044–1059. [CrossRef]
27. Koutroulis, A.; Kuehne, S.A.; Cooper, P.R.; Camilleri, J. The role of calcium ion release on biocompatibility and antimicrobial properties of hydraulic cements. *Sci. Rep.* **2019**, *9*, 19019. [CrossRef] [PubMed]
28. Verheijen, M.; Lienhard, M.; Schrooders, Y.; Clayton, O.; Nudischer, R.; Boerno, S.; Timmermann, B.; Selevsek, N.; Schlapbach, R.; Gmuender, H.; et al. DMSO induces drastic changes in human cellular processes and epigenetic landscape in vitro. *Sci. Rep.* **2019**, *9*, 4641. [CrossRef] [PubMed]
29. Khan, M.; Shaik, M.R.; Khan, S.T.; Adil, S.F.; Kuniyil, M.; Khan, M.; Al-Warthan, A.A.; Siddiqui, M.R.H.; Tahir, M.N. Enhanced Antimicrobial Activity of Biofunctionalized Zirconia Nanoparticles. *ACS Omega* **2020**, *5*, 1987–1996. [CrossRef]
30. Bannunah, A.M. Biomedical Applications of Zirconia-Based Nanomaterials: Challenges and Future Perspectives. *Molecules* **2023**, *28*, 5428. [CrossRef]
31. Borges, R.P.; Sousa-Neto, M.D.; Versiani, M.A.; Rached-Júnior, F.A.; De-Deus, G.; Miranda, C.E.S.; Pécora, J.D. Changes in the surface of four calcium silicate-containing endodontic materials and an epoxy resin-based sealer after a solubility test. *Int. Endod. J.* **2012**, *45*, 419–428. [CrossRef] [PubMed]

Disclaimer/Publisher's Note: The statements, opinions and data contained in all publications are solely those of the individual author(s) and contributor(s) and not of MDPI and/or the editor(s). MDPI and/or the editor(s) disclaim responsibility for any injury to people or property resulting from any ideas, methods, instructions or products referred to in the content.

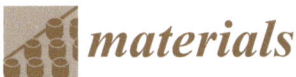

Article

In Vitro Assessment of a New Block Design for Implant Crowns with Functional Gradient Fabricated with Resin Composite and Zirconia Insert [†]

Nicolás Gutiérrez Robledo [1,2,*], Miquel Punset Fuste [3,4,5,6], Alejandra Rodríguez-Contreras [3,5,6], Fernando García Marro [5,7], José María Manero Planella [3,5,6], Oscar Figueras-Álvarez [1] and Miguel Roig Cayón [1]

1. School of Dentistry, Universitat Internacional de Catalunya (UIC), 08195 Barcelona, Spain; ofigueras@uic.es (O.F.-Á.); mroig@uic.es (M.R.C.)
2. Independent Research, 28028 Madrid, Spain
3. Biomaterials, Biomechanics and Tissue Engineering Group (BBT), Universitat Politècnica de Catalunya (UPC), 08019 Barcelona, Spain; miquel.punset@upc.edu (M.P.F.); alejandra.maria.rodriguez@upc.edu (A.R.-C.); jose.maria.manero@upc.edu (J.M.M.P.)
4. UPC Innovation and Technology Center (CIT-UPC), Universitat Politècnica de Catalunya (UPC), 08034 Barcelona, Spain
5. Barcelona Research Centre in Multiscale Science and Engineering, Universitat Politècnica de Catalunya (UPC), 08019 Barcelona, Spain; fernando.garcia.marro@upc.edu
6. Reserach Institute San Joan de Déu (IRSJD), 08950 Barcelona, Spain
7. Center for Structural Integrity, Reliability and Micromechanics of Materials Research Group (CIEFMA), Universitat Politècnica de Catalunya (UPC), 08019 Barcelona, Spain
* Correspondence: ngutierrez@uic.es
† In memoriam of Dr. Ralf Böhner.

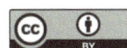

Abstract: This study aims to evaluate and compare the mechanical resistance, fatigue behavior and fracture behavior of different CAD/CAM materials for implant crowns. Eighty-eight implant crowns cemented-screwed with four sample groups: two monolithic G1 Zirconia (control) and G3 composite and two bi-layered G2 customized zirconia/composite and G4 prefabricated zirconia/composite. All static and dynamic mechanical tests were conducted at 37 °C under wet conditions. The fractographic evaluation of deformed and/or fractured samples was evaluated via electron microscopy. Statistical analysis was conducted using Wallis tests, which were performed depending on the variables, with a confidence interval of 95%, ($p < 0.05$). The Maximum Fracture Strength values displayed by the four groups of samples showed no statistically significant differences. The crown–abutment material combination influenced the failure mode of the restoration, transitioning from a fatigue fracture type located at the abutment–analog connection for monolithic materials (G1 and G3) to a brittle fracture located in the crown for bi-layered materials (G2 and G4). The use of layered crown materials with functional gradients appears to protect the crown/abutment connection area by partially absorbing the applied mechanical loads. This prevents catastrophic mechanical failures, avoiding long chairside time to solve these kinds of complications.

Keywords: ceramic-reinforced resin-composite blocks; monolithic dental crown; layered dental crown; zirconia insert; dental fatigue

1. Introduction

The absence of the periodontal ligament in the implant–prosthesis–bone set can frequently generate mechanical complications in implant prostheses. This occurs due to the mechanical overload caused by the lack of cushioning [1], especially in the unitary crowns of male molars [2,3]. The most frequent mechanical complications are the loosening of the fixation screw or the transepithelial abutment [4,5] and the fracture or delamination (chipping) of the esthetic coating material of the restoration [6].

The mechanical properties of the ceramic-reinforced resin composite with a dispersed filler microstructure (DFM) included in the new classification of ceramic materials [7], have considerably improved due to new industrial polymerization methods (atmospheric pressure and high temperature) [8,9], which replace intraoral photopolymerization [10]. A reduced monomer release and an increase in flexural strength, hardness, tenacity and even density of these materials have been observed [11–14]. The great stability achieved in resin-composite blocks (RCBs) allows excellent reproducibility by machining [15,16] and causes less wear on the opposing enamel compared to glass-matrix ceramics [17–20]. All these characteristics, together with the low flexural modulus, allow RCBs to achieve a cushioning effect on implant restorations by transmitting less stress to the prosthetic attachment and implant, which favors bone response [21–25]. On the other hand, when the implant–prosthesis–bone complex exceeds the limits of physiological adaptation, it produces bone overload, which, in turn, triggers osteoclastic activity and bone resorption [26–28]. This sometimes results in traumatic failure, diverging from infectious failure or bacterial peri-implantitis [29].

Marginal bone preservation is influenced by multiple factors, such as implant design, crown material, prosthetic abutment, connection and disconnection of the prosthetic abutment and the type of surgery performed. The correct selection of the restorative material, as well as the prosthetic abutment, is one of the keys to success in implant prosthesis [30–32]. Given that the masticatory force into the crown is then transmitted to the maxillary or mandibular bone through the prosthesis and implant [33], the use of resilient materials that function as a shock absorber to the implant–prosthesis set could help reduce stress and pressure on the bone [34]. It may reduce prosthetic complications derived from the overload received in the crown [35]. Currently, the prefabricated titanium abutment with a mesostructured zirconia to mask the grayish color of titanium has become the prosthetic abutment of choice for restorations on implants, given its excellent mechanical and esthetic properties as well as its biocompatibility with the tissues [36–38].

Functional gradient materials (FGMs) are a new concept in materials engineering [39], where both the material composition and structure gradually change. Their sole purpose is to dissipate or absorb stress or mechanical load.

FGMs have been used in several investigations in the dental field [40–42]. In this process, both the material composition and the structure gradually change throughout the volume, resulting in changes in the material's properties, chemical composition, physical state and geometric configuration. This has allowed us to explore optimal designs of bio-inspired or bio-mimetic materials in which different layers of materials achieve greater stress reduction and distribution. The best example is the human tooth, which consists of two main layers: enamel and dentin. The outer layer allows it to maintain its shape and resist fracture and wear upon loading. This quality is due to a variation of the transformation in its microstructure and chemical composition. Starting from the outermost layer, four well-differentiated histological layers are recognized until reaching the dentin–enamel junction (DEJ) [43,44]. This interface plays a crucial role in the fatigue resistance of the natural tooth, given the reliable connection between the different layers of the tooth [45,46]. This study is the first one in the field and is unique because it combines different materials perfectly bonded to produce a functional gradient implant crown, trying to emulate the natural tooth structure.

The reproducibility of the resin composite by machining and the feasibility of polishing or intraoral adjustment allow great control of the occlusion. Moreover, the favorable cutting properties lead to considerable savings in production time and reduce wear on manufacturing instruments, such as motors and diamond milling cutters; in contrast, materials with a ceramic matrix, when machined, often result in lower-quality margins and edges [16]. A layered design with an individualized zirconia mesostructure implies additional production costs, as the mesostructure must be designed and milled separately from an additional block and then requires an additional cementation to the resin composite crown. As a solution, a new resin-composite block design with an industrially bonded zirconia insert is proposed (Figure 1). The industrially manufactured insert, which is a component of the resin block, enables the masking of the metal's colors and ensures an optimal fit tolerance to the titanium base. In addition, it can be used for chair-side restorations on implants, as it can be machined within 12–14 min and does not require thermal processing.

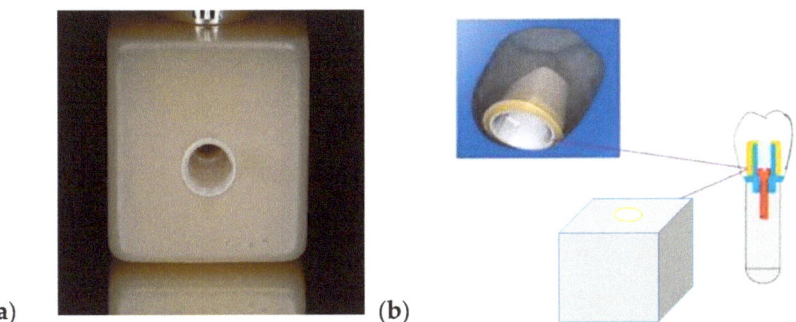

Figure 1. Experimental setup: (**a**) resin composite experimental block with prefabricated zirconia insert and (**b**) implant crown cemented over Ti-base and screwed on the implant analog.

The design of the new experimental block is composed of two materials commonly used today: resin composite with filler content of VOL % 51.5 and zirconia. These two materials are industrially bonded to ensure optimal and consistent tolerances. From a mechanical and an esthetic point of view, the experimental crown could be an effective prosthetic solution with the combination of prefabricated zirconia insert and resin-composite block [35,47]. Furthermore, it is easy to polish and repair in the mouth. Additionally, due to its low production cost, it could be affordable for most patients.

This study aims to evaluate the mechanical resistance of the resin-composite blocks for implant crowns under different scenarios. We will compare fracture behavior and failure mode with the control group monolithic zirconia, one of the most common materials for single-unit implant crowns under static and dynamic loads.

The study's main hypothesis suggests the presence of statistically significant differences in both maximum static strength and fatigue limit among the materials evaluated. However, the null hypothesis in this study proposes the absence of statistically significant disparities in these properties, regardless of the material's characteristics and the component's geometry.

2. Materials and Methods

2.1. Materials

Eighty-eight ASTRA EV implant analogs (Dentsply Sirona, Charlotte, NC, USA) with a diameter of XL 5.4 mm (Ref 25547 and LOT 456009) were prepared with the corresponding CEREC Ti-base (CEREC/inLab Ref 6586338 and LOT B200003054), onto which a crown of each group (n = 22) was previously cemented. The sample groups were designated as G1 (control group) and G3, which comprised monolithic crowns, whereas the sample groups G2 and G4 comprised layered crowns with customized or prefabricated mesostructured zirconia (Figure 2).

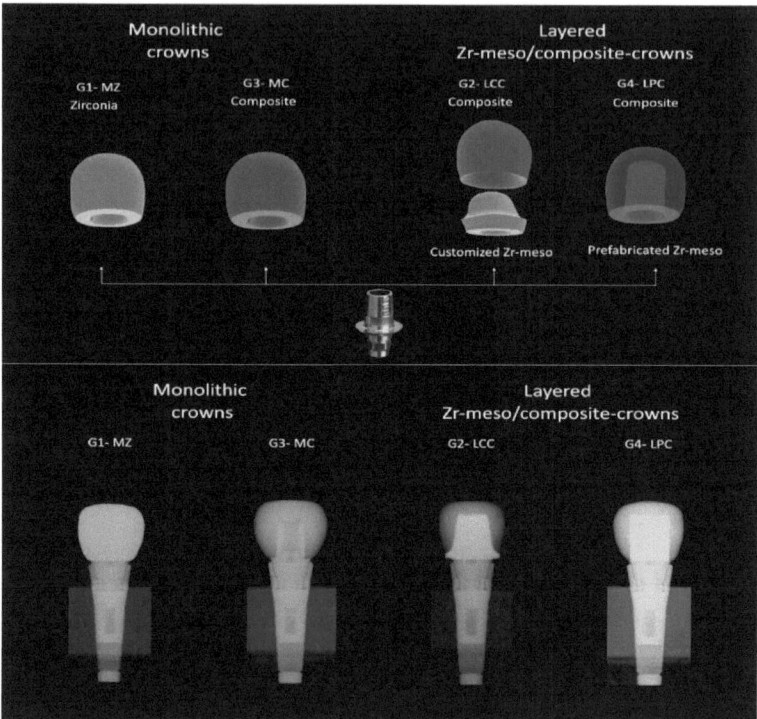

Figure 2. Different study groups and X-rays of samples tested: monolithic zirconia (G1-MZ), monolithic composite (G3-MC), layered customized composite (G2-LCC) and layered prefabricated composite (G4 LPC).

2.2. Sample Preparation

All samples were prepared and treated according to ISO 14801:2016 [48]. The preparation of the samples to be mechanically tested in this study was carried out in two consecutive and well-differentiated sequential stages. The first stage involved embedding the ASTRA EV implant analogs in a bone-like resin, followed by the second stage of fabricating and assembling the different crowns by cementation.

Before performing any static and dynamic mechanical testing, all titanium analogs were inserted into a bone-like polymeric resin to provide stable support, as well as to mimic oral conditions. Analog samples were embedded into a polymeric resin (Mecaprex MA2+, PRESI SAS, Eybens, France), leaving the implant 3 ± 0.1 mm above the implant nominal bone level determined by the implant manufacturer. All samples were embedded, resulting in a total set of 88 samples for the study. The resin discs with the embedded implants were subjected to rectifying operations, thus ensuring parallelism between the upper and lower faces.

The second phase of sample preparation included the fabrication of four distinct crown groups, along with their final embedment into the analog, which had been previously fixed in a resin-like bone material during the preceding stage. The Ti-base was scanned with a Dentsply Sirona Ineos X5 extraoral scanner (Dentsply Sirona, Charlotte, NC, USA) using the corresponding "L" scan-body for the Ti-base. Once scanned, a crown was designed using the InLab CAD 19 software (Dentsply Sirona, Charlotte, NC, USA). An STL model of the monolithic crown groups G1-MZ and G3-MC and the layered crown groups G2-LCC and G4-LPC was obtained. The material's characteristics are described in Table 1.

Table 1. General table of the material properties for each study sample group.

Materials	Manufacturers	Composition	Flexural Strength	Fracture Toughness	Modulus of Elasticity
Zirconia crown: CEREC Zirconia meso L A2 LOT 2017484418	Dentsply Sirona®	Yttria stabilized zirconia	>900 MPa	7.1 MPa$^{1/2}$	210 GPa
Composite crown: BRILLIANT Crios Disc A2 LT H18 LOT J52869	Coltene®	Barium glass < 1.0 μm, amorphous silica SiO_2 < 20 nm, cross linked methacrylic matrix and inorganic pigments	198 MPa	2.0 MPa m0.5	10.3 GPa
Customized meso structure: inCoris ZI meso F2 L LOT 3314000426	Dentsply Sirona®	Dentsply Sirona®	>900 MPa	5.8 MPa$^{1/2}$	210 GPa
Zirconia insert	Coltene®	Yttria stabilized zirconia (3 mol% Y2O3)	500–1000 MPa	5.8–10.5 MPa m0.5	210 GPa
TiBase CEREC/inLab AT EV 4,8 GH 1 "L" LOT B200003054	Dentsply Sirona®	Ti6Al4V, medical grade 5, ASTM 136	n.a	n.a	105–117 GPa
Implant Replica EV 5.4 LOT 456009	Dentsply Sirona®	Ti6Al4V Grade 5 ASTM F136	n.a	n.a	105–117 GPa
Cement: Solocem® LOT J64901	Coltene®	UDMA, TEGDMA, HEMA Methacrylate, zinc oxide, dental glass, MDP and 4-MET (A) monomers	120 MPa	n.a	7.2 GPa
Bonding: OneCoat 7 Universal® LOT J69945	Coltene®	Methacrylates including 10-MDP photoinitiators, ethanol, water	n.a	n.a	n.a

The single blocks for crowns of the G1-MZ, G2-LCC and G4-LPC groups were milled using the MCXL, a 4-axis milling machine (Dentsply Sirona, Charlotte, NC, USA), serial no. 106352, using the wet strategy and diamond burs. For the crowns of G3-MC, a 5-axis Imes icore 350 PRO milling machine (Imes Icore GmbH, Eiterfeld, Germany) was used. In addition, the Brilliant Crios Disc (Coltene Whaledent, Altstätten, Switzerland) was used and a CAM Mill Box software v5 SMART(CIM Systems s.r.l., Milan, Italy). Then, all the crowns were carefully separated from the blocks and discs using a cutting disk. Once the supports were polished, the zirconia crowns from G1 and the customized mesostructured from G2 were dried in a pre-drying oven (Imes Icore) for 15 min to remove the moisture from the wet milling. Subsequently, they were sintered in the corresponding program of the DEKEMA sintering furnace model AUSTROMAT 674 (DEKEMA Dental-Keramiköfen GmbH, Freilassing, Germany).

Before cementing all the crowns, the Ti-bases were attached to the implant analogs according to the manufacturer recommendations using a torque wrench with 25 Ncm, and then they were cemented over a Ti-base and finally, the crown holes were filled with Teflon tape and light-cure composite Brilliant EverGlow A2/B2 and One coat 7 Universal (Coltene Whaledent, Altstätten, Switzerland) as bonding. Lastly, the composite fillings were polished using silicon polishers DIATECH Shape guard (Coltene Whaledent, Altstätten,

Switzerland). The surface treatment during the cementation of the different crown samples is described in Table 2.

Table 2. Descriptive table of the surface treatments used for sample adhesion.

Surface Pre-Treatment Group	G1	G2	G3	G4
Ti-base	Sand-blasting 2.5 bar, Al_2O_3, particles, 50 μm			
Monolithic zirconia crown	Sand-blasting, 1 bar, Al_2O_3 particles, 50 μm,			
Composite crown	Sand-blasting, 2 bar, Al_2O_3 particles, 50 μm,			
Zirconia mesostructure		Sand-blasting, 1 bar, Al_2O_3 particles, 50 μm,		
Zirconia insert				Sand-blasting, 1 bar, Al_2O_3 particles, 50 μm,
Primer/Cement	OneCoat 7 universal and Solocem by Coltene®			

2.3. Observation by Field Emission Scanning Electron Microscope

Scanning Electron Microscopy (SEM) enables the surface-level and comprehensive evaluation of components and samples by acquiring high-resolution images using the interactions generated between an incident electron beam and the surface under analysis. A Field Emission Scanning Electron Microscope (FSEM) model JSM-7001F Scanning Microscope (JSM 7100, JEOL Ltd., Akishima, Japan) was used for fractographic evaluation of deformed and/or fractured specimens, operating at a potential of 20 kV and an approximate working distance ranging from 9 to 11 mm. This equipment is equipped with an Energy-Dispersive X-ray Spectroscopy (EDS) analysis probe, Oxford Xmax20 model, which allows for the identification of chemical composition by acquiring the characteristic X-ray emission of each chemical element.

Coating ceramic samples for SEM observation is essential to improve conductivity, prevent charge accumulation, protect the sample, and obtain higher quality and resolution images, enabling a more precise and detailed analysis of the properties and characteristics of this type of material. Once the samples had been fractured through fatigue testing, the fragments were positioned on pin-shaped holders to undergo a coating process using PVD-Sputtering techniques, specifically the LEICA EM ACE600 equipment (LEICA MICROSYSTEMS, Wetzlar, Germany). Using this equipment, a PVD-Sputtered Pt-Au conductive coating was applied to the samples prior to the SEM observation; this coating had an average thickness ranging from 5 to 10 nm.

2.4. Determination of the Maximum Compression Strength

A universal MTS model BIONIX-370 servo-hydraulic mechanical testing machine (MTS Bionix 370, Minneapolis, MN, USA) was used for the determination of the maximum compressive strength using a 2.5 kN load cell controlled by Telstar II software (Telstar, MTS System Corp., Eden Prairie, MN, USA). A total of 20 uniaxial static compression tests were carried out, divided into 5 tests for each of the 4 study sample groups to be evaluated. All static and dynamic mechanical tests were conducted at (37 ± 1) °C, fixing the specimen in the testing machine with a 30° angle of inclination and under wet conditions using Hank's salt solution as a liquid medium. All the analyses were carried out under the same test conditions. The implants were held with the same and unique clamping device, consisting of a clamping jaw made of stainless steel, which supports the resin block in which each implant has previously been encased (Figure 3). The compressive load was applied at a constant displacement rate of 1 mm/min on the loading device (cap) until system failure.

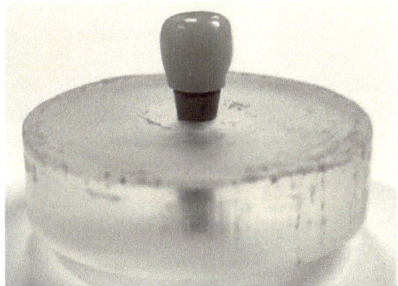

Figure 3. Image of the dental implant system embedded in the resin ready for testing.

All samples were prepared following ISO-14801:2017. According to the standard, the bone anchoring part of the sample must be fixed in a fixed anchoring device that must hold the sample at a distance of 3.0 ± 0.1 mm apically from the nominal bone level determined by the manufacturer (Figure 4); in this case, the company Astra implants by Detsply Sirona. This distance is internationally accepted as the average level of bone resorption after dental implant implantation. The ISO-14801:2017 standard also specifies the existence of a constant distance of 11.0 ± 0.1 mm from the implant support level to the center of the hemispherical free end. This distance must be measured parallel to the central longitudinal axis of the implant body, and it is counted from the surface of the resin to the center of the hemispherical dome.

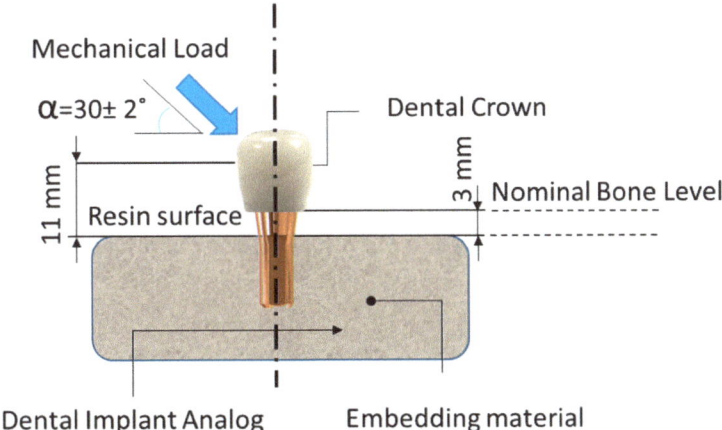

Figure 4. Schematic diagram of an embedded sample.

2.5. Determination of S-N Curve

Dental implant fracture is a critical concern in prosthetic dentistry. Cyclic loads experienced during mastication can potentially lead to structural failures, compromising the longevity and functionality of dental implants. Hence, it is crucial to evaluate the resistance of implants under varying cyclic load conditions to ensure their reliability and durability. The ISO14801 standard provides guidelines for testing the fatigue strength of dental implants, offering a standardized approach for assessing their performance. After conducting static compression-to-fracture tests, fatigue tests were carried out at various percentages of the previously obtained maximum breaking load. This allowed determining the number of cycles before fracture at each load level ($n \leq 4$), starting from an initial load of 80% according to ISO 14801 of the load to failure in a static test carried out with the same test geometry. Following this guideline, the implants were submitted to a sinusoidal compression–compression fatigue test at a frequency of 2 Hz and a stress variation of 10%.

The total number of cycles applied to each sample was fixed at 2×10^6, also defined as run-outs for fatigue tests performed in liquid immersion according to the ISO standard. Implants that survived this number of cycles were considered to have passed the test successfully. The force of the impact was performed on the distal cuspid of the implant-supported restoration for all groups of samples. Implants that endured this number of cycles were considered to have passed the test successfully. The fatigue test was run in liquid immersion using Hank's salt solution (Sigma Aldrich, St. Louis, MO, USA) as a liquid medium.

2.6. Characterization of Hardness and Fracture Toughness

The determination of hardness was analyzed by using a Vickers EMCO-Test micro-hardness tester (EMCO-TEST Prüfmaschinen Gmbh, Kuchl, Austria) equipped with a Vickers indenter, which consists of a diamond pyramid with a base angle of 136°. The standard used for the determination of the hardness of the materials under study was ASTM E384-17 [49].

The hardness measurements were carried out under a constant load of 5 kg applied for 15 s, making a total of three measurements for each of the four materials studied. The Vickers hardness number (VHN) (GPa) was obtained and compared. The Vickers hardness number (VHN) in GPa has been expressed following Equation (1). VHN as a function of the applied load (F) in N and the average of the diagonals of the indentation (d) in μm. The constant value, 1854.4, was obtained from the calculation of the contact area.

$$\text{VHN} 1854.4 \times \frac{P}{d^2} \quad (1)$$

The estimation of fracture toughness K_{Ic} [49–54] was achieved through the measurement of crack length nucleated at the corners of the residual imprint, utilizing indentation fracture toughness, following research by Niihara et al. [55]. Sample preparation was necessary to produce a polished cross-section for each pillar (Figure 5).

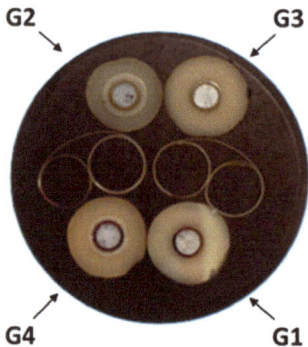

Figure 5. Picture of the polished cross-sections of G1, G2, G3 and G4 material.

The fracture toughness K_{Ic} [50] is a crucial mechanical parameter in brittle materials that quantifies their ability to resist crack propagation. The estimation of fracture toughness can be achieved through the measurement of crack length nucleated at the corners of the residual imprint, utilizing a technique known as indentation microfracture. Various mathematical formulations have been suggested to determine K_{Ic}, contingent upon the tip indenter geometry and crack morphology (such as radial, half a penny, or

Palmqvist). Among these, the expression most commonly employed for radial cracks is Equation (2) [51]:

$$K_{IC} = a\left(\frac{E}{H}\right)^{1/2} \times \left(\frac{P}{C^{3/2}}\right) \quad (2)$$

where a is a (dimensionless) empirical constant depending on the indenter geometry (a = 0016 for pyramidal tips), P (in mN) is the peak indentation load, and C (in mm) is the length of the radial cracks. For Palmqvist cracks, the following Equation (3) applies [52]:

$$K_{IC} = \left(\frac{a}{l}\right)^{1/2} \times \left(\frac{E}{H}\right)^{2/3} \times \left(\frac{P}{C^{3/2}}\right) \quad (3)$$

where xv is 0.016 for a Berkovich tip indenter, a (mm) is the length from the center of the imprint until one of the corners, and l (mm) is the crack length. The applicability of the different expressions for indentation microfracture tests performed with Berkovich indenters has been extensively discussed in [53,54].

2.7. Statistical Analysis

Statistical analysis has been carried out using the statistical software Minitab® 16.2.1 (Minitab Inc., State College, PA, USA). Parametric ANOVA or a non-parametric test with Kruskal–Wallis was performed, depending on the variables, with a confidence interval of 95% and considered statistically different when $p < 0.05$. Maximum compression strength results are set out as mean ± standard deviation.

All data were analyzed, beginning with a normal distribution test to determine if the data followed a normal distribution. If the values followed a normal distribution ($p > 0.05$) and two independent data groups were compared, the statistical study was conducted using the parametric t-test. If the values followed a normal distribution ($p > 0.05$) and three or more independent data groups were compared, the statistical study was conducted using the ANOVA test. In both studies, the initial hypothesis assumed that all means were equal. To accept this initial hypothesis as true, the probability was set within a 95% confidence interval, meaning the probability of it not being true was only 5%. Therefore, when the probability is less than 0.05, it indicates that the hypothesis is not met and that the means are not equal. Thus, if $p < 0.05$, the means are different, indicating statistically significant differences.

If the values did not follow a normal distribution ($p < 0.05$) and two independent data groups were compared, the study was conducted using the non-parametric Mann–Whitney test. If the values did not follow a normal distribution ($p < 0.05$) and three or more independent data groups were compared, the study was conducted using the non-parametric Kruskal–Wallis test. Therefore, when the Mann–Whitney and Kruskal–Wallis probability is $p < 0.05$, there are statistically significant differences between the variables and the factors analyzed.

3. Results

3.1. Uniaxial Flex-Compression Resistance

To obtain average values of the static compression strength for all tested implant sample groups, it is necessary to determine the starting point for the different levels of load required to create an S/N curve. In order to do this, compression tests were conducted on five different samples (n = 5) per sample group (Table 3). The comparative analysis of the maximum static fracture strength values suggested slightly higher maximum strength values in groups G3 and G1 in comparison to groups G4 and G2, respectively (Figure 6a). However, the statistical analysis of maximum fracture force results of the four sample groups did not reveal the presence of statistically significant differences ($p = 0.213$).

Table 3. General table of maximum compressive force and elongation at break values determined by static compression.

Properties/Group of Samples	N°	G1	G1	G3	G4
Fmax, N	1	1706.10	1699.50	1720.10	1572.20
	2	1578.60	1397.70	1717.10	1701.40
	3	1737.10	1439.70	1818.10	1487.40
	4	1565.00	1696.50	1523.00	1549.60
	5	1546.10	1317.60	1577.60	1457.10
	$\overline{X}$	1626.58	1510.20	1671.18	1553.54
	D. Std	88.19	176.96	119.17	94.74
Elongation at break, mm	1	1.25	0.95	1.32	0.67
	2	1.29	0.60	1.23	0.88
	3	1.17	1.06	1.28	1.16
	4	1.26	1.40	1.50	1.07
	5	1.31	0.94	1.35	0.80
	$\overline{X}$	1.26	0.99	1.34	0.92
	D. Std	0.05	0.29	0.10	0.20

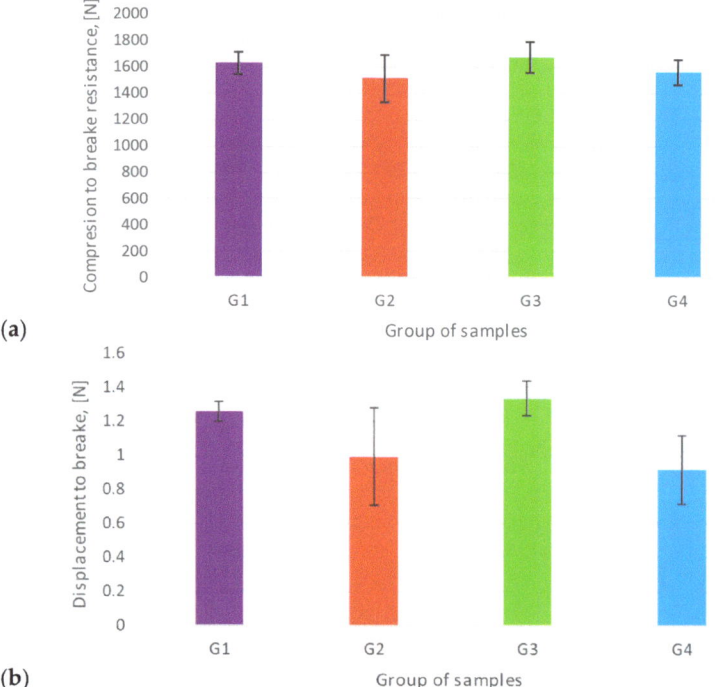

Figure 6. Comparative graphs of Fmax (**a**) and displacement to break (**b**).

Moreover, the comparative analysis of displacement at break proposed higher displacement values in groups G3 and G1 compared to groups G2 and G4, respectively (Figure 6b). Furthermore, the analysis conducted on the displacement-to-fracture outcomes within the four groups unveiled the existence of statistically significant disparities in displacement ($p = 0.005$). There were statistically significant differences from displacement-to-fracture between the G3 and G4 sample groups ($p = 0.006$) but not between G1 and G2 ($p = 0.71$). The four study groups showed different modes of fracture. They were characterized by a deformation of the neck of the analog and a fracture of the fixation screw in groups G1 and G3, and crown fracture in groups G2 and G4 (Figure 7).

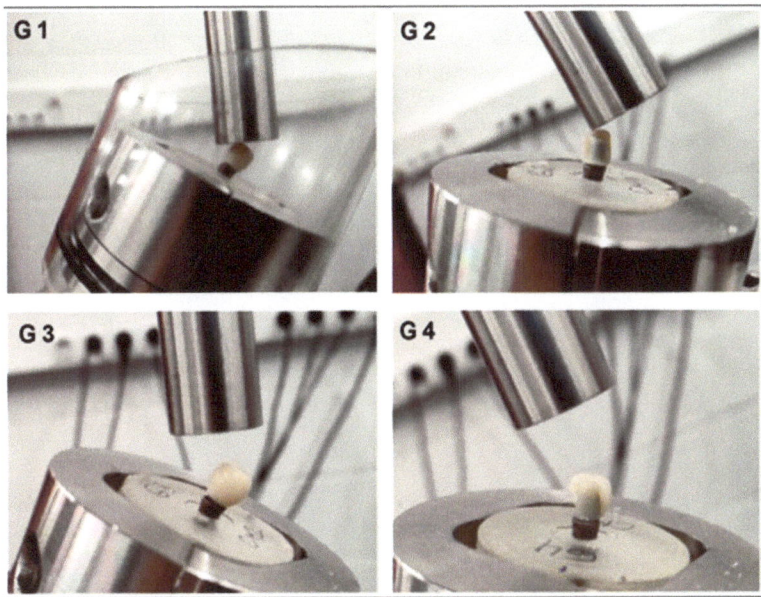

Figure 7. Photographic images of the fracture modes under static uniaxial compression.

The images in Figure 7 show the different modes of fracture exhibited by the analyzed samples of the four study groups. They are characterized by a crown fracture in groups G2 and G4, a deformation of the neck of the analog and the fracture of the fixation screw in groups G1 and G3.

3.2. Uniaxial Cyclic Fatigue Test

The S-N graphics obtained from the tests showed similar decreasing tendencies for all the groups (Figure 8). Moreover, the fatigue limit obtained was very similar for groups G2 and G4, whereas the G1 group showed the highest fatigue limit. Table 4 summarizes the fatigue limit (FL) for all sample groups.

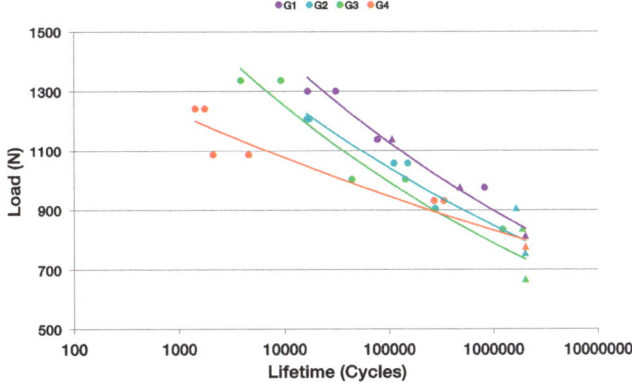

Figure 8. Comparative graph of S-N curves obtained for all groups of samples tested.

Table 4. Comparative table of fatigue limit values (FL) obtained for all groups of samples tested.

Property/Group of Samples	G1	G2	G3	G4
FL, N	813	755	668	777

Moreover, Table 5 indicates the loads supported by each group sample and shows up to eight different fracture modes, from T1 through T8, with the eighth being run out of the samples. Likewise, Figure 9 is the illustrative image of these fracture modes on the samples.

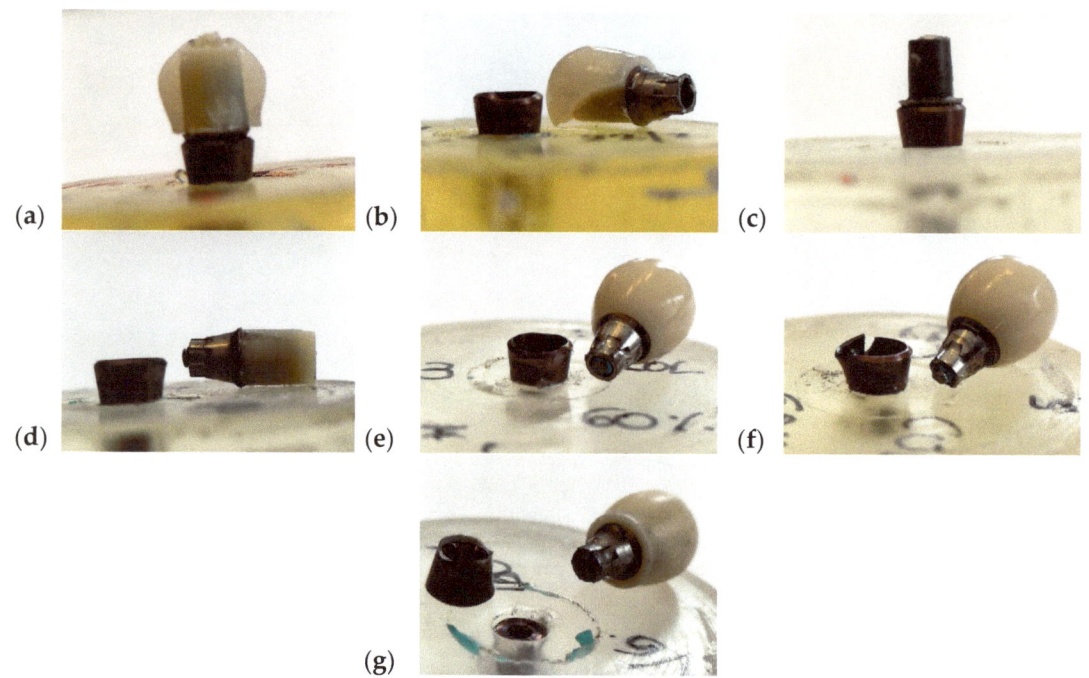

Figure 9. Photographic images of the different fracture modes identified: (**a**) T1, (**b**) T2, (**c**) T3, (**d**) T4, (**e**) T5, (**f**) T6 and (**g**) T7.

Table 5. Maximum and minimum loads supported by each group sample illustrating up to 8 distinct fracture modes.

Group of Samples	% Fmax	Fmax (N)	Fmin (N)	N° Cycles to Break	Failure Mode
G1	80	1301	130	16,314	T2
	80	1301	130	30,475	T4
	70	1139	114	105,522	T6
	70	1139	114	75,315	T5
	60	976	98	470,741	T7
	60	976	98	805,596	T8
	50	813	81	2,000,000	Run out
	50	813	81	2,000,000	Run out

Table 5. Cont.

Group of Samples	% Fmax	Fmax (N)	Fmin (N)	N° Cycles to Break	Failure Mode
G2	80	1208	121	16,028	T5
	80	1208	121	16,930	T5
	70	1057	106	109,106	T5
	70	1057	106	148,110	T6
	60	906	91	1,631,627	T5
	60	906	91	273,531	T6
	50	755	76	2,000,000	Run out
	50	755	76	2,000,000	Run out
G3	80	1337	134	3797	T5
	80	1337	134	9108	T6
	60	1003	100	43,309	T5
	60	1003	100	140,250	T6
	50	836	84	1,197,943	T5
	50	836	84	1,864,478	T6
	40	668	67	2,000,000	Run out
	40	668	67	2,000,000	Run out
G4	80	1243	124	1724	T1
	80	1243	124	1396	T5
	70	1087	109	2063	T3
	70	1087	109	4518	T2
	60	932	93	265,460	T1
	60	932	93	328,837	T4
	50	777	78	2,000,000	Run out
	50	777	78	2,000,000	Run out

Where: T1: (Partial fracture of the crown), T2: (Partial fracture of the crown and fracture of screw, with deformation of both implant and abutment), T3: (Total fracture of the crown, without deformation of either the implant or the abutment), T4: (Total fracture of the crown, with deformation of both implant and abutment), T5: (Fracture of the screw, with deformation of both implant and abutment), T6: (Fracture of the screw, with deformation of the abutment and partial fracture of the implant), T7: (Fracture of the screw, with deformation of the abutment and total fracture of the implant).

A comparative analysis of the failure modes observed in this study has also revealed discrepancies among the different groups of samples evaluated. The implants in groups G2 and G3 exhibited very similar fracture behaviors, characterized by the same types of fracture modes at equivalent percentages of applied cyclic load. However, the G1 and G4 groups of samples not only displayed variations in fracture modes between each other but also demonstrated distinct fracture behaviors compared to the remaining groups, along with a greater variability of fracture modes.

Figure 10 illustrates the fracture sections of fractured crowns pertaining to sample groups G2 and G4. A fractographic indicated a localized fracture initiation site at the crown's uppermost region, presumably at the point of interaction with the load application clamp. Both samples exhibited crack formation on the external surface.

The fracture surface of sample G2 displayed superior material adherence. In contrast, the fracture surface of sample G4 exhibited interfacial cracks and areas with inadequate adherence, suggesting the existence of air bubbles between the material and the zirconia insert surface.

Scanning Electron Microscopy (SEM) images of non-fractured crowns subjected to fatigue tests for sample groups G1 (images a and b) and G3 (images c and d) are presented in Figure 11, respectively.

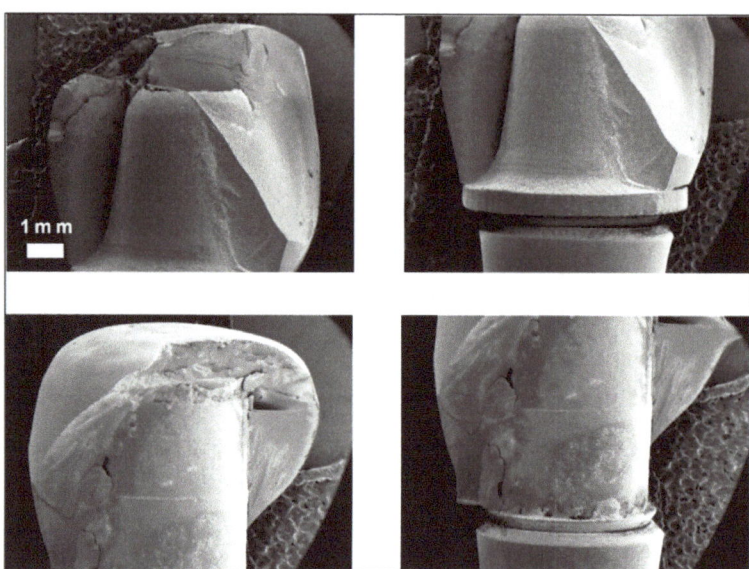

Figure 10. Fracture sections from sample group G2 (**upper** images) and G4 (**lower** images), respectively.

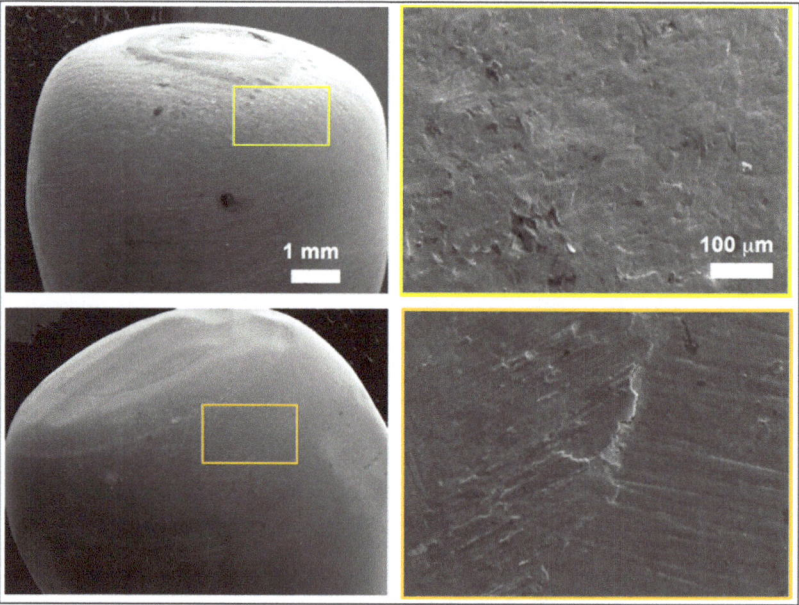

Figure 11. SEM images of unfractured samples of group G1 (**upper** images) and G3 (**lower** images).

Detailed fractographic analysis of both specimens at higher magnifications (images b and d) shows a minimal contact area between the clamp and crown with no evidence of fissures, cracks, delamination or material detachment in the crown.

The mechanical load applied to the top of the samples would have been efficiently transmitted to the crown/analog connection area without causing any adverse effects on the crown material beyond minor wear marks due to relative sliding between the clamp and crown at the contact point.

As shown in Figure 12, there was a significant level of plastic deformation experienced in the crown/abutment connection area (a and c), which transitioned from a spherical geometry to a completely oval shape. The components tested exhibited fracture along the loading direction and underwent significant levels of deformation in the same direction. Three fracture regions were identified (d): Region I, the initial nucleation crack zone, above the uppermost yellow striped line; Region II, the stable fatigue crack growth zone, between the yellow striped lines; and Region III, the catastrophic overload fracture zone, below the lower yellow striped line.

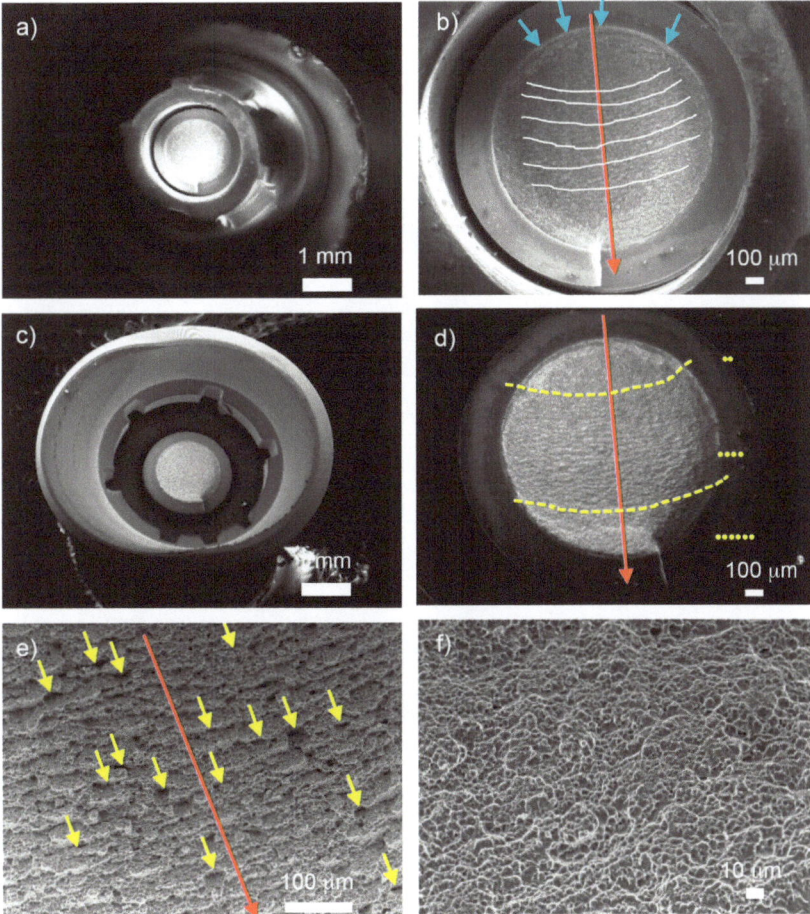

Figure 12. SEM images of fractured G1 samples, detailing: (**a**) abutment deformation, (**c**) fracture section of the screw with multiple crack initiation points, (**b**) analogous deformation, (**d**) detailed view of fracture regions within the screw's fracture section, (**e**) secondary cracking and fatigue striations. Red arrows denote the direction of fracture propagation and (**f**) micro-cavity "dimples".

The observation of Region II (d) revealed the presence of two characteristic aspects indicative of fatigue fracture processes: striations and secondary cracking. Striations appeared as cyclic fatigue loading patterns in the form of thin parallel lines (e), while secondary cracking manifested as arrays of parallel microcracks perpendicular to the main direction of fracture propagation. In the ultimate failure in Region III (f), the fracture became unstable, leading to an "overload fracture" characterized by significant plastic deformation and "dimple" micro-cavity formation on the fracture surface.

Figure 12 depicts the fractured sections of group G3, highlighting the same three fracture regions on the fracture surface (d), delineated by yellow dashed lines. Region I was located on the outer surface of the screw in the zone submitted to bending and tensile stresses. In addition, it exhibited a limited number of crack initiation points indicated by blue arrows (d). These initiation points were situated on the smooth outer surface of the screw near the body–head connection zone, specifically within the thread valley. Region II exhibited the largest fracture surface area among the three regions, in addition to the presence of typical fracture advancement beach marks: (c) indicated by white lines and typical secondary crack striations and (e) indicated by yellow arrows.

In Region II (Figure 13), beach marks were observed, and their positions are perpendicular to the path of fracture advancement, which helps locate the point of fracture initiation. The secondary cracks seemed to propagate in the same preferential direction perpendicular to both the fracture advancement direction and beach marks (e), gradually reducing the resistant section of the screw. Region III, situated in the lower section of the micrograph (d), displayed notable plastic deformation from mechanical overloading, leading to the formation of "dimple" micro-cavities (f). This rougher region featured granular morphology and numerous dimples characteristic of microvoid coalescence.

The indentation tests on the zirconia regions resulted in "small" imprints with a diameter of approximately 82 μm, while the same tests on the composite regions produced much larger imprints with a diameter of 355 μm (Figure 14). Contrarily, no cracks were observed in the composite regions at the corners of the imprints that prevented the determination of fracture toughness in these areas.

As shown in Table 6, the zirconia regions exhibited the standard hardness and fracture toughness values for dental zirconia ceramic grades, while the composite regions displayed lower hardness values.

Table 6. Summary of HV5 hardness and KIC fracture toughness characterization.

Sample Groups	Region	HV5 (GPa)	K_{IC} (MPa·m$^{1/2}$)
G1	Zirconia	13.7 ± 0.3	5.0 ± 0.3
G2	Zirconia (internal region)	13.6 ± 0.2	4.6 ± 0.4
	Composite (external region)	0.7 ± 0.1	-
G3	Composite	0.7 ± 0.1	-
G4	Zirconia (internal region)	13.8 ± 0.3	4.6 ± 0.4
	Composite (external region)	0.7 ± 0.1	-

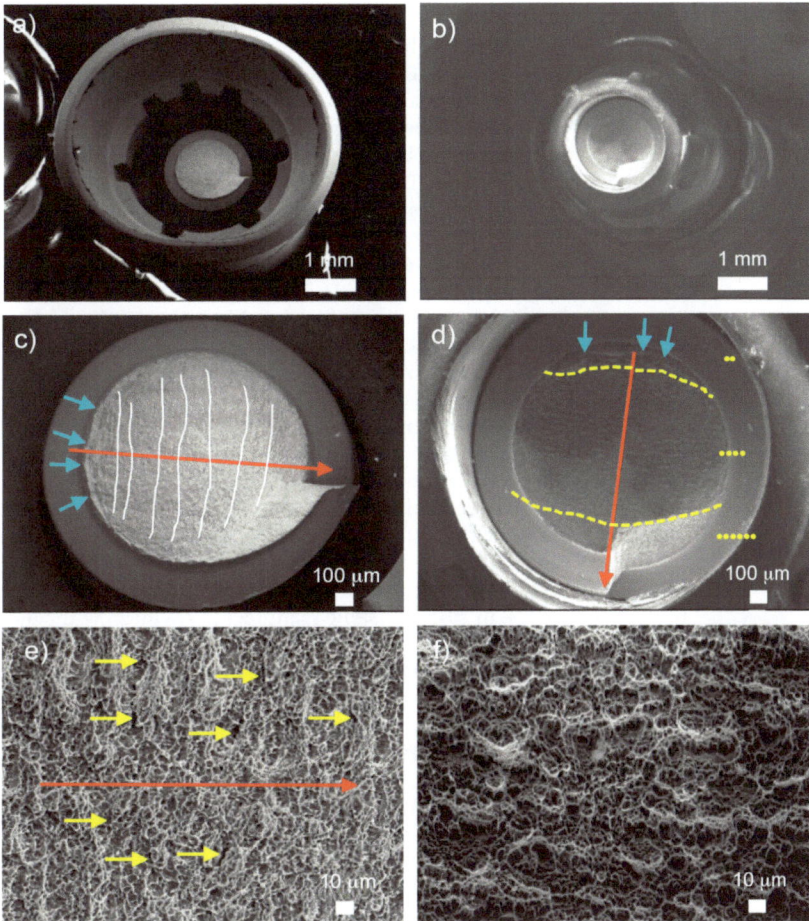

Figure 13. SEM images of fractured G3 samples. (**a**,**b**) Analogous and abutment deformation and screw's fracture sections. (**c**) Multiple crack initiation points (blue arrows). (**d**) Detailed view of fracture regions within the screw's fracture section. (**e**) Secondary cracking and fatigue striations Red arrows denote the direction of fracture propagation. (**f**) Micro-cavity "dimples".

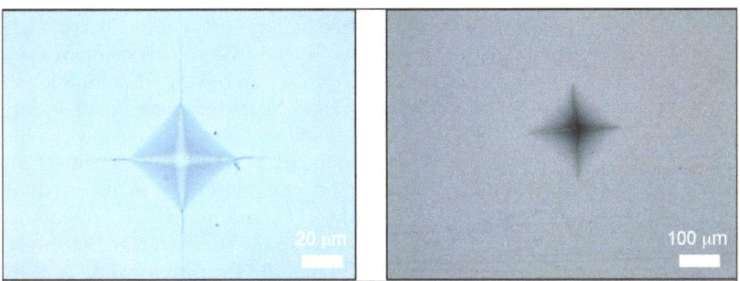

Figure 14. Images of indentations captured through optical microscopy. (**Right**) Low-magnification imprint obtained in a composite region of a dental abutment pillar. (**Left**) High-magnification imprint obtained in a zirconia region of a dental abutment pillar.

4. Discussion

The main objective was to evaluate the mechanical behavior of the different combinations of materials among the samples and see how it affects the failure mode under static and dynamic loading.

Since the beginning of dental implantology history, the lack of cushioning on the ankylosis of implants has been a great concern and represents a big challenge for industrial manufacturers. The first attempt was the IMZ implant with the intra-mobile element (IME) as its implant system, which was very popular in the 1980s [56]; another different prototype was presented in 2014 [57]. New developments in CAD/CAM materials, especially resin-based blocks, appeared on the market in the same decade. In 2012, the global manufacture of dental materials (3M ESPE, Seefeld, Germany) launched a new CAD/CAM restorative material: Lava Ultimate, based on Magne et al. [24] which was the first study that combined stiff ceramic and the resilient composite block. Despite the promising results of this combination of materials in emulating the Cushing effect of the periodontal ligament, the results from one clinical trial presented a higher failure rate, approximately 80% [58]. Two in vitro studies by Krejci et al. [59] and Lohbauer et al. [60] explained the reasons for the failures by demonstrating the high stress concentration at the bonding interface in between composite/zirconia and the reasons for debonding.

Thus, combining resilient composite on top of the implant crown with a low module of elasticity (around 10–15 Gpa of resin-composite blocks) and stiff ceramic with a high module of elasticity (210 Gpa of zirconia) on the base of the implant crown and bonded to the Ti-base abutment needs adequate bonding to work accordingly with the materials. Hence, in 2015, the same manufacturer withdrew the indication for implant and dental crowns, given the lack of a bonding strategy. Later, in 2016, a new resin block was launched in the dental market along with a new bonding strategy: Brilliant Crios and One Coat 7 Universal (Coltene Whaledent, Altstätten, Switzerland). The effectiveness of the new bonding protocol was confirmed by Reymus et al. [61] and Emsermann et al. [62], showing the disadvantages of using silane over resin-composite blocks and the benefits of monomers containing MDP.

Currently, the use of resin-composite blocks for implant crowns is well accepted because of the damping effect, considering the high occlusal forces of around 900 N required for molar areas [63–65]. Given the lack of evidence, it is unknown which is the best scenario for this material: either the monolithic bonded directly to the Ti-base (G3) or combined with mesostructured zirconia (G2 and G4), as proposed by Magne et al. [24]. According to our results, both scenarios—monolithic G2 or layered G3 and G4—demonstrated fracture strength in comparison to zirconia monolithic ceramic crowns G1, with no statistically significant differences in Fmax.

The key point of this study was focused on the damping effect and the failure mode of the material combination crown–abutment. This influenced the failure mode of the restoration, transitioning from a fatigue fracture type located at the abutment–analog connection for monolithic materials (G1 and G3) to a brittle fracture located in the crown for bi-layered materials (G2 and G4). This coincides with the research carried out by Elsayed et al. [35], where they demonstrated favorable failures, and Taha et al. [34], who concluded that with less rigid crown materials, a stiff substructure might be able to preserve their force absorption behavior.

This study was conducted to simulate the chewing function using cyclic loading and the humidity of the oral cavity conditions to ensure their reliability and durability. We also used prefabricated blocks and original Ti-base abutments with a conical abutment connection [66–68] to achieve the ideal tolerance, cement space and a proper bonding strategy between the Ti-base and the different layers of the implant crowns under study. Thus, to achieve the damping effect in resin implant restorations with a low module of elasticity, it is necessary to have support from a stiff material, such as a substructure or mesostructure, in contact with the titanium base, as demonstrated by Südbeck et al. [69].

Furthermore, a reliable bonding interface among the different materials is essential, as confirmed by Rosentritt et al. [23].

The main hypothesis of this study was validated twice through the experimental findings, as significant differences had been observed among the four assessed materials within implant–abutment–screw assemblies, both in terms of maximum fracture strength and fatigue limit values. Consequently, the null hypothesis was rejected due to the discernment of significant differences among the sample groups, as proved by the results of analyses of fracture resistance, fatigue survival, and fracture mode. This makes them potentially suitable as an alternative for restoring single implants, even in the posterior area of the mouth. The fatigue limits of the four tested groups have been determined, with the resistance arranged in the following decreasing order: G1 > G4 > G2 > G3.

Future research works are expected to focus on increasing the fracture and fatigue resistance of these bi-layered crowns through a geometric overhaul of the internal ceramic insert. This dual objective aims to amplify load-absorption capacity and refine internal load distribution, thereby concurrently reducing potential stress concentration effects.

The main limitations of the study are, among others, the use of implant replicas instead of real implants, the use of implant crowns with bigger prosthetic height and testing the wear of the implant composite block. Those aspects should be laboratory and clinically tested to evaluate the long-term performance of these restorations in the future scope of current work.

5. Conclusions

From the results obtained from both static and dynamic mechanical tests, the use of monolithic crowns would entail the direct and complete transmission of applied mechanical loads to the crown/abutment connection area, leading to progressive deformation of the abutment neck and eventual fatigue fracture of the connection screw. On the other hand, the use of bi-laminar crowns appears to protect the crown/abutment connection area by partially absorbing the applied mechanical loads, preventing deformation and fracture of the connection area at the expense of facing the final partial or total fracture of the crown.

The maximum fracture strength values obtained in this study greatly surpass the previously reported maximum beat occlusal forces, with mean Fmax values ranging from 1510.20 ± 176.96 N to 1671.18 ± 119.17 N, corresponding to the sample groups G2 and G3, respectively. Additionally, in a comparative context, the fatigue limit (LF) values obtained in this study, ranging between 668 N and 813 N, would be of a comparable magnitude, potentially indicative of infinite fatigue life resistance without failure.

Both monolithic and bi-laminar designs are approved for dental crown use, even in high-stress molar regions. Bi-laminar crowns, however, seem to safeguard the crown/abutment junction by absorbing mechanical loads, averting excessive deformation and implant fracture. This enables the crown repair of post-partial or full fractures without the need for implant removal.

In future studies, efforts are expected to improve the fracture and fatigue resistance of these bi-laminar crowns by geometrically redesigning the inner ceramic insert to enhance load distribution and reduce potential stress concentration.

6. Patents

The authors, Dr. Nicolas Gutierrez R. and Dr. Ralf Böhner (RIP), declare the rights as inventors of the "DENTAL BLANK WITH AN INSERT" by the European patent # 17175940.0-1126 on 19 September 2018 and US patent # 11.633,267 B2 in 25 April 2023.

Author Contributions: Conception and Design: N.G.R. and M.P.F. Drafting the article or revising: N.G.R., M.P.F., A.R.-C., F.G.M., J.M.M.P., O.F.-Á. and M.R.C. Final approval of the version submitted: N.G.R., M.P.F., A.R.-C., F.G.M., J.M.M.P., O.F.-Á. and M.R.C. All authors have read and agreed to the published version of the manuscript.

Funding: The authors acknowledge the financial support received from the Ministry of Science and Innovation of Spain for financial support through the PID2021- 125150OB-I00 project, cofounded by the EU through the European Regional Development Funds (MINECO-FEDER, EU). The authors are thankful to both Generalitat de Cataluña and the Agència de Gestioó d'Ajuts Universitaris i de Recerca (2021 SGR 01368) for financial support. The authors also wish to thank the Ministry of Science and Innovation of Spain for financial support through the María de Maeztu Program for Units of Excellence CEX2023-001300-M funded by MICIU/AEI/10.13039/501100011033.

Informed Consent Statement: Not applicable.

Data Availability Statement: The original contributions presented in the study are included in the article, further inquiries can be directed to the corresponding author.

Acknowledgments: The authors wish to thank COLTENE/WALEDENT for their financial support used in the in vitro assays and the material support and to DENTSPLY SIRONA for the material support. We also want to thank Ralf Böhner (RIP) for his contributions to the design and development of the new block patent.

Conflicts of Interest: The authors declare no conflict of interest.

References

1. Chang, H.H.; Yeh, C.L.; Wang, Y.L.; Huang, Y.C.; Tsai, S.J.; Li, Y.T.; Yang, J.H.; Lin, C.P. Differences in the biomechanical behaviors of natural teeth and dental implants. *Dent. Mater.* **2021**, *37*, 682–689. [CrossRef] [PubMed]
2. Murakami, H.; Igarashi, K.; Fuse, M.; Kitagawa, T.; Igarashi, M.; Uchibori, S.; Komine, C.; Gotouda, H.; Okada, H.; Kawai, Y. Risk factors for abutment and implant fracture after loading. *J. Oral Sci.* **2021**, *63*, 92–97. [CrossRef] [PubMed]
3. Yi, Y.; Heo, S.J.; Koak, J.Y.; Kim, S.K. Mechanical complications of implant-supported restorations with internal conical connection implants: A 14-year retrospective study. *J. Prosthet. Dent.* **2023**, *129*, 732–740. [CrossRef] [PubMed]
4. Jung, R.E.; Zembic, A.; Pjetursson, B.E.; Zwahlen, M.; Thoma, D.S. Systematic review of the survival rate and the incidence of biological, technical, and aesthetic complications of single crowns on implants reported in longitudinal studies with a mean follow-up of 5 years. *Clin. Oral Implants Res.* **2012**, *23* (Suppl. S6), 2–21. [CrossRef] [PubMed]
5. Jung, R.E.; Pjetursson, B.E.; Glauser, R.; Zembic, A.; Zwahlen, M.; Lang, N.P. A systematic review of the 5-year survival and complication rates of implant-supported single crowns. *Clin. Oral Implants Res.* **2008**, *19*, 119–130. [CrossRef] [PubMed]
6. Pjetursson, B.E.; Sailer, I.; Latyshev, A.; Rabel, K.; Kohal, R.J.; Karasan, D. A systematic review and meta-analysis evaluating the survival, the failure, and the complication rates of veneered and monolithic all-ceramic implant-supported single crowns. *Clin. Oral Implants Res.* **2021**, *32* (Suppl. S21), 254–288. [CrossRef] [PubMed]
7. Gracis, S.; Thompson, V.P.; Ferencz, J.L.; Silva, N.R.; Bonfante, E.A. A New Classification System for All-Ceramic and Ceramic-like Restorative Materials. *Int. J. Prosthodont.* **2015**, *28*, 227–235. [CrossRef] [PubMed]
8. Nguyen, J.F.; Migonney, V.; Ruse, N.D.; Sadoun, M. Resin composite blocks via high-pressure high-temperature polymerization. *Dent. Mater.* **2012**, *28*, 529–534. [CrossRef] [PubMed]
9. Ruse, N.D.; Sadoun, M.J. Resin-composite blocks for dental CAD/CAM applications. *J. Dent. Res.* **2014**, *93*, 1232–1234. [CrossRef] [PubMed]
10. Mainjot, A.K.; Dupont, N.M.; Oudkerk, J.C.; Dewael, T.Y.; Sadoun, M.J. From Artisanal to CAD-CAM Blocks: State of the Art of Indirect Composites. *J. Dent. Res.* **2016**, *95*, 487–495. [CrossRef]
11. Mourouzis, P.; Andreasidou, E.; Samanidou, V.; Tolidis, K. Short-term and long-term release of monomers from newly developed resin-modified ceramics and composite resin CAD-CAM blocks. *J. Prosthet. Dent.* **2020**, *123*, 339–348. [CrossRef]
12. Hampe, R.; Theelke, B.; Lümkemann, N.; Eichberger, M.; Stawarczyk, B. Fracture toughness analysis of ceramic and resin composite CAD/CAM material. *Oper. Dent.* **2019**, *44*, E190–E201. [CrossRef]
13. Naffah, N.; Ounsi, H.; Ozcan, M.; Bassal, H.; Salameh, Z. Evaluation of the adaptation and fracture resistance of three CAD-CAM resin ceramics: An in vitro study. *J. Contemp. Dent. Pract.* **2019**, *20*, 571–576.
14. Lauvahutanon, S.; Takahashi, H.; Shiozawa, M.; Iwasaki, N.; Asakawa, Y.; Oki, M.; Finger, W.J.; Arksornnukit, M. Mechanical properties of composite resin blocks for CAD/CAM. *Dent. Mater. J.* **2014**, *33*, 705–710. [CrossRef]
15. Awada, A.; Nathanson, D.; Coldea, A.; Swain, M.V.; Thiel, N.; Della Bona, A. Mechanical properties of resin-ceramic CAD/CAM restorative materials. *J. Prosthet. Dent.* **2015**, *114*, 587–593. [CrossRef]
16. Chavali, R.; Nejat, A.H.; Lawson, N.C. Machinability of CAD-CAM materials. *J. Prosthet. Dent.* **2017**, *118*, 194–199. [CrossRef] [PubMed]
17. Lauvahutanon, S.; Takahashi, H.; Oki, M.; Arkornnukit, M.; Kanehira, M.; Finger, W.J. In vitro evaluation of the wear resistance of composite resin blocks for CAD/CAM. *Dent. Mater. J.* **2015**, *34*, 495–502. [CrossRef] [PubMed]
18. Zaim, B.; Kalay, T.S.; Purcek, G. Friction, and wear behavior of chairside CAD-CAM materials against different types of antagonists: An in vitro study. *J. Prosthet. Dent.* **2022**, *128*, 803–813. [CrossRef] [PubMed]
19. Stawarczyk, B.; Liebermann, A.; Eichberger, M.; Güth, J.F. Evaluation of mechanical and optical behavior of current esthetic dental restorative CAD/CAM composites. *J. Mech. Behav. Biomed. Mater.* **2015**, *55*, 1–11. [CrossRef]

20. Stawarczyk, B.; Özcan, M.; Trottmann, A.; Schmutz, F.; Roos, M.; Hämmerle, C. Two-body wear rate of CAD/CAM resin blocks and their enamel antagonists. *J. Prosthet. Dent.* **2013**, *109*, 325–332. [CrossRef]
21. Gracis, S.E.; Nicholls, J.I.; Chalupnik, J.D.; Yuodelis, R.A. Shock-absorbing behavior of five restorative materials used on implants. *Int. J. Prosthodont.* **1991**, *4*, 282–291. [CrossRef] [PubMed]
22. Niem, T.; Youssef, N.; Wöstmann, B. Energy dissipation capacities of CAD-CAM restorative materials: A comparative evaluation of resilience and toughness. *J. Prosthet. Dent.* **2019**, *121*, 101–109. [CrossRef] [PubMed]
23. Rosentritt, M.; Schneider-Feyrer, S.; Behr, M.; Preis, V. In Vitro Shock Absorption Tests on Implant-Supported Crowns: Influence of Crown Materials and Luting Agents. *Int. J. Oral Maxillofac. Implants* **2018**, *33*, 116–122. [CrossRef] [PubMed]
24. Magne, P.; Silva, M.; Oderich, E.; Boff, L.L.; Enciso, R. Damping behavior of implant-supported restorations. *Clin. Oral Implants Res.* **2013**, *24*, 143–148. [CrossRef] [PubMed]
25. Menini, M.; Conserva, E.; Tealdo, T.; Bevilacqua, M.; Pera, F.; Signori, A.; Pera, P. Shock Absorption Capacity of Restorative Materials for Dental Implant Prostheses: An In Vitro Study. *Int. J. Prosthodont.* **2013**, *26*, 549–556. [CrossRef] [PubMed]
26. Han, J.Y.; Hou, J.X.; Zhou, G.; Wang, C.; Fan, Y.B. A histological and biomechanical study of bone stress and bone remodeling around immediately loaded implants. *Sci. China Life Sci.* **2014**, *57*, 618–626. [CrossRef] [PubMed]
27. Frost, H.M. Wolff's Law and bone's structural adaptation to mechanical usage: An overview for clinicians. *Angle Orthod.* **1994**, *64*, 175–188. [PubMed]
28. Fu, J.H.; Hsu, Y.T.; Wang, H.L. Identifying occlusal overload and how to deal with it to avoid marginal bone loss around implants. *Eur. J. Oral Implantol.* **2012**, *5*, S91–S103.
29. Rossenberg, E.S.; Torosian, J.P.; Slots, J. Microbial differences in 2 clinically distinct types of failures of osseointegrated implants. *Clin. Oral Implants Res.* **1991**, *2*, 135–144. [CrossRef]
30. Delgado-Ruiz, R.A.; Calvo-Guirado, J.L.; Romanos, G.E. Effects of occlusal forces on the peri-implant-bone interface stability. *Periodontol. 2000* **2019**, *81*, 179–193. [CrossRef]
31. Mish, C.E. *Contemporary Implant Dentistry*, 3rd ed.; Elsevier: St. Louis, MO, USA, 2008.
32. Korabi, R.; Shemtov-Yona, K.; Dorogoy, A.; Rittel, D. The Failure Envelope Concept Applied to the Bone-Dental Implant System. *Sci. Rep.* **2017**, *7*, 2051. [CrossRef]
33. Atkinson, S.R. Balance-the magic word. *Am. J. Orthod.* **1964**, *50*, 189–202. [CrossRef]
34. Taha, D.; Cesar, P.F.; Sabet, A. Influence of different combinations of CAD-CAM crown and customized abutment materials on the force absorption capacity in implant supported restorations—In Vitro study. *Dent. Mater.* **2022**, *38*, e10–e18. [CrossRef] [PubMed]
35. Elsayed, A.; Yazigi, C.; Kern, M.; Chaar, M.S. Mechanical behavior of nano-hybrid composite in comparison to lithium disilicate as posterior cement-retained implant-supported crowns restoring different abutments. *Dent. Mater.* **2021**, *37*, e435–e442. [CrossRef]
36. Mascarenhas, F.; Yilmaz, B.; McGlumphy, E.; Clelland, N.; Seidt, J. Load to failure of different zirconia implant abutments with titanium components. *J. Prosthet. Dent.* **2017**, *117*, 749–754. [CrossRef] [PubMed]
37. Guilherme, N.M.; Chung, K.H.; Flinn, B.D.; Zheng, C.; Raigrodski, A.J. Assessment of reliability of CAD/CAM tooth-colored implant custom abutments. *J. Prosthet. Dent.* **2016**, *116*, 206–213. [CrossRef]
38. Moris, I.C.M.; Chen, Y.C.; Faria, A.C.L.; Ribeiro, R.F.; Fok, A.S.L.; Rodrigues, R.C.S. Fracture loads and failure modes of customized and non-customized zirconia abutments. *Dent. Mater.* **2018**, *34*, e197–e204. [CrossRef]
39. Miyamoto, Y.; Kaysser, W.A.; Rabin, B.H.; Kawasaki, A.; Ford, R.G. *Functionally Graded Materials; Design, Processing and Applications*; Springer Science + Business Media: New York, NY, USA, 1999; pp. 2–9.
40. Cui, C.; Sun, J. Optimizing the design of bio-inspired functionally graded material (FGM) layer in all-ceramic dental restorations. *Dent. Mater. J.* **2014**, *33*, 173–178. [CrossRef] [PubMed]
41. Petrini, M.; Ferrante, M.; Su, B. Fabrication and characterization of biomimetic ceramic/polymer composite materials for dental restoration. *Dent. Mater.* **2013**, *29*, 375–381. [CrossRef]
42. Chen, Y.C.; Fok, A. Stress distributions in human teeth modeled with a natural graded material distribution. *Dent. Mater.* **2014**, *30*, e337–e348. [CrossRef]
43. He, L.H.; Yin, Z.H.; Van Vuuren, L.J.; Carter, E.A.; Liang, X.W. A natural functionally graded biocomposite coating-human enamel. *Acta Biomater.* **2013**, *9*, 6330–6337. [CrossRef] [PubMed]
44. He, L.H.; Swain, M.V. Enamel—A "metallic-like" deformable biocomposite. *J. Dent.* **2007**, *35*, 431–437. [CrossRef] [PubMed]
45. Arola, D. Fatigue testing of biomaterials and their interfaces. *Dent. Mater.* **2017**, *33*, 367–381. [CrossRef] [PubMed]
46. Wang, Z.; Wang, K.; Xu, W.; Gong, X.; Zhang, F. Mapping the mechanical gradient of human dentin-enamel-junction at different intratooth locations. *Dent. Mater.* **2018**, *34*, 376–388. [CrossRef]
47. Joda, T.; Huber, S.; Bürki, A.; Zysset, P.; Brägger, U. Influence of Abutment Design on Stiffness, Strength, and Failure of Implant-Supported Monolithic Resin Nano Ceramic (RNC) Crowns. *Clin. Implant. Dent. Relat. Res.* **2015**, *17*, 1200–1207. [CrossRef]
48. *ISO 14801-2016*; Dentistry—Implants—Dynamic Loading Test for Endosseous Dental Implants. International Organization for Standardization: Geneva, Switzerland, 2016.
49. *ASTM-E-384-17*; Standard Test Method for Microindentation Hardness of Materials. ASTM International: West Conshohocken, PA, USA, 2017.
50. Anderson, T.L. *Fracture Mechanics: Fundamentals and Applications*; Taylor & Francis: Abingdon, UK, 2005; ISBN 978-0-8493-1656-2.

51. Marshall, D.B.; Lawn, B.R.; Evans, A.G. Elastic/plastic indentation damage in ceramics: The lateral crack system. *J. Am. Ceram.* **1980**, *574*. [CrossRef]
52. Laugier, M.T. Load bearing capacity of TiN coated WC–Co cemented carbides. *J. Mater. Sci. Lett.* **1983**, *2*, 419–421. [CrossRef]
53. Dukino, R.D.; Swain, M.V. Comparative measurement of indentation fracture toughness with Berkovich and Vickers indenters. *J. Am. Ceram. Soc.* **1992**, *75*, 3299–3304. [CrossRef]
54. Casellas, D.; Caro, J.; Molas, S.; Prado, J.M.; Valls, I. Fracture toughness of carbides in tool steels evaluated by nanoindentation. *Acta Mater.* **2007**, *55*, 4277–4286. [CrossRef]
55. Niihara, K.; Morena, R.; Hasselman, D.P.H. Evaluation of KIc of brittle solids by the indentation method with low crack-to-indent ratios. *J. Mater. Sci.* **1982**, *1*, 13–16.
56. Mautsch, C.; Wolfard, S.; Mautsch, W.; Rittich, A. Long-term outcome of the IMZ implant system: A retrospective clinical study with a follow-up between 23 and 34 years. *Int. J. Implant. Dent.* **2022**, *8*, 54. [CrossRef] [PubMed]
57. Chena, Y.Y.; Chena, W.P.; Chang, H.H.; Huang, S.H.; Lin, C.P. A novel dental implant abutment with micro-motion capability—Development and biomechanical evaluations. *Dent. Mater.* **2014**, *30*, 131–137. [CrossRef] [PubMed]
58. Schepke, U.; Meijer, H.J.; Vermeulen, K.M.; Raghoebar, G.M.; Cune, M.S. Clinical Bonding of Resin Nano Ceramic Restorations to Zirconia Abutments: A Case Series within a Randomized Clinical Trial. *Clin. Implant. Dent. Relat. Res.* **2016**, *18*, 984–992. [CrossRef] [PubMed]
59. Krejci, I.; Daher, R. Stress distribution difference between Lava Ultimate full crowns and IPS e. *max CAD full crowns on a natural tooth and on tooth-shaped implant abutments*. Odontology **2017**, *105*, 254–256. [PubMed]
60. Lohbauer, U.; Belli, R.; Cune, M.S.; Schepke, U. Fractography of clinically fractured, implant-supported dental computer- aided design and computer-aided manufacturing crowns. *SAGE Open Med. Case Rep.* **2017**, *5*, 2050313X17741015. [CrossRef]
61. Reymus, M.; Roos, M.; Eichberger, M.; Edelhoff, D.; Hickel, R.; Stawarczyk, B. Bonding to new CAD/CAM resin composites: Influence of air abrasion and conditioning agents as pretreatment strategy. *Clin. Oral Investig.* **2019**, *23*, 529–538. [CrossRef]
62. Emsermann, I.; Eggmann, F.; Krastl, G.; Weiger, R.; Amato, J. Influence of Pretreatment Methods on the Adhesion of Composite and Polymer Infiltrated Ceramic CAD-CAM Blocks. *J. Adhes. Dent.* **2019**, *21*, 433–443.
63. Ferrario, V.F.; Sforza, C.; Serrao, G.; Dellavia, C.; Tartaglia, G.M. Single tooth bite forces in healthy young adults. *J. Oral Rehabil.* **2004**, *31*, 18–22. [CrossRef]
64. Varga, S.; Spalj, S.; Lapter Varga, M.; Anic Milosevic, S.; Mestrovic, S.; Slaj, M. Maximum voluntary molar bite force in subjects with normal occlusion. *Eur. J. Orthod.* **2011**, *33*, 427–433. [CrossRef] [PubMed]
65. Padma, S.; Umesh, S.; Asokan, S.; Srinivas, T. Bite Force Measurement Based on Fiber Bragg Grating Sensor. *J. Biomed. Opt.* **2017**, *22*, 107002. [CrossRef]
66. Ramalho, I.S.; Bergamo, E.T.P.; Witek, L.; Coelho, P.G.; Lopes, A.C.O.; Bonfante, E.A. Implant-abutment fit influences the mechanical performance of single-crown prostheses. *J. Mech. Behav. Biomed. Mater.* **2020**, *102*, 103506. [CrossRef] [PubMed]
67. Alonso-Pérez, R.; Bartolomé, J.F.; Ferreiroa, A.; Salido, M.P.; Pradíes, G. Original vs. non-original abutments for screw-retained single implant crowns: An in vitro evaluation of internal fit, mechanical behaviour and screw loosening. *Clin. Oral Implants Res.* **2018**, *29*, 1230–1238. [CrossRef] [PubMed]
68. Schmitt, C.M.; Nogueira-Filho, G.; Tenenbaum, H.C.; Lai, J.Y.; Brito, C.; Doering, H.; Nonhoff, J. Performance of conical abutment (Morse Taper) connection implants: A systematic review. *J. Biomed. Mater. Res. A* **2014**, *102*, 552–574. [CrossRef] [PubMed]
69. Südbeck, S.; Hoffmann, M.; Reymus, M.; Buser, R.; Edelhoff, D.; Stawarczyk, B. Bending moment of implants restored with CAD/CAM polymer-based restoration materials with or without a titanium base before and after artificial aging. *Dent. Mater.* **2022**, *38*, e245–e255. [CrossRef] [PubMed]

Disclaimer/Publisher's Note: The statements, opinions and data contained in all publications are solely those of the individual author(s) and contributor(s) and not of MDPI and/or the editor(s). MDPI and/or the editor(s) disclaim responsibility for any injury to people or property resulting from any ideas, methods, instructions or products referred to in the content.

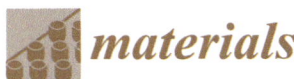

Article

Alendronate as Bioactive Coating on Titanium Surfaces: An Investigation of CaP–Alendronate Interactions

Ines Despotović [1,*], Željka Petrović [2,*], Jozefina Katić [3] and Dajana Mikić [3]

[1] Division of Physical Chemistry, Ruđer Bošković Institute, Bijenička Cesta 54, 10002 Zagreb, Croatia
[2] Division of Materials Chemistry, Ruđer Bošković Institute, Bijenička Cesta 54, 10002 Zagreb, Croatia
[3] Department of Electrochemistry, Faculty of Chemical Engineering and Technology, University of Zagreb, Marulićev Trg 19, 10000 Zagreb, Croatia; jkatic@fkit.unizg.hr (J.K.); dmikic@fkit.unizg.hr (D.M.)
* Correspondence: ines.despotovic@irb.hr (I.D.); zeljka.petrovic@irb.hr (Ž.P.)

Abstract: The surface modification of dental implants plays an important role in establishing a successful interaction of the implant with the surrounding tissue, as the bioactivity and osseointegration properties are strongly dependent on the physicochemical properties of the implant surface. A surface coating with bioactive molecules that stimulate the formation of a mineral calcium phosphate (CaP) layer has a positive effect on the bone bonding process, as biomineralization is crucial for improving the osseointegration process and rapid bone ingrowth. In this work, the spontaneous deposition of calcium phosphate on the titanium surface covered with chemically stable and covalently bound alendronate molecules was investigated using an integrated experimental and theoretical approach. The initial nucleation of CaP was investigated using quantum chemical calculations at the density functional theory (DFT) level. Negative Gibbs free energies show a spontaneous nucleation of CaP on the biomolecule-covered titanium oxide surface. The deposition of calcium and phosphate ions on the alendronate-modified titanium oxide surface is governed by Ca^{2+}–phosphonate (-PO_3H) interactions and supported by hydrogen bonding between the phosphate group of CaP and the amino group of the alendronate molecule. The morphological and structural properties of CaP deposit were investigated using scanning electron microscopy, energy dispersive X-ray spectroscopy, X-ray diffraction and attenuated total reflectance Fourier transform infrared spectroscopy. This integrated experimental–theoretical study highlights the spontaneous formation of CaP on the alendronate-coated titanium surface, confirming the bioactivity ability of the alendronate coating. The results provide valuable guidance for the promising forthcoming advancements in the development of biomaterials and surface modification of dental implants.

Keywords: titanium dental implant; alendronate coating; calcium phosphate CaP; bioactivity; DFT quantum chemical calculations

Citation: Despotović, I.; Petrović, Ž.; Katić, J.; Mikić, D. Alendronate as Bioactive Coating on Titanium Surfaces: An Investigation of CaP–Alendronate Interactions. *Materials* **2024**, *17*, 2703. https://doi.org/10.3390/ma17112703

Academic Editors: Evgeny Levashov and Csaba Balázsi

Received: 9 April 2024
Revised: 6 May 2024
Accepted: 30 May 2024
Published: 3 June 2024

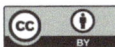

Copyright: © 2024 by the authors. Licensee MDPI, Basel, Switzerland. This article is an open access article distributed under the terms and conditions of the Creative Commons Attribution (CC BY) license (https://creativecommons.org/licenses/by/4.0/).

1. Introduction

Titanium-based materials are the most commonly used for the manufacture of medical implants [1–5], mainly due to their suitable mechanical properties [6]. In addition, titanium and most of its alloys have shown excellent tissue compatibility [7]. However, these materials have been shown to be highly bioinert due to poor contact with the living body upon implantation [8,9]. Since the effectiveness of the osseointegration process with the surrounding tissue depends on the interactions that occur at the outermost surface layer with few atomic distances, the titanium surface has been specifically modified to improve integration with the surrounding tissue and minimize the risks associated with the release of metal ions into the body. Among a number of established approaches to surface modification (functionalization) [10], the formation of a biocompatible and bioactive layer that irreversibly adheres to the surface has attracted particular attention [11–14].

Organophosphorus compounds such as phosphonates have proven to be effective agents for the functionalization of titanium surfaces by forming homogeneous self-assembled monolayers. In particular, alendronate, a nitrogen-containing bisphosphonate, exhibits good coating properties on titanium surfaces [15–17], and the effect of immobilizing alendronate on the titanium surface to stimulate new bone formation and improve bone-implant integration after implantation has been widely reported [17–20]. On the titanium surface, alendronate molecules are covalently bound to the TiO_2 layer via phosphonate groups (-PO_3H) [15]. At the same time, those unbound phosphonate groups (-PO_3H), together with the amine groups (-NH_2) and hydroxyl groups (-OH) of the alendronate molecules, remain free and can participate in the chemical reactions during new bone growth. These reactions include the spontaneous precipitation of different calcium phosphate phases (CaP), including hydroxyapatite (HAp), a naturally occurring form of calcium phosphate that is an essential component for the formation of new bone matrix. The CaP deposit has an important role in initial cell attachment since it can adsorb proteins from the surrounding tissue, promoting cell adhesion and the recruitment of osteogenic cells to the implant surface and facilitating the new bone mineralization process [21–24]. As known from the literature, the chemical precipitation and nucleation of calcium phosphate (CaP) are strongly influenced by self-assembled monolayers carrying different functional groups [25–28]. Specifically, different monolayers with phosphonate (-PO_3H), amino (-NH_2) or hydroxyl (-OH) groups were investigated [29–35], and they were found to promote the mineralization process and affect the texture of the CaP deposit. These results sparked our interest in investigating the potential of alendronate coating as a promoter of CaP formation in the contents of the enhanced bioactivity of the underlying titanium.

In our previous publications, the mechanism of the formation of the alendronate coating on the titanium surface and its chemical stability when exposed to artificial saliva was reported in detail [15,16]. Since the alendronate-modified titanium surface has been shown to exhibit good chemical stability, which is the basic prerequisite for its biocompatibility, it was of great importance to investigate bioactivity as an essential property for successful osseointegration. In this study, the bioactivity potential of the alendronate coating was monitored via the spontaneous formation of CaP deposits on the alendronate-coated titanium surface. To the best of our knowledge, a combined experimental and theoretical approach was used for the first time to fully elucidate the formation of CaP. Quantum chemical DFT calculations provided insights into the interactions of the calcium and phosphate ions with alendronate molecules on the titanium surface in the early phase of the CaP nucleation process. The results indicated spontaneous CaP formation, which was confirmed experimentally using scanning electron microscopy (SEM), energy dispersive X-ray spectroscopy (EDS), X-ray diffraction (XRD) and attenuated total reflection Fourier transform infrared spectroscopy (ATR-FTIR). The phase analysis of the CaP deposit confirmed the mixture of the phases, beta-tricalcium phosphate (β-TCP) and calcium-deficient HAp, having beneficial properties from an application point of view.

2. Materials and Methods
2.1. Quantum Chemical Calculations

Density functional theory (DFT) quantum chemical calculations have been carried out, employing the M06 functional developed by Truhlar's group [36–38]. The 6-31+G(d,p) + LANL2DZ basis set was utilized for geometry optimization. Pople's 6-31+G(d,p) double-ξ basis set was chosen for the H, C, O, N, Ca, and P atoms, and the LANL2DZ basis set was chosen for the transition metal (Ti) atoms [39]. The vibrational frequency analysis under the harmonic oscillator approximation was used to verify all calculated structures to be true minima on the potential energy surface. In addition, the thermal correction to the Gibbs free energy was derived from the same vibrational analysis. To refine the energy, a highly flexible 6-311++G(2df,2pd) basis set was utilized for H, C, O, N, Ca and P atoms, while the same LANL2DZ ECP-type basis set was used for the titanium atoms. The polarizable continuum solvation model SMD (solvation model based on density) [40] was used to model the solvation effects. The solvent water is represented by a dielectric constant of ε = 78.3553. To account for the specific interaction of the metal cation with the water solvent, the first solvation shell [41], represented by a specific number of water molecules coordinating the calcium ion, is explicitly included in the quantum chemical region, and the remaining bulk solvent is approximated by a polarizable continuum, leading to the cluster continuum method [42]. All calculations were performed with the program package Gaussian 09 (revision D.01) [43].

The topological analysis of the charge density distribution was performed through means of Bader's quantum theory of atoms in molecules (QTAIM) [44] using the AIMALL [45] program package (version 17.01.25) and utilizing the SMD/M06/6-31+G(d,p) + LANL2DZ wave function obtained from the optimization.

The Gibbs free energy of the interactions, ΔG^*_{INT}, was calculated according to the formula $\Delta G^*_{INT} = G^*_{AB} - G^*_A - G^*_B$, where G^*_{AB} is the total free energy of the resulting AB structure and G^*_A and G^*_B are the total free energies of the associating units A and B, respectively. A detailed description of the computational modeling can be found in the Supplementary Materials.

2.2. Materials, Chemicals and Solutions

The substrates whose surfaces were functionalized were the titanium discs (Ti, 99.9%, ϕ = 12 mm, thickness 1.5 mm, Alfa Aesar®, Karlsruhe, Germany).

The following chemicals were used as received: sodium alendronate trihydrate (≥97%, Merck Sharp & Dohme, Rahway, NJ, USA), acetone (p.a., Gram-Mol, Zagreb, Croatia) and absolute ethanol (p.a., Gram-Mol, Zagreb, Croatia).

The powder of sodium alendronate trihydrate was dissolved in Milli-Q® water (Millipore, Merck, Darmstadt, Germany) via ultrasonic stirring for 10 min to obtain a 10 mmol dm^{-3} solution. The phosphate-buffered solution (10.0530 g $Na_2HPO_4 \cdot 7H_2O$ + 1.9501 g $NaH_2PO_4 \cdot 2H_2O$ were dissolved in 0.5 dm^3 water; pH = 7.4) was used to prepare an oxide layer on the Ti substrate. The Fusayama artificial saliva, prepared via dissolving 0.4 g NaCl, 0.4 g KCl, 0.6 g $CaCl_2 \cdot 2H_2O$, 0.58 g $Na_2HPO_4 \cdot 2H_2O$ and 1 g urea in 1 dm^3 water [46], was used as a model solution to monitor spontaneous CaP formation. All solutions were prepared with Milli-Q® water.

2.3. Functionalisation of the Titanium Samples

The titanium sample covered using electrochemically formed oxide film coated with alendronate (Ti/oxide/alendronate) was prepared.

Prior to modification, the surface of Ti samples was abraded with 240, 500 and 600 grit SiC emery paper, ultrasonically cleaned with absolute ethanol, acetone and Mili-Q® water and dried with nitrogen (99.999%, Messer®, Bad Soden, Germany). To create the oxide layer on the Ti surface (Ti/oxide), a potential of 2.5 V vs. Ag|AgCl, 3.0 mol dm^{-3} KCl was applied to the Ti in a phosphate-buffered solution for 5 h. The oxide layer formation was performed on the Ti disc, which was placed in a Teflon holder so that an area of 1 cm^2 was exposed to the electrolyte. The measurement was performed in a three-electrode cell with the Ti as the working electrode, the Ag|AgCl, 3.0 mol dm^{-3} KCl (E = 0.210 V vs. standard hydrogen electrode, SHE) as the reference and the graphite rod as the counter electrode using the Autolab 128N potentiostat/galvanostat (Metrohm Autolab BV, Utrecht, The Netherlands) controlled using Nova 2.1.6® software (Metrohm Autolab BV, Utrecht, The Netherlands). The Ti/oxide samples were then rinsed and dried with nitrogen. Functionalization with an alendronate layer was performed on the Ti sample with oxide layer (Ti/oxide), according to the following procedure. The Ti/oxide samples were immersed in the prepared alendronate solution at 22 ± 1 °C for 24 h. The functionalized samples were then dried at 70 °C for 7 h to ensure the chemical stability of the coating [47]. Samples were then rinsed with Milli-Q® water and absolute ethanol and dried in a nitrogen stream.

2.4. Spontaneous Formation of Calcium Phosphates (CaP) on the Titanium Samples

To investigate potential bioactivity of the Ti/oxide/alendronate sample, samples were immersed in the Fusayama artificial saliva (pH 6.8) at 22 ± 2 °C for a period of 100 days. After this period, white deposits were visible on the surface of the sample, which was characterized in more detail.

2.5. Characterisation of the Titanium Samples

The phase composition of the samples was recorded in the 2θ range between 10° and 90°, and 45 kV and 40 mA on the Empyrean powder X-ray diffractometer (PXRD) (Malvern Pananalytical B.V., Almelo, The Netherlands) with CuKα radiation (0.1542 mm).

Morphology and elemental analysis was performed using the field emission scanning electron microscope (FE-SEM, model JSM-7000F, Jeol Ltd., Tokyo, Japan) in conjunction with the energy dispersive X-ray analyzer EDS/INCA 350, (Oxfore Instruments, High Wycombe, UK). Micrographs were recorded at 5 kV accelerating voltage and 10 mm working distance. The EDS analysis was performed with an accelerating voltage of 10 kV, a working distance of 10 mm, acquisition time of 180 s and a dead time of 16%.

The attenuated total reflectance Fourier transform infrared (ATR-FTIR) spectra were measured with the IRTracer-100 spectrometer (Shimadzu, Kyoto, Japan) during 45 cycles in the range of 4000 to 450 cm^{-1} with a scan resolution of 4 cm^{-1}.

The results shown in this study are the average of three measurements.

3. Results and Discussion

3.1. The Mechanism of Interaction of Calcium and Phosphate Ions with Ti/Oxide/Alendronate

To gain insight into the possible interactions between calcium and phosphate ions present in body fluids with Ti/oxide/alendronate at the molecular level, a detailed theoretical study using quantum chemical DFT calculations was performed. The interaction of calcium and phosphate ions with the alendronate-coated surface was analyzed in terms of the interaction pattern and interaction energy. Herein, the aim of the theoretical simulations was not to investigate the entire nucleation route for calcium phosphate, but rather the initial stage of the aggregation of calcium and phosphate ions at the alendronate coating. The hydrogen phosphate anion HPO_4^{2-} was considered for the simulation as it is the main phosphate species present in the solution at pH = 6.5. Also, it is important to point out that the ion association process between Ca^{2+} and HPO_4^{2-} occurs immediately at the beginning of the deposition process, forming a $CaHPO_4$ ion pair which interacts with alendronate coating.

Since the TiO_2 layer is present on the titanium surface, the TiO_2 nanocluster was selected for the simulation of the metal oxide layer. For the sake of computational efficiency, the $(TiO_2)_{10}$ nanocluster used by Qu and Kroes [48] was selected to serve for cluster modeling.

Previously reported results for the alendronate–coated titanium surface [15] showed that it is most likely the result of two energetically competing structures, one in which the alendronate molecule is bound to the TiO_2 surface via both the amine and phosphonate groups, while in the other the alendronate molecule is bound only via the phosphonate group, with the former being slightly more favorable by 3.48 kcal mol^{-1}. Therefore, to model the $(TiO_2)_{10}$-alendronate-CaP structure, both $(TiO_2)_{10}$-alendronate structures are taken into account.

In the case of the more stable $(TiO_2)_{10}$–alendronate structure, the formation of the CaP deposit can be initiated by the following two structures. In one, $(TiO_2)_{10}$-alendronate–CaP–I (Figure 1a), which is more favorable, the calcium ion binds to the two phosphonate groups of the alendronate molecule, releasing the Gibbs free energy of $\Delta G^*_{INT} = -31.14$ kcal mol^{-1}.

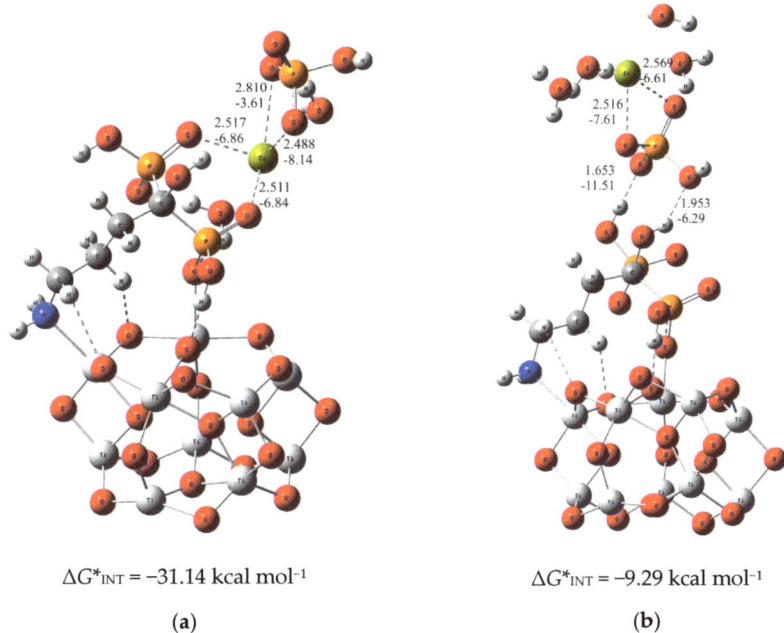

$\Delta G^*_{INT} = -31.14$ kcal mol^{-1} $\Delta G^*_{INT} = -9.29$ kcal mol^{-1}

(a)   (b)

Figure 1. The most stable structures predicted using DFT calculations: (a) (TiO$_2$)$_{10}$–alendronate–CaP–I and (b) (TiO$_2$)$_{10}$–alendronate–CaP–II. The bond lengths are given in Å, the bond energies are given in kcal mol^{-1}. Ti—light gray, O—red, C—gray, N—blue, P—orange, H—white, Ca—yellow-green.

The interaction between the phosphonate groups and the calcium ion is achieved by two strong coordinate P–O–Ca bonds ($d_{Ca\cdots O}$ = 2.517 Å and 2.511 Å; $E_{Ca\cdots O}$ = −6.84 kcal mol^{-1} and −6.86 kcal mol^{-1}; Figure 1a), where a free electron pair from the oxygen atom of the phosphonate group of the alendronate molecule is involved in the binding with the calcium ion. In addition, the HPO$_4^{2-}$ ion binds to the calcium ion via Ca–O bonds ($d_{Ca\cdots O}$ = 2.810 Å and 2.488 Å; $E_{Ca\cdots O}$ = −3.61 kcal mol^{-1} and −8.14 kcal mol^{-1}; Figure 1a) in bidentate fashion, and is aligned in the upper part of the (TiO$_2$)$_{10}$–alendronate–CaP–I structure. The formed Ca–O bonds are attributed to an ionic interaction type according to $\nabla^2\rho(rc) > 0$ and $H(rc) > 0$ from the topological analysis of the electronic density distribution. In addition, two water molecules are found in the first coordination shell of the Ca^{2+} ion.

When the formation of CaP is accomplished via the phosphate group of the CaHPO$_4$ ion pair, the considerably less stable structure ((TiO$_2$)$_{10}$–alendronate–CaP–II) with $\Delta G^*_{INT} = -9.29$ kcal mol^{-1} is obtained (Figure 1b). In this structure, the phosphate group binds to the alendronate molecule at the phosphonate site via two strong hydrogen O···H–O bonds ($d_{O\cdots H}$ = 1.653 Å and 1.953 Å; $E_{O\cdots H}$ = −11.51 kcal mol^{-1} and −6.29 kcal mol^{-1}; Figure 1b). The remaining two oxygen atoms of the phosphate group coordinate the calcium in a bidentate manner ($d_{Ca\cdots O}$ = 2.516 Å and 2.569 Å; $E_{Ca\cdots O}$ = −7.61 kcal mol^{-1} and −6.61 kcal mol^{-1}; Figure 1b). The critical point of the formed Ca–O bonds was characterized by positive values of the electron density Laplacian, $\nabla^2\rho(rc) > 0$, and by a positive value of the electron energy density, $H(rc) > 0$, which assigns the Ca–O bonds to an ionic interaction type.

The calculated Gibbs free energies of the interactions for the (TiO$_2$)$_{10}$–alendronate–CaP structures selected above point to the spontaneous formation ($\Delta G^*_{INT} < 0$) for both structures. However, the binding is found to be much more exergonic in the case of (TiO$_2$)$_{10}$–alendronate–CaP–I (Figure 1a), leading to the conclusion that CaP deposition on the alendronate coatings occurs mainly through the calcium (CaHPO$_4$)–phosphonate (alendronate) interactions.

For the thermodynamically less stable but highly competitive $(TiO_2)_{10}$–alendronate structure, two modes of binding of calcium and phosphate ions to alendronate molecule are also obtained (Figure 2). In the one, thermodynamically more stable structure, the calcium and phosphate ions interact with the alendronate molecule via the calcium ion, which binds to two oxygen atoms of the phosphonate group of the alendronate molecule ($(TiO_2)_{10}$–alendronate–CaP–III, $d_{Ca \cdots O}$ = 2.478 Å and 2.450 Å; $E_{Ca \cdots O}$ = −7.50 kcal mol^{-1} and −8.11 kcal mol^{-1}; Figure 2a). The phosphate ion binds to the calcium ion via two oxygen atoms with $d_{Ca \cdots O}$ = 2.507 Å and 2.663 Å and $E_{Ca \cdots O}$ = −7.79 kcal mol^{-1} and −5.19 kcal mol^{-1}, respectively (Figure 2a). The additional interaction of the phosphate ion with the amino group is established through the strong O···H–N hydrogen bond ($d_{O \cdots H}$ = 2.192 Å; $E_{O \cdots H}$ = −4.00 kcal mol^{-1}; Figure 2a). It can be considered, according to the QTAIM analysis, as a partially ionic and partially covalent interaction in accordance with the positive value of Laplacian, $\nabla^2 \rho(rc) > 0$, and the negative value of the electron energy density, $H(rc) < 0$, at the bond critical point. The Gibbs free energy of interaction for the structure under consideration is calculated as ΔG^*_{INT} = −34.65 kcal mol^{-1}.

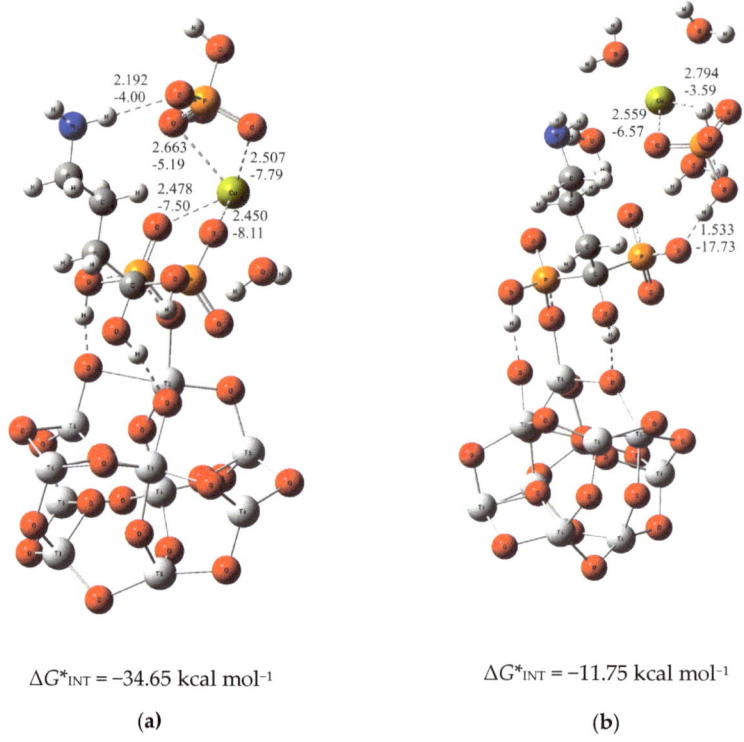

ΔG^*_{INT} = −34.65 kcal mol^{-1} ΔG^*_{INT} = −11.75 kcal mol^{-1}

(a) (b)

Figure 2. The most stable structures predicted using DFT calculations: (**a**) $(TiO_2)_{10}$–alendronate–CaP–III and (**b**) $(TiO_2)_{10}$–alendronate–CaP–IV. The bond lengths are given in Å, the bond energies are given in kcal mol^{-1}. Ti—light gray, O—red, C—gray, N—blue, P—orange, H—white, Ca—yellow-green.

In the alternative structure, $(TiO_2)_{10}$–alendronate–CaP–IV (Figure 2b), the binding of the CaP ion pair via the phosphate group, leads to a less stable structure with a Gibbs free interaction energy of −11.75 kcal mol^{-1}. In this structure, the phosphate ion of the CaHPO$_4$ ion pair interacts with the phosphonate group of the alendronate molecule, resulting in an anchoring hydrogen O···H–O bond with a corresponding bond length of 1.533 Å and an energy of $E_{O \cdots H}$ = −17.73 kcal mol^{-1}. The phosphate group coordinates the calcium ion through two bonds with a corresponding bond length of $d_{Ca \cdots O}$ = 2.559 Å and 2.794 Å and energies of $E_{Ca\cdots O}$ = −6.57 kcal mol^{-1} and −3.59 kcal mol^{-1}, respectively (Figure 2b). It is worth mentioning that no interaction of the CaP ion pair with the NH$_2$ group of alendronate molecule was found.

In summary, the deposition of calcium and phosphate ions on the alendronate modified titanium oxide surface is governed by Ca^{2+}–phosphonate interaction. It is supported by the hydrogen bond between the phosphate group of CaP and the amino group of the alendronate molecule, as found in the structure (TiO$_2$)$_{10}$–alendronate–CaP–III. Those interactions ensure a thermodynamically strong favorable binding pattern with a released Gibbs free interaction energy of ΔG^*_{INT} = −34.65 kcal mol^{-1}.

To put the above results in perspective, the DFT calculations of the interactions of bare TiO$_2$ clusters with calcium phosphate ions were carried out. The most stable structure for each of the considered binding modes (analogous to the previous ones with alendronate coating) were determined and demonstrated in Figure 3.

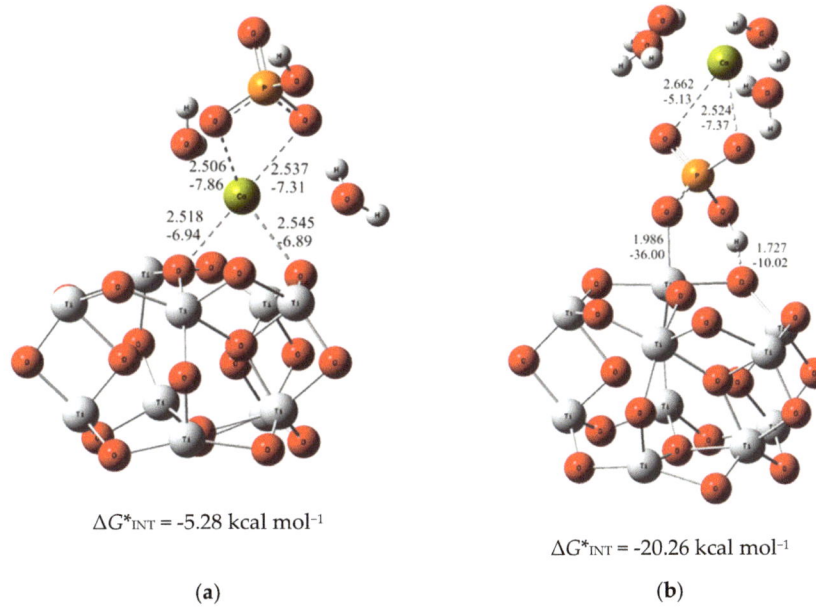

Figure 3. The most stable structures predicted using DFT calculations: (**a**) (TiO$_2$)$_{10}$–CaP–I and (**b**) (TiO$_2$)$_{10}$–CaP–II. The bond lengths are given in Å, the bond energies are given in kcal mol^{-1}. Ti—light gray, O—red, C—gray, P—orange, H—white, Ca—yellow-green.

As can be seen from the DFT results, the binding established through the interaction of the phosphate ion of CaP (ΔG^*_{INT} = −20.26 kcal mol^{-1}; Figure 3b) with the TiO$_2$ surface is more exergonic than the binding achieved through the Ca^{2+} − O$_{(TiO2)10}$ (ΔG^*_{INT} = −5.28 kcal mol^{-1}; Figure 3a) interactions. However, compared to the most favorable binding of calcium phosphate ions to the alendronate modified titanium oxide surface, it appeared significantly less exergonic ($\Delta(\Delta G^*_{INT})$ = 14.39 kcal mol^{-1}). These findings clearly indicate the positive effects of alendronate coating on the formation of CaP which is fully in line with the experimental observations.

3.2. Experimental Evidence for the Spontaneous Formation of Calcium Phosphates (CaP) on the Ti/oxide/Alendronate Surface

Since the DFT results clearly showed that the spontaneous formation of CaP on the alendronate-modified Ti/oxide surface is possible, experimental evidence was obtained using SEM, EDS, ATR-FTIR and XRD techniques. The prepared Ti/oxide/alendronate samples were immersed for 100 days in Fusayama artificial saliva solution as simulated body fluid to test alendronate coating's bioactivity on the basis of monitoring the spontaneous CaP deposit formation.

Morphology, Chemical and Phase Analysis of Ti/Oxide/Alendronate Samples after 100 Days Immersion in Artificial Saliva

SEM measurements were performed to gain insight into the morphology of the Ti/oxide/alendronate sample before and after immersion in the artificial saliva for 100 days. The results are shown in Figure 4. The inhomogeneous-layered structure is evident for the Ti/oxide/alendronate surface (Figure 4a), as a consequence of the presence of electrochemically prepared oxide film on the Ti surface. It is well-known that the alendronate coating has no significant effect on the morphology due to its low thickness (one monolayer) [47].

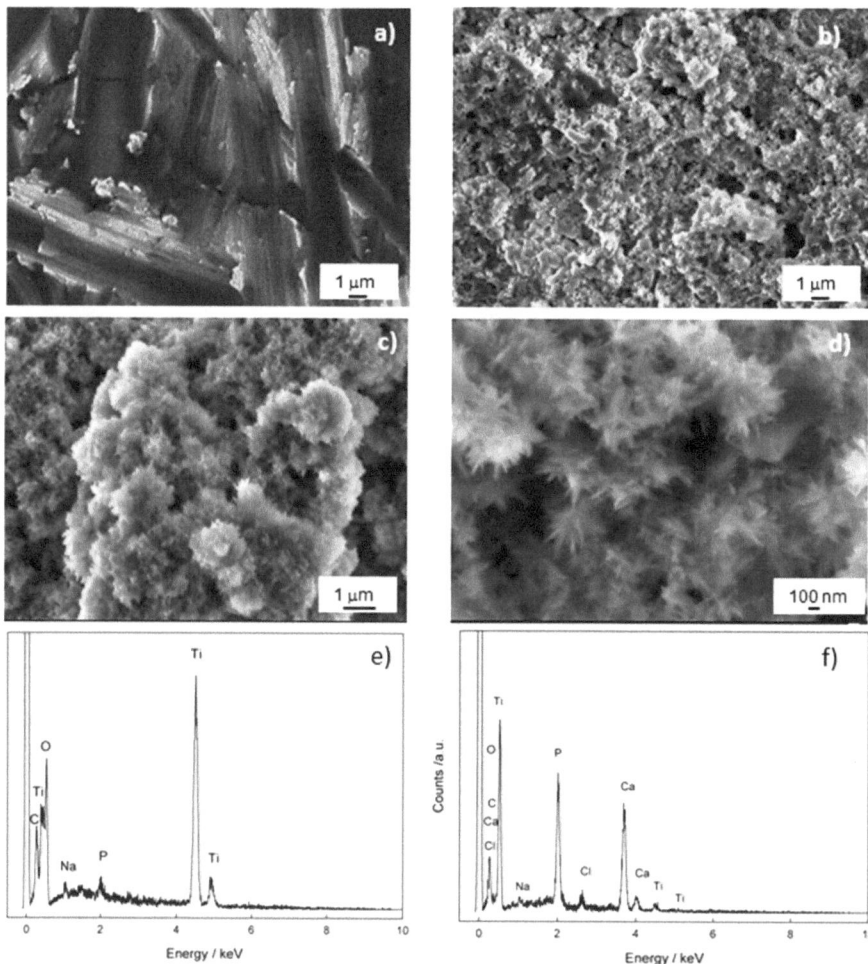

Figure 4. The FE-SEM images of Ti/oxide/alendronate (**a**) before and (**b**–**d**) after immersion in artificial saliva. The images were taken at (**a**,**b**) 5000×, (**c**) 10,000× and (**d**) 33,000× magnification. The chemical composition of the Ti/oxide/alendronate sample (**e**) before and (**f**) after immersion in artificial saliva.

The immersion of the sample in the artificial saliva over a period of 100 days changed the morphology of the Ti/oxide/alendronate surface significantly and resulted in the spontaneous formation of agglomerates over almost the entire surface (Figure 4b,c). A deeper look into the spontaneously formed deposit (Figure 4d) revealed a flower agglomerate consisting of nanoneedles. The morphology obtained is one of the possible forms of CaP structures such as nanosheets, microrods, and microplates, which are influenced by the precipitation conditions (temperature, pH, reactants and their concentrations) [49,50]. Nanoneedles are also observed under similar pH conditions [50–52].

To check the chemical composition of the Ti/oxide/alendronate sample before and after immersion in artificial saliva, the samples were analyzed using EDS. The results are shown in Table 1 and Figure 4e,f, and indicate that the alendronate coating (Na and P were detected) was present over the oxide layer on the titanium before immersion in artificial saliva. As can be seen after 100 days of immersion, the elements Na, Ca, P and Cl were detected on the surface of the sample, whereby the amount of the element P increased significantly and the other elements Ca and Cl were incorporated into the structure of the deposit (Table 1). The Ca/P atomic ratio is 1.51 and may indicate the presence of calcium-deficient hydroxyapatite (CDHAp) [53]. Furthermore, due to the presence of the elements Cl and Na, it can be concluded that the apatite formed is biocompatible, closely resembling the natural bone composition, which could have a positive effect on bone metabolism [54].

Table 1. Chemical composition of the Ti/oxide/alendronate sample before and after the immersion in artificial saliva (the average of three measurements).

Sample	Ti K	C K	O K	Na K	P K	Ca K	Cl K
			Element, at. %				
Before immersion	40.76	12.18	45.16	0.99	0.91	/	/
After immersion	1.41	16.68	54.22	0.49	10.41	15.74	1.05

It should be emphasized that atmospheric carbon contamination is possible, which could influence the EDS results. The prompt gamma-ray activation analysis (PGAA) can be useful for the accurate determination of elemental composition, as shown by A. Nespoli et al. [55].

The surface characterization (composition) of Ti/oxide/alendronate samples before and after immersion was performed using ATR-FTIR (Figure 5). Prior to sample immersion, weak bands around 1000 cm^{-1} are visible characteristics for the P–O and P=O bands present in the alendronate molecule [16,56,57]. On the other hand, after immersion bands were detected in the spectral range from 900 to 1100 cm^{-1}, typical for the symmetric and asymmetric P–O stretching modes in the phosphate group [58–60]. The noticeable strong bands are indicative of phosphate layer deposits; i.e., dominant ν_3 PO$_4^{3-}$ absorption bands in the range 1080–1000 cm^{-1} (P–O asymmetric stretching vibrations), the ν_1 PO$_4^{3-}$ band at 961 cm^{-1} (P–O symmetric stretching vibrations) and the bending mode bands (O–P–O vibrations) in range from 560 to 630 cm^{-1} [58–60]. The visible band at 1645 cm^{-1} is assigned to the ν_2 bending mode of adsorbed water associated with the hydroxyapatite phase [58], accompanied with bands at 3456 and 3344 cm^{-1} typical for the hydroxyl stretching present in hydroxyapatite [59].

Additionally, the bands at 1464, 862 and 774 cm^{-1} are attributed to the ν_1 CO$_3^{2-}$ band (asymmetric stretching mode of carbonate group), the ν_2 CO$_3^{2-}$ band (symmetric stretching mode of carbonate group) and the ν_4 CO$_3^{2-}$ band (asymmetric stretching mode of carbonate group) and point to the carbonate content present in the calcium phosphate deposit [58,59], which is due to the atmospheric conditions during spontaneous deposition. Carbonate ions replace hydroxyl or phosphate ions in the hydroxyapatite coating, resulting in the formation of calcium-deficient hydroxyapatite with a decreased Ca/P ratio in comparison to the Ca/P ratio of hydroxyapatite [21]. This was the case for the deposit investigated, with the Ca/P ratio of 1.51. Hence, the results obtained are in accordance with the SEM/EDS results discussed previously in this section. The detected carbonate content should not be considered detrimental or unwanted since it allows for a closer resemblance to the natural bone composition [22,61].

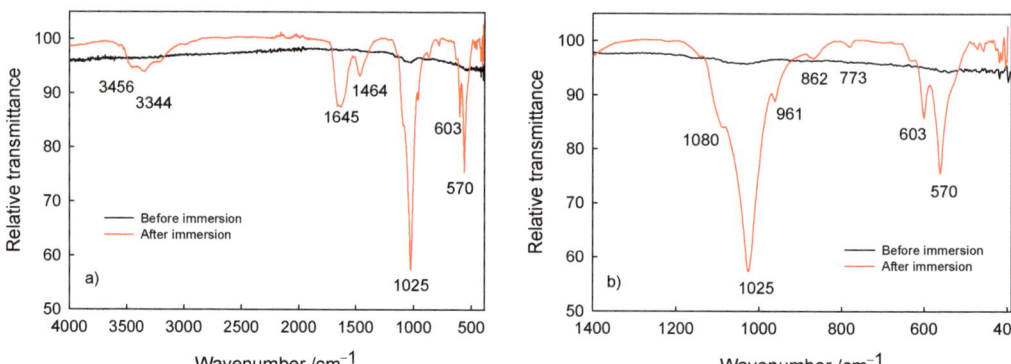

Figure 5. The ATR-FTIR of Ti/oxide/alendronate before and after immersion in artificial saliva: (a) wide range spectra and (b) P–O bands in the fingerprint region of the spectra.

The obtained ATR-FTIR spectra confirm the spontaneous formation of a calcium phosphate deposit on the Ti/oxide/alendronate sample during immersion in the artificial saliva solution, corroborating the enhanced bioactivity of the titanium implant material upon alendronate coating formation.

The phase analysis of the samples before and after immersion in artificial saliva solution was performed using XRD and the results are shown in Figure 6. Figure 6a shows the XRD data for the Ti/oxide/alendronate before immersion in artificial saliva solution. The comparison of the experimental data with the reference card for titanium (JCPDS #00-044-1294) [62] clearly shows the dominance of the titanium substrate as a single phase. Since the electrochemically formed oxide layer is obviously very thin, the oxide phase was not detected in the XRD pattern.

The XRD pattern of the Ti/oxide/alendronate sample after immersion in artificial saliva solution contains characteristic peaks for hydroxyapatite (HAp, JCPDS # 00-009-0432) [53] and beta-tricalcium phosphate (β-TCP, JCPDS # 00-009-0169) [21,63], (Figure 6b,c). The peaks of the titanium substrate are also visible. The results are in accordance with the ATR-FTIR results. The experimental conditions (artificial saliva with a pH of 6.5, room temperature and 100 days immersion) lead to the formation of a mixture of β-TCP and HAp in the form of floral deposits of nanoneedles. The result is consistent with the EDS results, where the Ca/P ratio also indicates the formation of HAp, i.e., calcium-deficient HAp. The formed mixture of HAp and β-TCP can be very useful from an application point of view, as this combination is an important material for tissue engineering and a process of bone formation [64].

In summary, the formation of calcium-deficient hydroxyapatite was spontaneously induced on the titanium covered with electrochemically prepared oxide film and was subsequently modified by the alendronate coating, as was validated using XRD, EDS and ATR-FTIR characterization methods. Spontaneous formation points to the bioactivity of the alendronate coating, resulting in the development of a calcium phosphate phase with beneficial properties. Since, the presence of hydroxyapatite plays a crucial role in various phases of new bone growth, including cell adhesion, the bone formation phase, also serving as a scaffold for new bone deposition, the mineralization phase and bone remodeling, its presence facilitates and is the essential for the successful implant integration [21–24].

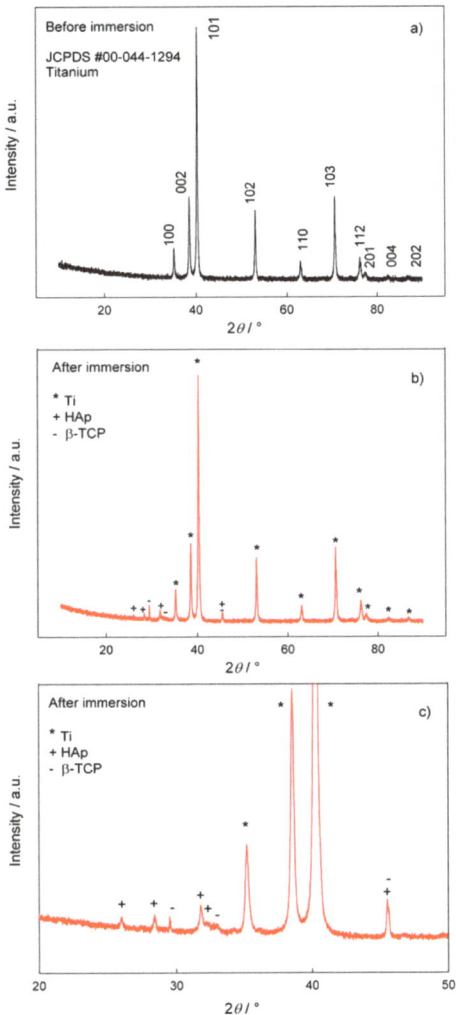

Figure 6. The XRD patterns of the Ti/oxide/alendronate sample (**a**) before and (**b**,**c**) after immersion in artificial saliva. (**c**) Pattern from figure (**b**) in the narrower 2θ region, 20–50°.

4. Conclusions

In this study, the spontaneous calcium phosphate deposition onto an alendronate modified TiO_2 surface was investigated both in silico by means of DFT quantum chemical calculations and in vitro by a simple immersion procedure in artificial saliva.

The DFT results showed that the molecular interactions between the alendronate–coated Ti/oxide surface and the calcium and phosphate ions were spontaneous according to the calculated negative Gibbs free interaction energy. It has been shown that the deposition of calcium and phosphate ions on the alendronate-modified titanium surface is determined by the interaction of Ca^{2+} with the phosphonate group (-PO_3H) of the alendronate molecule and is strongly supported by the O···H–N hydrogen bonding between the phosphate (HPO_4^{2-}) and the amino group (-NH_2) of the alendronate molecule. The formation of the most stable $(TiO_2)_{10}$–alendronate–CaP structure proves to be a highly exergonic process with a calculated Gibbs free interaction energy of $\Delta G^*_{INT} = -34.65$ kcal mol^{-1}.

The results of scanning electron microscopy, energy dispersive X-ray spectroscopy and attenuated total reflectance Fourier transform infrared spectroscopy confirmed spontaneous calcium phosphate deposition on the Ti/oxide/alendronate surface after 100 days of exposure of the sample to artificial saliva. The spontaneously formed deposit is a mixture of two phases, beta-tricalcium phosphate and calcium-deficient hydroxyapatite, according to the X-ray diffraction phase analysis. The presence of trace elements (Na, Cl) and carbonate ions in the hydroxyapatite structure, detected using energy dispersive X-ray spectroscopy and attenuated total reflectance Fourier transform infrared spectroscopy, indicates the biological hydroxyapatite, which is also confirmed by the Ca/P ratio of 1.51 (energy dispersive X-ray spectroscopy).

These results indicate the potential bioactivity of functionalized titanium and provide fundamental information useful for the development of dental implants with improved osseointegrity. For further clinical testing, biological studies in a medium similar to the complex oral environment followed by in vivo studies are required.

Supplementary Materials: The following supporting information can be downloaded at: https://www.mdpi.com/article/10.3390/ma17112703/s1, Computational modeling, Figure S1: Optimized structures of the selected systems (bond distances in Å, bond energies in kcal mol^{-1}), Table S1: Formation of CaP layer. Standard state (1M) free energies of interaction $\Delta_r G^*_{INT}$ computed by using the SMD solvation model at the M06/6-311++G(2df,2pd) + LANL2DZ// M06/6-31+G(d,p) + LANL2DZ level of theory (in kcal mol^{-1}), Table S2: Total electronic energy, E^{Tot}_{soln}, obtained at the SMD/M06/6-311++G(2df,2pd) + LANL2DZ//SMD/M06/6-31+G(d,p) + LANL2DZ level of theory, thermal correction to the Gibbs free energy, $\Delta G^*_{VRT,soln}$, obtained at the SMD/M06/6-31+G(d,p) + LANL2DZ level of theory, and total free energy, G^*_X, ($G^*_X = E^{Tot}_{soln} + \Delta G^*_{VRT,soln}$) in water media of the investigated species (all energies in hartree), Table S3: Bond lengths (d), energies (E) and QTAIM properties of the selected bonds in the investigated systems, Cartesian coordinates of the calculated systems. Refs. [65–75] are cited in the Supplementary Materials.

Author Contributions: Conceptualization, I.D.; methodology, I.D., Ž.P. and J.K.; software, I.D.; validation, I.D., Ž.P. and J.K.; formal analysis, I.D., J.K. and Ž.P.; investigation, I.D., Ž.P. and D.M.; resources, I.D. and Ž.P.; data curation, I.D. and Ž.P.; writing—original draft preparation, I.D., J.K. and Ž.P.; writing—review and editing, I.D., Ž.P. and J.K.; visualization, I.D., Ž.P. and J.K.; supervision, I.D., Ž.P. and J.K.; project administration, I.D.; funding acquisition, I.D. and Ž.P. All authors have read and agreed to the published version of the manuscript.

Funding: This research was partially funded by the Croatian Academy of Sciences and Arts Foundation for 2023: "Mechanism of hydroxyapatite layer formation on the surface of a titanium implant modified with an organic nano-coating".

Institutional Review Board Statement: Not applicable.

Informed Consent Statement: Not applicable.

Data Availability Statement: The original contributions presented in the study are included in the article/Supplementary Materials, further inquiries can be directed to the corresponding authors.

Acknowledgments: The authors would like to thank the Zagreb University Computing Centre (SRCE) for generously granting computational resources on the ISABELLA cluster (isabella.srce.hr). The authors would like to thank Đurđica Brlek for her technical support with the XRD measurements.

Conflicts of Interest: The authors declare no conflicts of interest.

References

1. Brunete, D.M.; Tangvall, P.; Textor, M.; Thomsen, P. *Titanium in Medicine*, 1st ed.; Springer: Berlin, Germany, 2001.
2. Salernitano, E.; Migliaresi, C. Composite Materials for Biomedical Applications: A Review. *J. Appl. Biomater. Biomech.* **2003**, *1*, 3–18. [CrossRef] [PubMed]
3. Breme, J.; Biehl, V.; Hoffman, A. Tailor-Made Composites Based on Titanium for Medical Devices. *Adv. Eng. Mater.* **2000**, *2*, 270–275. [CrossRef]
4. Ngadiman, N.H.A.; Saman, M.Z.M. A Comprehensive Review of Biomaterials and Its Characteristics for Bone Tissue Engineering Scaffold. *J. Med. Device Technol.* **2023**, *2*, 56–62. [CrossRef]

5. Qu, H.; Fu, H.; Han, Z.; Sun, Y. Biomaterials for bone tissue engineering scaffolds: A review. *RSC Adv.* **2019**, *45*, 26252–26262. [CrossRef] [PubMed]
6. Wu, H.; Chen, X.; Kong, L.; Liu, P. Mechanical and Biological Properties of Titanium and Its Alloys for Oral Implant with Preparation Techniques: A Review. *Materials* **2023**, *16*, 6860. [CrossRef] [PubMed]
7. Hanawa, T. Biocompatibility of titanium from the viewpoint of its surface. *Sci. Technol. Adv. Mater.* **2022**, *23*, 457–472. [CrossRef] [PubMed]
8. Chen, Q.; Thouas, G.A. Metallic implant biomaterials. *Mater. Sci. Eng. R* **2015**, *87*, 1–57. [CrossRef]
9. Kaur, M.; Singh, K. Review on titanium and titanium-based alloys as biomaterials for orthopaedic applications. *Mater. Sci. Eng. C* **2019**, *102*, 844–862. [CrossRef] [PubMed]
10. Xue, T.; Attarilar, S.; Liu, S.; Liu, J.; Song, X.; Li, L.; Zhao, B.; Tang, Y. Surface Modification Techniques of Titanium and its Alloys to Functionally Optimize Their Biomedical Properties: Thematic Review. *Front. Bioeng. Biotechnol.* **2020**, *8*, 603072. [CrossRef]
11. Petrović, Ž.; Katić, J.; Šarić, A.; Despotović, I.; Matijaković, N.; Kralj, D.; Leskovac, M.; Petković, M. Influence of Biocompatible Coating on Titanium Surface Characteristics. *ICMS* **2020**, *10*, 37–46. [CrossRef]
12. Vyas, V.; Kaur, T.; Kar, S.; Thirugnanam, A. Biofunctionalization of commercially pure titanium with chitosan/hydroxyapatite biocomposite via silanization: Evaluation of biological performances. *J. Adhes. Sci. Technol.* **2017**, *31*, 1768–1781. [CrossRef]
13. Sharma, A.; Kokil, G.R.; He, Y.; Lowe, B.; Salam, A.; Altalhi, T.A.; Ye, Q.; Kumeria, T. Inorganic/organic combination: Inorganic particles/polymer composites for tissue engineering applications. *Bioact. Mater.* **2023**, *24*, 535–550. [CrossRef]
14. Nayak, G.S.; Carradò, A.; Masson, P.; Pourroy, G.; Mouillard, F.; Migonney, V.; Falentin-Daudre, C.; Pereira, C.; Palkowski, H. Trends in Metal-Based Composite Biomaterials for Hard Tissue Applications. *JOM* **2022**, *74*, 102–125. [CrossRef]
15. Petrović, Ž.; Šarić, A.; Despotović, I.; Katić, J.; Peter, R.; Petravić, M.; Petković, M. A New Insight into Coating's Mechanism Between TiO_2 and Alendronate on Titanium Dental Implant. *Materials* **2020**, *13*, 3220. [CrossRef]
16. Petrović, Ž.; Šarić, A.; Despotović, I.; Katić, J.; Peter, R.; Petravić, M.; Ivanda, M.; Petković, M. Surface Functionalisation of Dental Implants with a Composite coating of Alendronate and Hydrolysed Collagen: DFT and EIS Studies. *Materials* **2022**, *15*, 5127. [CrossRef]
17. Rojo, L.; Gharibi, B.; McLister, R.; Meenan, B.; Deb, S. Self-assembled monolayers of alendronate on Ti_6Al_4V alloy surfaces enhance osteogenesis in mesenchymal stem cells. *Sci. Rep.* **2016**, *6*, 30548. [CrossRef] [PubMed]
18. Meraw, S.J.; Reeve, C.M.; Wollan, P.C. Use of alendronate in peri-implant defect regeneration. *J. Periodontol.* **1999**, *70*, 151–158. [CrossRef] [PubMed]
19. Meraw, S.J.; Reeve, C.M. Qualitative analysis of peripheral peri-implant bone and influence of alendronate sodium on early bone regeneration. *J. Periodontol.* **1999**, *70*, 1228–1233. [CrossRef]
20. Abtahi, J.; Tengvall, P.; Aspenberg, P. A bisphosphonate-coating improves the fixation of metal implants in human bone. A randomized trial of dental implants. *Bone* **2012**, *50*, 1148–1151. [CrossRef]
21. Eliaz, N.; Metoki, N. Calcium Phosphate Bioceramics: A Review of Their History, Structure, Properties, Coating Technologies and Biomedical Applications. *Materials* **2017**, *10*, 334. [CrossRef]
22. Jeong, J.; Kim, J.H.; Shim, J.H.; Hwanf, N.S.; Heo, C.Y. Bioactive calcium phosphate materials and applications in bone regeneration. *Biomater. Res.* **2019**, *23*, 4. [CrossRef] [PubMed]
23. Xiao, D.; Zhang, J.; Zhang, C.; Barbieri, D.; Yuan, H.; Moroni, L.; Feng, G. The role of calcium phosphate surface structure in osteogenesis and the mechanisms involved. *Acta Biomater.* **2020**, *106*, 22–33. [CrossRef] [PubMed]
24. Hou, X.; Zhang, L.; Zhou, Z.; Luo, X.; Wang, T.; Zhao, X.; Lu, B.; Chen, F.; Zheng, L. Calcium Phosphate-Based Biomaterials for Bone Repair. *J. Funct. Biomater.* **2022**, *13*, 187. [CrossRef] [PubMed]
25. Liu, Q.; Ding, J.; Mante, F.K.; Wunder, S.L.; Baran, G.R. The role of surface functional groups in calcium phosphate nucleation on titanium foil: A self-assembled monolayer technique. *Biomaterials* **2002**, *23*, 3103–3111. [CrossRef] [PubMed]
26. Li, H.; Huang, W.; Zhang, Y.; Zhong, M. Biomimetic synthesis of enamel-like hydroxyapatite on self-assembled monolayers. *Mater. Sci. Eng. C* **2007**, *27*, 756–761. [CrossRef]
27. Majewski, P.J.; Allidi, G. Synthesis of hydroxyapatite on titanium coated with organic self-assembled monolayers. *Mater. Sci. Eng. A* **2006**, *420*, 13–20. [CrossRef]
28. Tanahashi, M.; Matsuda, T. Surface functional group dependence on apatite formation on self-assembled monolayers in a simulated body fluid. *J. Biomed. Mater. Res.* **1997**, *34*, 305–315. [CrossRef]
29. Zeller, A.; Musyanovych, A.; Kappl, M.; Ethirajan, A.; Dass, M.; Markova, D.; Klapper, M.; Landfester, K. Nanostructured Coatings by Adhesion of Phosphonated Polystyrene Particles onto Titanium Surface for Implant Material Applications. *ACS Appl. Mater. Interfaces* **2010**, *2*, 2421–2428. [CrossRef] [PubMed]
30. Liu, L.; Zheng, Y.; Zhang, Q.; Yu, L.; Hu, Z.; Liu, Y. Surface phosphonation treatment shows dose-dependent enhancement of the bioactivity of polyetheretherketone. *RSC Adv.* **2019**, *9*, 30076–30086. [CrossRef]
31. Chang, R.; Liu, Y.-J.; Zhang, Y.-L.; Zhang, S.-Y.; Han, B.-B.; Chen, F.; Chen, Y.-X. Phosphorylated and Phosphonated Low-Complexity Protein Segments for Biomimetic Mineralization and Repair of Tooth Enamel. *Adv. Sci.* **2022**, *9*, 2103829. [CrossRef]
32. Liu, C.; Liu, C.; Gao, Y.; Cheng, F.; Xiao, G.G.; Wang, J.; Jian, X. Apatite Formation on Poly(aryl ether sulfone ketone) Surfaces by Means of Polydopamine Layers Functionalized with Phosphonate Groups. *Adv. Mater. Interfaces* **2018**, *5*, 1800003. [CrossRef]

33. Tan, G.; Ouyang, K.; Wang, H.; Zhou, L.; Wang, X.; Liu, Y.; Zhang, L.; Ning, C. Effect of Amino-, Methyl- and Epoxy-Silane Coupling as a Molecular Bridge for Formatting a Biomimetic Hydroxyapatite Coating on Titanium by Electrochemical Deposition. *J. Mater. Sci. Technol.* **2016**, *32*, 956–965. [CrossRef]
34. Yakufu, M.; Wang, Z.; Wang, Y.; Jiao, Z.; Guo, M.; Liu, J.; Zhang, P. Covalently functionalized poly(etheretherketone) implants with osteogenic growth peptide (OGP) to improve osteogenesis activity. *RSC Adv.* **2020**, *10*, 9777–9785. [CrossRef] [PubMed]
35. Sánchez-Bodón, J.; Andrade Del Olmo, J.; Alonso, J.M.; Moreno-Benítez, I.; Vilas-Vilela, J.L.; Pérez-Álvarez, L. Bioactive Coatings on Titanium: A Review on Hydroxylation, Self-Assembled Monolayers (SAMs) and Surface Modification Strategies. *Polymers* **2021**, *31*, 165. [CrossRef] [PubMed]
36. Zhao, Y.; Thrular, D.G. The M06 suite of density functionals for main group thermochemistry, thermochemical kinetics, noncovalent interactions, excited states, and transition elements: Two new functionals and systematic testing of four M06-class functionals and 12 other functionals. *Theor. Chem. Acc.* **2008**, *120*, 215–241. [CrossRef]
37. Zhao, Y.; Truhlar, D.G. Density Functionals with Broad Applicability in Chemistry. *Acc. Chem. Res.* **2008**, *41*, 157–167. [CrossRef] [PubMed]
38. Zhao, Y.; Truhlar, D.G. Density Functional Theory for Reaction Energies: Test of Meta and Hybrid Meta Functionals, Range-Separated Functionals, and Other High-Performance Functionals. *J. Chem. Theory Comput.* **2011**, *7*, 669–676. [CrossRef]
39. Wadt, W.R.; Hay, P.J. Ab initio effective core potentials for molecular calculations. Potentials for main group elements Na to Bi. *J. Chem. Phys.* **1985**, *82*, 284–298. [CrossRef]
40. Marenich, A.V.; Cramer, C.J.; Truhlar, D.G. Universal Solvation Model Based on Solute Electron Density and on a Continuum Model of the Solvent Defined by the Bulk Dielectric Constant and Atomic Surface Tensions. *J. Phys. Chem. B* **2009**, *113*, 6378–6396. [CrossRef]
41. Srinivasa Rao, J.; Dinadayalane, T.C.; Leszczynski, J.; Sastry, N. Comprehensive Study on the Solvation of Mono- and Divalent Metal Cations: Li^+, Na^+, K^+, Be^{2+}, Mg^{2+} and Ca^{2+}. *J. Phys. Chem. A* **2008**, *112*, 12944–12953. [CrossRef]
42. Pliego, J.R.; Riveros, J.M. The Cluster-Continuum Model for the Calculation of the Solvation Free Energy of Ionic Species. *J. Phys. Chem. A* **2001**, *105*, 7241–7247. [CrossRef]
43. Frisch, M.J.; Trucks, G.W.; Schlegel, H.B.; Scuseria, G.E.; Robb, M.A.; Cheeseman, J.R.; Scalmani, G.; Barone, V.; Mennucci, B.; Petersson, G.A.; et al. *Gaussian 09, Revision D.01*; Gaussian, Inc.: Wallingford, CT, USA, 2013.
44. Bader, R.F.W. *Atoms in Molecules: A Quantum Theory*; Oxford University Press: Oxford, NY, USA, 1994.
45. Keith, T.A. *AIMAll, Version 17.01.25*; TK Gristmill Software; Overland Park: Johnson County, KS, USA, 2017. Available online: https://aim.tkgristmill.com/ (accessed on 18 January 2024).
46. Mellado-Valero, A.; Muñoz, A.I.; Pina, V.G.; Sola-Ruiz, M.F. Electrochemical Behaviour and Galvanic Effects of Titanium Implants Coupled to Metallic Suprastructures in Artificial Saliva. *Materials* **2018**, *11*, 171. [CrossRef] [PubMed]
47. Katić, J.; Šarić, A.; Despotović, I.; Matijaković, N.; Petković, M.; Petrović, Ž. Bioactive Coating on Titanium Dental Implants for Improved Anticorrosion Protection: A Combined Experimental and Theoretical Study. *Coatings* **2019**, *9*, 612. [CrossRef]
48. Qu, Z.; Kroes, G.-J. Theoretical Study of Stable, Defect-Free $(TiO_2)n$ Nanoparticles with n = 10−16. *J. Phys. Chem. C* **2007**, *111*, 16808–16817. [CrossRef]
49. Katić, J.; Krivačić, S.; Petrović, Ž.; Mikić, D.; Marciuš, M. Titanium Implant Alloy Modified by Electrochemically Deposited Functional Bioactive Calcium Phosphate Coatings. *Coatings* **2023**, *13*, 640. [CrossRef]
50. Dorozhkin, S.V. Calcium orthophosphate deposits: Preparation, properties and biomedical applications. *Mater. Sci. Eng. C* **2015**, *55*, 272–326. [CrossRef] [PubMed]
51. Lu, X.; Wang, Y.; Wang, J.; Qu, S.; Weng, J.; Xin, R.; Leng, Y. Calcium phosphate crystal growth under controlled environment through urea hydrolysis. *J. Cryst. Growth* **2006**, *297*, 396–402. [CrossRef]
52. Kobayashi, T.; Ono, S.; Hirakura, S.; Oaki, Y.; Imai, H. Morphological variation of hydroxyapatite grown in aqueous solution based on simulated body fluid. *CrystEngComm* **2012**, *14*, 1143–1149. [CrossRef]
53. Beaufils, S.; Rouillon, T.; Millet, P.; Le Bideau, J.; Weiss, P.; Chopart, J.P.; Daltin, A.L. Synthesis of calcium-deficient hydroxyapatite nanowires and nanotubes performed by template-assisted electrodeposition. *Mater. Sci. Eng. C* **2019**, *98*, 333–346. [CrossRef]
54. Lin, K.; Zhou, Y.; Zhou, Y.; Qu, H.; Chen, F.; Zhu, Y.; Chang, J. Biomimetic hydroxyapatite porous microspheres with co-substituted essential trace elements: Surfactant-free hydrothermal synthesis, enhanced degradation and drug release. *J. Mater Chem* **2011**, *21*, 16558–16565. [CrossRef]
55. Nespoli, A.; Passaretti, F.; Szentmiklósi, L.; Maróti, B.; Placidi, E.; Cassetta, M.; Yada, R.Y.; Farrar, D.H.; Tian, K.V. Biomedical NiTi and β-Ti Alloys: From Composition, Microstructure and Thermo-Mechanics to Application. *Metals* **2022**, *12*, 406. [CrossRef]
56. Ochiuz, L.; Grigoras, C.; Popa, M.; Stoleriu, I.; Munteanu, C.; Timofte, D.; Profire, L.; Grigoras, A.G. Alendronate-Loaded Modified Drug Delivery Lipid Particles Intended for Improved Oral and Topical Administration. *Molecules* **2016**, *21*, 858. [CrossRef] [PubMed]
57. Albano, C.S.; Gomes, A.M.; da Silva Feltran, G.; da Costa Fernandes, C., Jr.; Trino, L.D.; Zambuzzi, W.F.; Lisboa-Filho, P.N. Biofunctionalization of titanium surfaces with alendronate and albumin modulates osteoblast performance. *Heliyon* **2020**, *6*, e04455. [CrossRef] [PubMed]
58. Koutsopoulos, S. Synthesis and characterization of hydroxyapatite crystals: A review study on the analytical methods. *J. Biomed. Mater. Res.* **2002**, *62*, 600–612. [CrossRef] [PubMed]

59. Berzina-Cimdina, L.; Borodajenko, N. Research of Calcium Phosphates Using Fourier Transform Infrared Spectroscopy. In *Infrared Spectroscopy—Materials Science, Engineering and Technology*; Theophanides, T., Ed.; IntechOpen: Rijeka, Croatia, 2012; pp. 123–148.
60. Chukanov, N.V.; Chervonnyi, A.D. IR Spectra of Minerals and Related Compounds, and Reference Samples' Data. In *Infrared Spectroscopy of Minerals and Related Compounds*; Chukanov, N.V., Chervonnyi, A.D., Eds.; Springer: Cham, Switzerland, 2015; pp. 51–1047.
61. LeGeros, R.Z. Calcium Phosphate-Based Osteoinductive Materials. *Chem. Rev.* **2008**, *108*, 4742–4753. [CrossRef] [PubMed]
62. Han, M.-K.; Im, J.-B.; Hwang, M.-J.; Kim, B.-J.; Kim, H.-Y.; Park, Y.-J. Effect of Indium Content on the Microstructure, Mechanical Properties and Corrosion Behavior of Titanium Alloys. *Metals* **2015**, *5*, 850–862. [CrossRef]
63. Lee, S.W.; Kim, Y.; Rho, H.T.; Kim, S. Microhardness and microstructural properties of a mixture of hydroxyapatite and b-tricalcium phosphate. *J. Asian Ceram. Soc.* **2023**, *11*, 11–17. [CrossRef]
64. Vallet-Regı́, M.; Gonza'lez-Calbet, J.M. Calcium phosphates as substitution of bone tissues. *Prog. Solid State Chem.* **2004**, *32*, 1–31. [CrossRef]
65. Allard, M.M.; Merlos, S.N.; Springer, B.N.; Cooper, J.; Zhang, G.; Boskovic, D.S.; Kwon, S.R.; Nick, K.E.; Perry, C.C. Role of TiO_2 Anatase Surface Morphology on Organophosphorus Interfacial Chemistry. *J. Phys. Chem. C* **2018**, *122*, 29237–29248. [CrossRef]
66. Bader, R.F.W. A Bond Path: A Universal Indicator of Bonded Interactions. *J. Phys. Chem. A* **1998**, *102*, 7314–7323. [CrossRef]
67. Bader, R.F.W.; Essén, H. The characterization of atomic interactions. *J. Chem. Phys.* **1984**, *80*, 1943–1960. [CrossRef]
68. Cremer, D.; Kraka, E. A Description of the Chemical Bond in Terms of Local Properties of Electron Density and Energy. *Croat. Chem. Acta* **1984**, *57*, 1259–1281.
69. Espinosa, E.; Molins, E.; Lecomte, C. Hydrogen bond strengths revealed by topological analyses of experimentally observed electron densities. *Chem. Phys. Lett.* **1998**, *285*, 170–173. [CrossRef]
70. Espinosa, E.; Alkorta, I.; Rozas, I.; Elguero, J.; Molins, E. About the evaluation of the local kinetic, potential and total energy densities in closed-shell interactions. *Chem. Phys. Lett.* **2001**, *336*, 457–461. [CrossRef]
71. Borissova, A.O.; Antipin, M.Y.; Karapetyan, H.A.; Petrosyan, A.M.; Lyssenko, K.A. Cooperativity effects of H-bonding and charge transfer in an L-nitroarginine crystal with Z' > 1. *Mendeleev Commun.* **2010**, *20*, 260–262. [CrossRef]
72. Baryshnikov, G.V.; Minaev, B.F.; Minaeva, V.A.; Nenajdenko, V.G. Single crystal architecture and absorption spectra of octathio[8]circulene and *sym*-tetraselenatetrathio[8]circulene: QTAIM and TD-DFT approach. *J. Mol. Model.* **2013**, *19*, 4511–4519. [CrossRef] [PubMed]
73. Baryshnikov, G.V.; Minaev, B.F.; Korop, A.A.; Minaeva, V.A.; Gusev, A.N. Structure of zinc complexes with 3-(pyridin-2-yl)-5-(arylideneiminophenyl)-1HH-1,2,4-triazoles in different tautomeric forms: DFT and QTAIM study. *Russ. J. Inorg. Chem.* **2013**, *58*, 928–934. [CrossRef]
74. Shahangi, F.; Chermahini, A.N.; Farrokhpour, H.; Teimouri, A. Selective complexation of alkaline earth metal ions with nanotubular cyclopeptides: DFT theoretical study. *RSC Adv.* **2014**, *5*, 2305–2317. [CrossRef]
75. Puntus, L.N.; Lyssenko, K.A.; Antipin, M.Y.; Bünzli, J.C.G. Role of Inner- and Outer-Sphere Bonding in the Sensitization of EuIII-Luminescence Deciphered by Combined Analysis of Experimental Electron Density Distribution Function and Photophysical Data. *Inorg. Chem.* **2008**, *47*, 11095–11107. [CrossRef]

Disclaimer/Publisher's Note: The statements, opinions and data contained in all publications are solely those of the individual author(s) and contributor(s) and not of MDPI and/or the editor(s). MDPI and/or the editor(s) disclaim responsibility for any injury to people or property resulting from any ideas, methods, instructions or products referred to in the content.

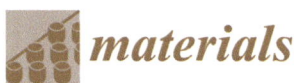 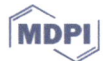

Article

Novel Strategy for Surface Modification of Titanium Implants towards the Improvement of Osseointegration Property and Antibiotic Local Delivery

Isabela da Rocha Silva [1], Aline Tavares da Silva Barreto [2], Renata Santos Seixas [1], Paula Nunes Guimarães Paes [3], Juliana do Nascimento Lunz [4], Rossana Mara da Silva Moreira Thiré [1,*] and Paula Mendes Jardim [1,*]

1. COPPE/Program of Metallurgical and Materials Engineering (PEMM), Universidade Federal do Rio de Janeiro (UFRJ), Rio de Janeiro 21941-598, RJ, Brazil
2. Graduation Program in Nanobiosystems, Universidade Federal do Rio de Janeiro (UFRJ), Duque de Caxias 25240-005, RJ, Brazil
3. Faculdade de Odontologia, Universidade do Estado do Rio de Janeiro (UERJ), Rio de Janeiro 20551-030, RJ, Brazil
4. Divisão de Metrologia de Materiais, Instituto Nacional de Metrologia, Qualidade e Tecnologia (Inmetro), Xerem 25250-020, RJ, Brazil
* Correspondence: rossana@metalmat.ufrj.br (R.M.S.M.T.); pjardim@metalmat.ufrj.br (P.M.J.); Tel.: +55-21-3938-8500 (R.M.S.M.T.)

Abstract: The topography and chemical composition modification of titanium (Ti) implants play a decisive role in improving biocompatibility and bioactivity, accelerating osseointegration, and, thus, determining clinical success. In spite of the development of surface modification strategies, bacterial contamination is a common cause of failure. The use of systemic antibiotic therapy does not guarantee action at the contaminated site. In this work, we proposed a surface treatment for Ti implants that aim to improve their osseointegration and reduce bacterial colonization in surgery sites due to the local release of antibiotic. The Ti discs were hydrothermally treated with 3M NaOH solution to form a nanostructured layer of titanate on the Ti surface. Metronidazole was impregnated on these nanostructured surfaces to enable its local release. The samples were coated with poly(vinyl alcohol)—PVA films with different thickness to evaluate a possible control of drug release. Gamma irradiation was used to crosslink the polymer chains to achieve hydrogel layer formation and to sterilize the samples. The samples were characterized by XRD, SEM, FTIR, contact angle measurements, "in vitro" bioactivity, and drug release analysis. The alkaline hydrothermal treatment successfully produced intertwined, web-like nanostructures on the Ti surface, providing wettability and bioactivity to the Ti samples (Ti + TTNT samples). Metronidazole was successfully loaded and released from the Ti + TTNT samples coated or not with PVA. Although the polymeric film acted as a physical barrier to drug delivery, all groups reached the minimum inhibitory concentration for anaerobic bacteria. Thus, the surface modification method presented is a potential approach to improve the osseointegration of Ti implants and to associate local drug delivery with dental implants, preventing early infections and bone failure.

Keywords: titanium; hydrothermal treatment; surface modification; local drug delivery system; osseointegration

Citation: Silva, I.R.; Barreto, A.T.S.; Seixas, R.S.; Paes, P.N.G.; Lunz, J.N.; Thiré, R.M.S.M.; Jardim, P.M. Novel Strategy for Surface Modification of Titanium Implants towards the Improvement of Osseointegration Property and Antibiotic Local Delivery. *Materials* 2023, 16, 2755. https://doi.org/10.3390/ma16072755

Academic Editor: Ines Despotović

Received: 13 February 2023
Revised: 20 March 2023
Accepted: 22 March 2023
Published: 29 March 2023

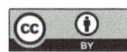

Copyright: © 2023 by the authors. Licensee MDPI, Basel, Switzerland. This article is an open access article distributed under the terms and conditions of the Creative Commons Attribution (CC BY) license (https://creativecommons.org/licenses/by/4.0/).

1. Introduction

Titanium implants are a safe and predictable alternative for rehabilitation treatments in dental surgeries, and their success is related to osseointegration. Titanium is considered the material of choice for the manufacture of implants due to its mechanical properties, chemical stability, and biocompatibility [1,2]. Surface treatments such as alkaline hydrothermal treatment have been developed and improved to modify and optimize the physical–chemical properties of the surface, such as roughness, topography, wettability, and its composition, influencing cellular events during the healing process [3,4]. Such treatment enables the growing of a layer of titanate nanostructures on the Ti surface, increasing its roughness, and consequently its surface area, and hydrophilicity, favoring protein adsorption and cell adhesion and proliferation [4]. The morphology of nanostructures is directly dependent on the experimental conditions used for hydrothermal treatment.

Infections associated with the surgical procedures during dental implantation are one of the causes of osseointegration failure, leading to its loss [5]. Such infections can be caused by contamination of bacteria that already exist at the surgical site, especially in patients with pre-existing periodontal disease [6]. The most critical moment regarding early loss induced by infection is when the implant comes into contact with human cells and local microorganisms in the initial moments after its installation [7]. Prophylactic antibiotic therapy has been proposed to decrease bacterial levels at the site to be instrumented. The pre-established biofilm restricts the diffusion of molecules and bacterial sensitivity to antibiotics, meaning that the systemic prophylactic antibiotic therapy will not have the desired effectiveness [8]. Therefore, it is desirable to develop strategies with a local antibiotics release approach as an alternative to systemic oral antimicrobial therapy [9]. The use of biodegradable material in combination with titanium implants as a local drug delivery system is an interesting approach.

Hydrogels have gained considerable attention in recent years for their unique physical–chemical properties, which are similar to those of living tissues and include high water content, soft and rubbery consistency, and low interfacial tension with water or biological fluids [10]. These materials can be defined as a 3D network formed from physical or chemical crosslinked hydrophilic polymers. They can swell in contact with water or biological fluids without losing their structural integrity [11]. Poly(vinyl alcohol)—PVA is a biodegradable, non-toxic, water-soluble, and hydrogel-forming polymer [12]. Due to its particular properties, such as chemical versatility, great biocompatibility to different cell lines, and high swelling capacity, PVA hydrogel has been recognized as potential biomaterial for various pharmaceuticals and biomedical applications, including as a matrix for drug delivery systems and as scaffolds for bone tissue engineering. Furthermore, PVA can only be solubilized in pure water, without needing any acid or alkaline solution, which could be a potential risk for cells [13,14].

Metronidazole is an antibacterial compound belonging to the class of imidazoles, a subgroup of nitroimidazoles, which acts against a wide variety of microorganisms [15]. It is clinically effective in the treatment of periodontitis and peri-implantitis caused by anaerobic bacteria [16]. It presents a good therapeutic response, but its high toxicity after continuous systemic doses can, for example, manifest gastrointestinal disorders, dizziness, and headaches, among others, often causing the patient to discontinue treatment [15]. Thus, the local delivery of metronidazole could reduce the systemic toxicity of the antibiotic and increase its efficiency even with lower doses.

In the present work, we propose a surface treatment methodology to titanium implants aiming to provide antimicrobial properties by the local release of metronidazole and the improvement of the osseointegration capacity obtained by the incorporation of nanostructures on the titanium surface. The proposed system consists of a Grade 4 Ti sample functionalized with a nanostructured titanate layer produced by hydrothermal treatment, impregnated with metronidazole and coated with PVA hydrogel to control antibiotic release. Grade 4 Ti has been the industry standard for dental implants for years due to its high strength and low malleability. The great advantage of surface modification is that the external layers of the materials can be modified without affecting its volumetric characteristics, such as mechanical properties. In other words, it is possible to change biomaterial–cell interaction without changing physical and chemical bulk properties.

2. Materials and Methods

2.1. Preparation of Titanate Nanostructured Coating

Grade 4 Ti circular cross-section bars (Titanews Industria e Comercio de Titanio LTDA, Barueri, Brazil) were used in the alkaline hydrothermal treatment as a surface substrate for the growth of the titanate layer. Before treatment, the Ti bars were cut in a cutting machine (ISOMET 4000 model, Buehler), forming discs 12 mm in diameter and 2 mm in thickness, which were mechanically polished with abrasive silicon carbide sandpaper of different grades (220, 400, 600, and 1500) using a metallographic polisher/sander machine (Aropol 2V—Arotec, Cotia, Brazil), followed by ultrasonic cleaning for 10 min with acetone, ethanol, and distilled water, sequentially. The alkaline hydrothermal treatment was carried out in a high-pressure reactor (BR-500–Berghof, Eningen, Germany) under 3M NaOH solution at 150 °C for 6 h. After the synthesis reaction, the samples were washed by immersion in distilled water four times for 10 min, as will be described below.

2.2. Loading of Metronidazole in Nanostructures

Metronidazole (MNZ) (0.5% (m/v) metronidazole injection solution, Fresenius Kabi Brasil Ltd. (Mount Kuring-gai, NSW, Australia) was added to the coated Ti discs to interact with the nanostructures and to compose the drug delivery system. The MNZ concentration was selected based on the Minimum Inhibitory Concentration to eliminate anaerobic bacteria, on the concentration range that could avoid cytotoxicity, and on the minimum concentration that could be read by a UV-Vis spectrophotometer. Firstly, a 25 µL-drop of MNZ was pipetted on to the discs and allowed to dry at room temperature. After drying, another drop was added. This procedure was repeated eight times until 22.2 µg/mL of MNZ had been deposited. In the case of systems with a thicker layer of PVA coating, it was necessary to deposit a higher volume of MNZ (33.3 µg/mL) in order to maintain the released amount of MNZ within the range of the sensitivity of the method.

2.3. Polymeric Coating of Nanostructured Samples

Poly(vinyl alcohol) (PVA) (Mw 85.000–124.000 g/mol, degree of hydrolysis > 99%, Sigma–Aldrich, Saint Louis, MO, USA) was used to coat the MNZ-loaded samples in order to control the drug release. Two different groups were produced by this procedure for comparative purposes, a group with one layer and a group with six layers of polymeric coating. For the production of one PVA layer, the PVA was dissolved in distilled water at 90 ± 2 °C for 4 h under magnetic stirring to obtain 10% (m/v) PVA aqueous solution. Then, the solution was cooled under stirring to 50 °C, and 0.2 mL of PVA solution was pipetted onto the samples. The spin coating technique was performed at a rotational speed of 400 rpm for 10 s, followed by a rotational speed of 4000 rpm for 60 s, to ensure even coverage. In the case of the group with six layers, this procedure was repeated six times. After the coating procedure, all the samples were left in a ventilated oven for 20 h at 50 °C.

2.4. Crosslinking of Polymeric Coating

In order to crosslink the polymeric films, the PVA-coated samples (TTNT + MNZ + 1PVA, TTNT + MNZ + 6PVA groups) were irradiated with gamma rays of Cobalt-60 at a dose of 25 KGy. By using this procedure, the samples could be sterilized concomitantly with PVA chain crosslinking [17]. The experimental groups were named as shown in Table 1.

Table 1. Experimental groups.

Groups	Description
TTNT	Titanate nanostructures on Ti disc surface via hydrothermal synthesis
TTNT + MNZ	Titanate nanostructures on Ti disc surface via hydrothermal synthesis + Metronidazole
TTNT + MNZ + 1PVA	Titanate nanostructures on Ti disc surface via hydrothermal synthesis + Metronidazole + 1 layer of irradiated PVA film
TTNT + MNZ + 6PVA	Titanate nanostructures on Ti disc surface via hydrothermal synthesis + Metronidazole + 6 layers of irradiated PVA film

2.5. Microstructural Characterization

After hydrothermal treatment, the samples were analyzed by Grazing Incidence X-ray diffraction (GIXRD) and Scanning Electron Microscopy (SEM). The GIXRD (X'pert PRO/PANalytical, Malvern, UK) patterns were collected using CuKα radiation (λ = 1.5418 Å) and the incidence angle of the beam in relation to the samples' surface of 1°. The surface morphology of the samples was examined by SEM using a Versa 3D microscope (Thermo Fisher, Helios/Thermo Fisher, Waltham, MA, USA) operating at an accelerating voltage of 20 kV. The samples were gold-coated prior to the analysis. The chemical bonds of the samples were analyzed by a FTIR spectrometer (Nicolet 6700, Thermo Scientific, Waltham, MA, USA) equipped with an ATR (Attenuated Total Reflection) accessory and using a resolution of 4 cm^{-1} in the region of 4000–650 cm^{-1}, with an average of 32 scans. The signal of the obtained spectra was processed with the Origin Pro version 9.1 software using the Savitzky–Golay algorithm (five smoothing points) and normalized to [0, 1].

2.6. Apatite Deposition—"In Vitro" Bioactivity Assay

The samples were soaked in simulated body fluid (SBF) to assess their bioactivity by examining the formation of calcium phosphate crystals on the surface. SBF was prepared according to Kokubo's formulation, and the bioactivity test was performed in accordance with ISO/FDIS 23317 (Implants for surgery—In vitro evaluation for apatite-forming ability of implant materials). The alkaline hydrothermally treated Ti samples and the untreated Ti (control sample) were soaked in SBF at pH = 7.4 and a constant temperature of 36.5 °C [18] for 14 days. After the soaking period, the samples were gently washed with distilled water and dried in a desiccator at room temperature. The formation of calcium phosphate crystals after the soaking period was investigated by means of SEM (Vega/Tescan operating at an acceleration voltage of 20 kV) and GIXRD (X'pert PRO/PANalytical, Malvern, UK). The samples were gold-coated prior to SEM analysis.

2.7. "In Vitro" Cytotoxicity Assay

To evaluate the influence of the hydrothermal treatment on the samples, a standardized cytocompatibility assay was performed (ISO 10993-5:2009—Biological evaluation of medical devices—Part 5: Tests for in vitro cytotoxicity). The 3-(4,5-dimethylthiazol-2-yl)-2,5-diphenyltetrazolium bromide (MTT) assay was performed with MG-63 cells (human fibroblast from osteosarcoma, Code 0173, Cell Bank of Rio de Janeiro, Brazil).

Ti and Ti + TTNT discs were separately soaked in no supplemented DMEM for 24 h to produce the extracts. Concomitantly, cells were seeded in a 96-well plate at a density of 2×10^4 cells/well and incubated in 200 µL of high-glucose Dulbecco's modified Eagle's medium GlutaMAX (hgDMEM) supplemented with 10% v/v of fetal bovine serum (FBS), penicillin (100 U·mL^{-1})/streptomycin (100 µg·mL^{-1}) (all Gibco Biosciences, Waltham, MA, USA), and 2.5µg·mL^{-1} amphotericin B (Sigma–Aldrich, Saint Louis, MO, USA)—XPAN mediun—at 37 °C, in an atmosphere of 5% CO_2. After overnight incubation (approximately 24 h), the EXPAN medium was replaced by the extracts, and the cells were incubated for a further 24 h. Latex extract was used as the positive control and polystyrene extract as the negative control. At the end of the incubation, the extracts were replaced by 100 µL of fresh EXPAN medium and 15 µL of 5 mg/mL MTT solution and incubated for 3.5 h. The MTT reaction was stopped by removing the MTT/EXPAN and adding 100 µL of dimethyl sulfoxide (DMSO) and stirring for 5 min. The absorbance of formazan solubilized in each well was read with a Synergy 2 microplate reader (BioTek, Winooski, VT, USA) at a wavelength of 550 nm. The measured absorbance of the samples was then normalized to the absorbance of the control cells, which had not received the extract.

2.8. "In Vitro" Drug Release

The release of metronidazole from the samples was investigated for 14 days by immersion in 45 mL of phosphate-buffered saline (PBS, pH 7.4, composition: 8.0 g NaCl,

1.1 g Na$_2$HPO$_4$, 0.2 g KCl, 0.2 g KH$_2$PO$_4$) at 37 °C and a rotational speed of 100 rpm. Measurement of the initial release was performed after 20 min of immersion, followed by 1, 1.8, 24, 48, 96, 168, 216, 264, and 336 h. At each interval, 4 mL of PBS was withdrawn, and the same fresh amount was replaced. In order to disregard the effects of this dilution, the following mathematical correction was made:

$$Correction\ Factor = \left(\frac{45}{45-4}\right)^{n-1}$$

where n is the sequential number of the sample, 45 is the volume in milliliters of the PBS solution, and 4 is the volume in milliliters of the removed aliquot. To perform the correction, the volume of antibiotic release measured in the spectrophotometry was multiplied by this factor [19].

The amount of drug released was measured by Ultraviolet/Visible Spectroscopy (UV/Vis) equipment (mod. SP-220, Biospectro, Curitiba, Brazil). To determine the concentrations of the metronidazole in the collected solution, a standard curve of absorbance at wavelength 320 nm versus known concentrations was used.

The surface of samples before and after the drug release experiment was analyzed by SEM (Vega/Tescan, Brno, Czech Republic) microscope operating at an acceleration voltage of 15 kV in low vacuum mode.

2.9. Statistical Analysis

The MNZ release data were analyzed using a commercially available statistical program (SigmaPlot for Windows version 11.0). Data are reported as mean ± standard deviation. If the difference was determined to be significant after the analysis of variance, pairwise comparisons were performed using a Holm–Sidak post-hoc test, and $p < 0.05$ was considered statistically significant. The experiment was performed in triplicate with all readings for each point of the release.

3. Results and Discussion

3.1. Titanate Nanostructured Coating

The speed and quality of osseointegration are directly linked to the surface roughness and chemical composition created in the titanium. Surface treatments such as alkaline hydrothermal modifies the topography of titanium on a nanoscale [20] to generate a surface that accommodates host cells, promoting an environment conducive to cell growth and enhancing the osseointegration process [21]. Besides that, the presence of Na+ ions on the titanate surface plays an important role in the formation of apatite and therefore its bioactivity [22,23]. The alkaline hydrothermal treatment consists of submerging the sample in an alkaline solution under certain conditions of high temperature, pressure, and time to form a titanate layer with nanoscale architecture [20]. The topography resulting from this process is determined by the combination of these parameters, being attractive due to its simplicity, cost-effectiveness, and potential for large-scale manufacturing [20,24].

Figure 1 shows a comparison of SEM images from the top view of the Ti surface before and after alkaline hydrothermal treatment under the proposed conditions (3M NaOH, 150 °C, 6 h). The hydrothermal synthesis condition chosen was based on a work by this group to be published, in which the bioactivity of different microstructures was evaluated. The Ti surface before hydrothermal treatment shows parallel grooves produced by polishing without any specific nanoscale topography (Figure 1a). On the other hand, the sample surface after treatment (Figure 1b,c) presented a microstructure composed by the intertwining of nanofibers approximately 83 nm in diameter, giving rise to micropores about 500 nm in size. This web-like morphology resembles that of the extracellular matrix of bone tissue, which can stimulate cell adhesion, proliferation, and differentiation.

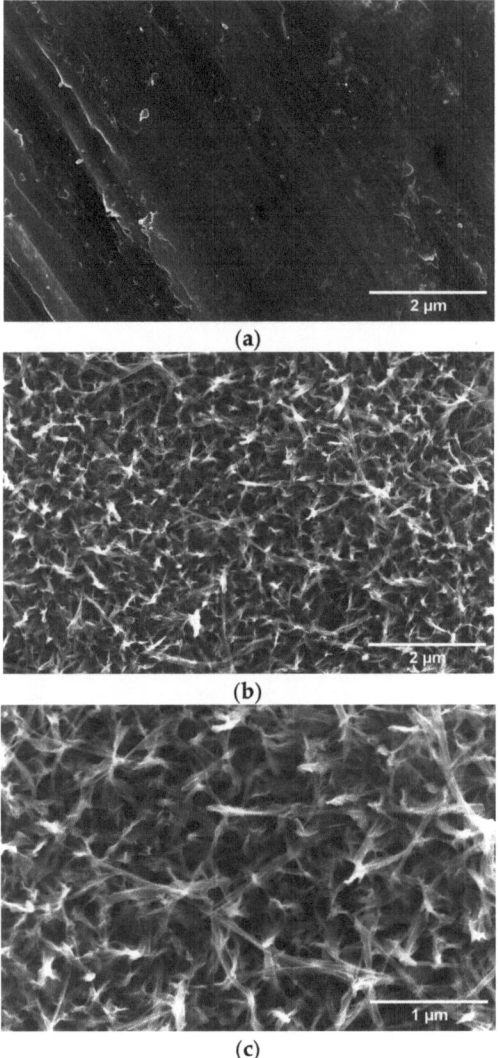

Figure 1. Top-view SEM image of Ti surface before (**a**) and after (**b**) alkaline hydrothermal treatment, and alkaline hydrothermal treatment at higher magnification (**c**).

Bone healing around an implant begins through cellular communication. Bone marrow mesenchymal cells interact with the implant surface, and surface properties, such as morphology, wettability, and mechanical and chemical properties, influence this process. Thus, the implant must function as a bioactive and biocompatible scaffold, with osteogenic characteristics that enable the migration, adhesion, and proliferation of cells of the osteogenic lineage [25]. The presence of a nanoscale framework that allows vascular proliferation and the passage of signaling molecules induces a desired cellular response, since interactions between cells and biomaterials occur at the nanoscale. Titanium surfaces hydrothermally treated with sodium hydroxide produce a nanoporous architecture that promotes appropriate cellular interaction with the surface, promoting the osteoblastic lineage [21].

The formation of a titanate layer was also confirmed by Grazing Incidence X-ray Diffraction (GIXRD). This is a surface sensitive technique that utilizes a small incident angle X-ray beam, which is very useful for analyzing the crystalline microstructure of thin films. Figure 2 shows the GIXRD pattern of the resulting nanostructured film, revealing typical diffraction peaks (attenuated and broadened by the nanoscale and anisotropic morphology) of layered sodium trititanate, $Na_2Ti_3O_7$ (at 2θ = 9.6°, 24.5°, 28.7°, and 48.4°). The strong broad peak at 2θ = 9.6° can be attributed to the interlayer distance [26]. The peaks at 2θ = 35.2°, 38.6°, 40.3°, 53.2°, 63.1°, and 70.8° correspond to the Ti substrate.

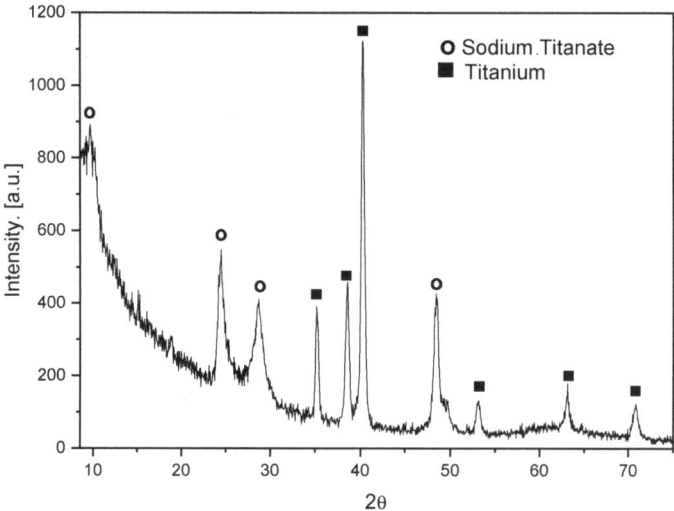

Figure 2. GIXRD diffractogram of Ti surface after hydrothermal treatment (TTNT).

3.2. "In Vitro" Bioactivity Assay

When an artificial material is implanted in a living body, it can be considered a bioactive material if it is able to connect to the living bone through a thin layer rich in calcium and phosphorus (apatite layer) without a distinct boundary. According to ISO/FDIS 23317 Standard, the formation of a bone-like apatite layer can be "in vitro" reproduced when a material is immersed in an acellular and protein-free simulated body fluid (SBF) with ion concentrations nearly equal to those of human blood plasma. Thus, under this condition, the formation of an apatite layer on the material surface is indicative of its in vivo bone-bonding ability.

Figure 3 shows SEM images of the surface of Ti discs with (TTNT) and without hydrothermal treatment after 14 days of incubation in SBF solution (pH 7.4, 37 °C). The uniform layer of the flake-like apatite crystals can only be identified covering the sodium titanate structure (Figure 3b). The apatite formation capacity of Ti discs submitted to hydrothermal treatment can be explained by the exchange of titanate Na^+ ions with H_3O^+ ions in the SBF solution to form a Ti–OH bond on the surface. In response, the surface becomes negatively charged, reacting with the calcium ions present in the SBF. These Ca^+ ions are accumulated, making the surface positively charged and reacting with the negatively charged phosphate ions, which causes an increase in the rate of apatite nucleation [22,23].

Figure 4 shows the GIXRD diffractograms of hydrothermally treated (TTNT) Ti before and after immersion in SBF. The typical peaks of apatite at 2θ = 26° and 2θ = 32° (ICSD 9-432) were observed, and the TTNT peaks are not visible in the diffractogram of TTNT after immersion in SBF, confirming the formation of apatite's uniform layer on the TTNT surface, thus indicating that hydrothermal treatment provides bioactivity to Ti samples.

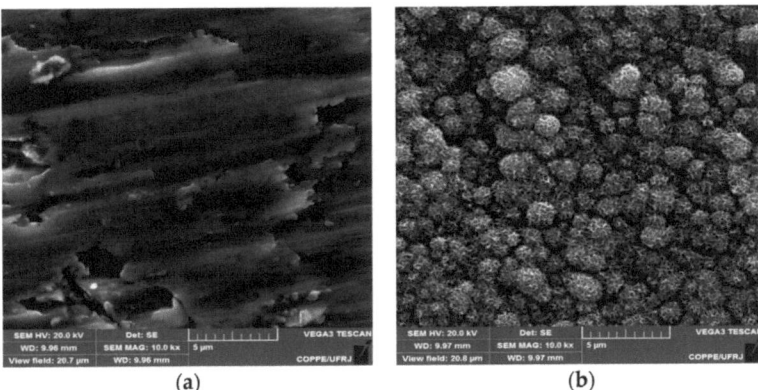

Figure 3. SEM images of samples' surface after 14 days of bioactivity assay comparing polished Ti without (**a**) and with alkaline hydrothermal treatment (**b**).

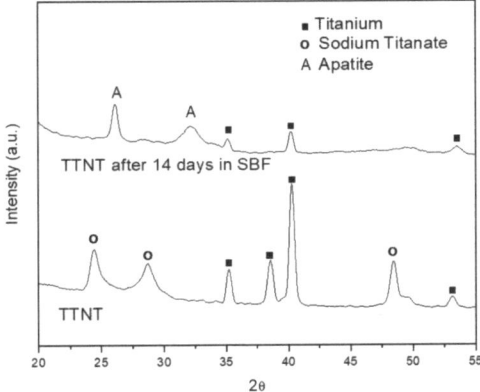

Figure 4. Diffractograms of Ti hydrothermally treated surface before and after immersion in SBF for 14 days.

3.3. Surface Wettability

Wettability influences the cascade of biological events that initiates osseointegration [27]. A hydrophilic surface results in closer contact between the titanium surface and the blood clot and cells by means of the increased availability of serum proteins with binding energy. The increase in the cell adhesion capacity by these proteins improves the adherence of the fibrin network and its retention to the surfaces of implants, as they mediate cell adhesion, followed by the cascade of coagulation and migration of undifferentiated cells and osteoblastic precursors [25,27].

Figure 5 presents images of a water droplet obtained during the contact angle measurements to evaluate the modification of surface wettability due to the surface treatment of Ti discs. In this context, the experimental group TTNT + MNZ + 1PVA was subjected to the analysis of the contact angle (Figure 5c) to monitor the change in wettability suffered after the deposition of the PVA layer when compared to the Ti pure samples (Figure 5a) and the Ti samples after hydrothermal treatment (TTNT, Figure 5c).

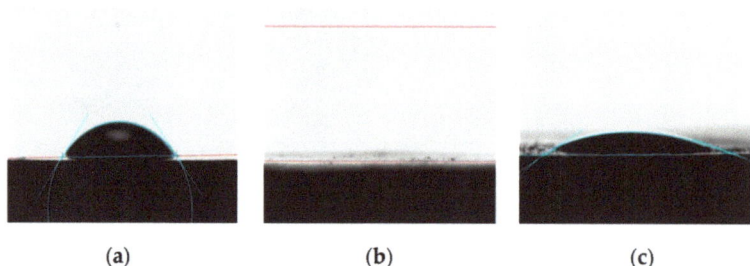

Figure 5. Contact angle measurements (blue lines indicate the angles). Images of a water droplet on the surface of (**a**) pure Ti surface, (**b**) Ti disc after alkaline hydrothermal treatment (TTNT), (**c**) Ti disc after addition of metronidazole (MNZ) and a layer of PVA (TTNT + MNZ + 1PVA).

The contact angle of the water drop on the surface of the pure titanium samples presented the highest value ($\theta_c = 46°$), indicating the less hydrophilic character of these samples. After the hydrothermal treatment, the water droplet spread out on the TTNT surface, indicating superhydrophilic behavior ($\theta_c = 0°$). This could be explained considering the increase in the surface area and the formation of pores due to the presence of the titanate layer, so the decrease in contact angle may be related to the drop absorption by capillarity. Additionally, although PVA molecules present a hydrophilic character, the contact angle value increased a little after MNZ addition and PVA coating. However, the TTNT + MNZ + 1PVA samples also presented a highly hydrophilic character with $\theta_c = 22°$. This fact could be explained by the smoothing of surface roughness by coating with the PVA layer, which probably hindered the water absorption by capillarity through the TTNT nanostructures. The hydrophilicity of the drug delivery system after PVA deposition for osseointegration purposes is important and indicates that this coated device could play a positive and significant role in the early stages of osseointegration.

3.4. "In Vitro" Metronidazole Release Evaluation

For osseointegration to occur, four stages are required: hemostasis, an inflammatory phase, a proliferative phase, and a remodeling phase. These must occur in a coordinated and organized manner [28,29], resulting in impeccable healing. The misalignment of this healing can occur in the initial inflammatory phase, which begins about 10 min after the implant is installed, creating a toxic environment. Host defense systems are activated at this stage by nonspecific molecules of bacterial origin. Polymorphonuclear leukocytes (PMN) and macrophages, and a group of glycoproteins that form membrane-perforating channels (perforins), which damage bacterial cells, are activated [30]. Therefore, the abundance of bacteria, as is the case with patients with active periodontal disease, for example, prolongs and amplifies the cellular immune response. PMNs kill bacteria through reactive radicals (oxygen species and hydroxylated groups, chlorine radicals and hypochlorite) that are also toxic to the host's cells and to the healthy tissue around the wound. Thus, a fulminant neutrophil response can induce the loss of healthy surrounding tissues [30].

To limit the inflammatory phase, antibacterial measures are needed, such as antibiotic therapy and local disinfection. The local and controlled release of the drug directly from the surface of the implant could act to combat bacteria, preventing their adhesion, exacerbating the inflammatory process, and failing the osseointegration process. To propose a release restriction the use of PVA with different numbers of layers was suggested to compare the release in different systems.

Figure 6 shows the evolution with time of the cumulative release of metronidazole from TTNT + MNZ samples with and without PVA coating during their immersion in PBS (pH 7.4, 37 °C). Table 2 shows the accumulated percentage of MNZ released during the first 48 h.

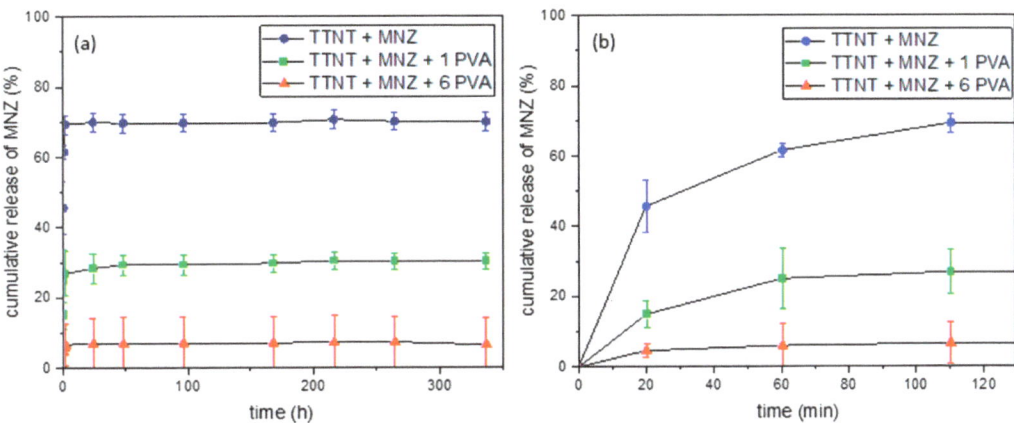

Figure 6. Cumulative release of MNZ with time: (**a**) whole experiment (14 days); (**b**) first 110 min.

Table 2. Percentage of MNZ released in each measurement during the assay and statistical difference (different upper-case letters within a column indicate significant differences among experimental groups, different lowercase letters within a row indicate significant differences among time).

% of MNZ Released	20 Min	60 Min	110 Min	24 h	48 h
TTNT + MNZ	45.7 ^{cA}	61.5 ^{bA}	69.3 ^{aA}	69.9 ^{aA}	69.6 ^{aA}
TTNT + MNZ + 1PVA	14.9 ^{bB}	25.0 ^{aB}	26.9 ^{aB}	28.4 ^{aB}	29.3 ^{aB}
TTNT + MNZ + 6PVA	4.66 ^{aC}	6.01 ^{aC}	6.72 ^{aC}	7.01 ^{aC}	7.02 ^{aC}

For all groups, the total amount of MNZ was not released in the medium. The maximum release of the drug was 70%, observed for the TTNT + MNZ group. This can be justified by a possible interaction between sodium titanate and metronidazole, which would prevent these molecules from being released by diffusion during the test, a suggestion that was confirmed by FTIR analyses. The samples coated with PVA, TTNT + MNZ + 1PVA and the TTNT + MNZ + 6PVA group presented a significant reduction in the total percentage of MNZ released, at about 27% and 6%, respectively. For these groups, besides the titanate–metronidazole interaction, PVA coating acted as a physical barrier, limiting the amount of MNZ released.

The hypothesis that there is no difference among group means was rejected by Two Way Repeated Measures ANOVA (One Factor Repetition) that assumed a statistically significant interaction between MNZ released by each experimental group and time ($p \leq 0.001$). In Table 2, a statistical treatment with all pairwise multiple comparison procedures (Holm-Sidak method) with overall significance level = 0.05 was carried out to observe, in a more reliable way, the difference between the release times, comparing the different groups. According to the data, the TTNT + MNZ + 6PVA group reached its release constant in just 20 min, which could be justified by the efficiency of a physical barrier formed by the six layers of PVA deposited on the surface. The TTNT + MNZ + 1PVA group had its constant release in 60 min, while the TTNT + MNZ sample continued to release until 110 min. These results imply that drug release profiles can be designed according to the thickness of the PVA coating.

Although the PVA coating did not promote a gradual and prolonged release of MNZ, as expected, the metronidazole concentrations released for all groups (1.6–15.5 µg/mL) were higher than the Minimum Inhibitory Concentration (MIC) of this drug for anaerobic bacteria. MIC is the lowest antibiotic concentration required for inhibiting the growth of a specific microorganism. Previous studies [31] reported the MIC of metronidazole to eliminate anaerobic bacteria without distinction as 0.06 to 32 µg/mL. Moreover, as discussed before, the local delivery of MNZ in an immediate regime could reduce early implant complication by removing the bacterial contamination of the surgical site and, thus, avoiding disturbance in the initial inflammatory phase of wound healing, which begins 10 min after the implantation.

3.5. Chemical Composition Evaluation after "In Vitro" Metronidazole Release Analysis

The samples were analyzed by FTIR before and after the drug release experiment. For a better interpretation of the FTIR spectra of the groups with MNZ, the FTIR spectra of nanostructured Ti samples after alkaline hydrothermal treatment (TTNT) and pure PVA film, shown in Figures 7 and 8 respectively, were previously analyzed.

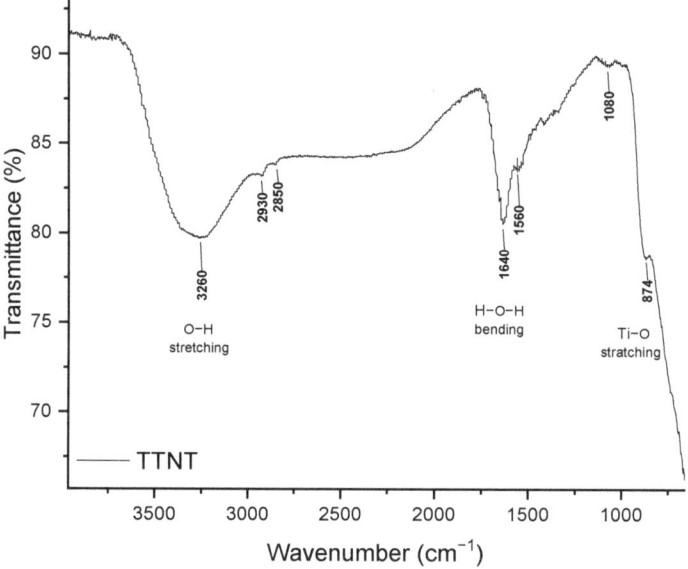

Figure 7. FTIR spectra of Ti sample after alkaline hydrothermal treatment (TTNT).

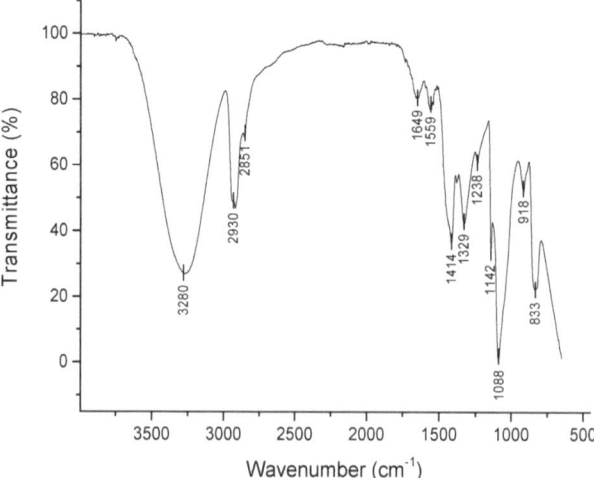

Figure 8. FTIR spectra of a PVA film produced by casting technique and irradiated with gamma rays at 25 KGy.

In the spectrum of the TTNT sample (Figure 7), a broad band between 3000 and 3500 cm^{-1} is observed, which can be attributed to fundamental stretching vibrations in different hydroxyl groups O-H (free or linked) [2,32,33]. This may be due to the absorption of water from the atmosphere [33] and the formation of the Ti-OH bond. The band at 1630 cm^{-1} can be attributed to bending vibrations in -OH [32,33] and can indicate water absorption in the titanate when exposed to the atmosphere [2]. The set of overlapping bands in the 800 to 400 cm^{-1} range may be related to the Ti-O and Ti-O-Ti groups [32].

PVA gamma-irradiated film was used as a reference in identifying the characteristic absorption bands of the TTNT + MNZ-coated samples. The FTIR spectrum of PVA film (Figure 8) shows the following bands and their respective vibration modes: 3280 cm^{-1}, hydroxyl group stretching vibration; 2930 cm^{-1} and 2851 cm^{-1}, C–H stretching vibration in CH$_2$ groups [34,35]; 1649 cm^{-1} and 1559 cm^{-1}, C=O stretching vibration and C=C stretching vibration, respectively, of the non-hydrolyzed acetate groups [35]; 1414 cm^{-1}, C–H wagging vibration in CH$_2$ groups [34,35]; 1329 cm^{-1}, (CH+OH) bending vibration; 1238 cm^{-1}, C–C stretching vibration; 1088 cm^{-1}, C–O stretching vibration; 918 cm^{-1}, CH$_2$ stretching vibration; 833 cm^{-1}, C–C stretching vibration [35] and C–H out-of-plane vibration.

The band observed at 1142 cm^{-1} is associated with the stretching of the C–O–C bond and can be an indicator of polymer crosslinking due to gamma irradiation [17]. According to the findings of Zainuddin et al. [36], it can be suggested that alkoxy radicals were formed in the PVA chains (~CH$_2$–CHO•–CH$_2$~) when radiation reached the polymer. Then, these radicals underwent further transformations, leading to the formation of C–O–C bindings between mers within the same chain or between those of different chains. These crosslinking reactions in PVA during radiolysis formed a three-dimensional network of the hydrogel without the need of a chemical crosslinking agent, which could have induced cytotoxicity to the system.

Figure 9 shows the FTIR spectra of the samples loaded with MNZ. The TTNT + MNZ spectrum is very similar to that of the samples after hydrothermal treatment (Figure 7), excepted by the presence of the absorption bands characteristic of MNZ, confirming the impregnation of MNZ in the titanate nanostructures. These MNZ bands were assigned to: anti-symmetric N-O and symmetrical elongation associated with the NO$_2$ group (1533 cm^{-1} and 1371 cm^{-1}, respectively); elongation N = O (1475 cm^{-1}); elongation C-O (1267 cm^{-1}); elongation C-N (1081 cm^{-1}); OH stretching (3214 cm^{-1}) [37,38]. A band at 877 cm^{-1} is also detected, which can be related both to the elongation of C-NO$_2$, characteristic of MNZ, and to the elongation of Ti-O, characteristic of titanate nanostructures.

Meanwhile, absorption bands of MNZ or of titanate were not detected in the FTIR spectra of the samples coated with PVA (TTNT + MNZ + 1PVA and TTNT + MNZ + 6PVA), which suggested that the MNZ molecules and titanate nanostructure were completely covered by PVA films, corroborating the contact angle analysis. Although the spectrometer's chamber was well purged by nitrogen, traces of gaseous carbon dioxide can be observed in some spectra. The double band at 2350 cm^{-1} presented in these spectra is assigned to asymmetric stretching modes of CO$_2$ [39].

Figure 10 shows the FTIR spectra of samples after 14 days of immersion in PBS solution at 37 °C. In all spectra, a large band centered at about 3250 cm^{-1} (-OH stretching) and a band at 1637 cm^{-1} (H-O-H bending) can be visualized, although their intensity is higher in TTNT + MNZ + 6PVA. These can be related to the –OH group stretching vibration of PVA and also to the absorption of water from PBS solution. Characteristic bands of PVA are clearly visualized in TTNT + MNZ + 6PVA, while no characteristic vibration band of MNZ was identified. This could indicate the presence of the coating layer even after 14 days of immersion. As proposed before, probably a thick PVA coating acted as a strong physical barrier and obstructed the release of the drug.

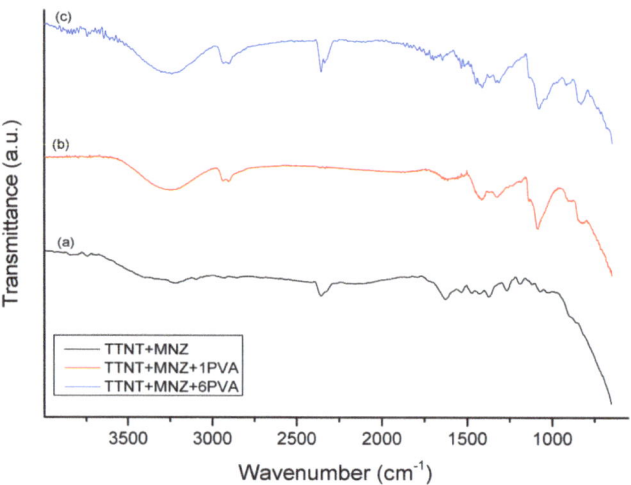

Figure 9. FTIR spectra of TTNT samples loaded with metronidazole: (a) TTNT + MNZ, (b) TTNT + MNZ + 1PVA and (c) TTNT + MNZ + 6PVA.

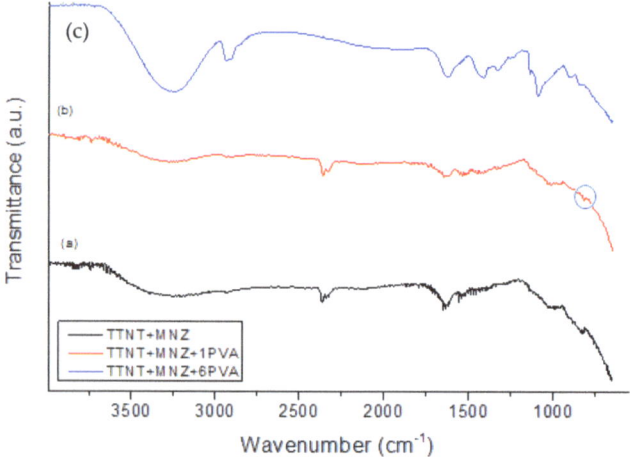

Figure 10. FTIR spectra of TTNT samples loaded with metronidazole, (a) TTNT + MNZ, and coated with PVA, (b) TTNT + MNZ + 1PVA and (c) TTNT + MNZ + 6PVA, after 14 days of immersion in PBS solution at 37 °C.

The spectra of TTNT + MNZ and TTNT + MNZ + 1PVA after MNZ release (Figure 10a,b) are very similar to that of pure TTNT (Figure 7), except for the presence of a small band at 1538 cm^{-1} that can be assigned to N-O antisymmetric stretching in the MNZ molecules. In the TTNT + MNZ spectrum, a shift in the band observed at 874 cm^{-1} (due to Ti-O stretching) to a lower wavenumber (835 cm^{-1}), and consequently to lower energy, may be attributed to the formation of an intermolecular interaction between TTNT and MNZ in an aqueous environment. This shifted band was also observed in the TTNT + MNZ + 1PVA spectrum as a small shoulder (circled in Figure 10b). This interaction can explain the partial release of MNZ molecules from these systems, as proposed in item 3.3. The intense band at 1088 cm^{-1} related to C–O stretching vibration in the PVA molecules was not present in the TTNT + MNZ + 1PVA spectra. It can be inferred that this layer of PVA in

TTNT + MNZ + 1PVA degraded in the PBS solution at least in the sample region analyzed by FTIR.

To confirm this assumption, SEM was used to analyze the surface of the TTNT + MNZ + 1PVA group, before and after the "in vitro" metronidazole release assay (Figure 11). An SEM image of the TTNT + MNZ + 1PVA group before the release test (Figure 11a) shows a homogeneous coating of PVA on the entire surface. The titanate nanostructure was not visualized due to the polymeric coating. The images after the MNZ release test (Figure 11b,c) reveal regions where the PVA coating has been degraded. In these regions, it is possible to observe tears in the polymeric coating and the morphology of the nanostructured film under the coating having kept intact. This partial degradation of the PVA film is in accordance with the FTIR results. Although PVA is soluble in water solution, most of its molecules remain insoluble due to crosslinking, forming a hydrogel. Thus, the much higher content of MNZ released by TTNT + MNZ + 1PVA when compared to the system with six layers of PVA may be attributed to the erosion of the coating.

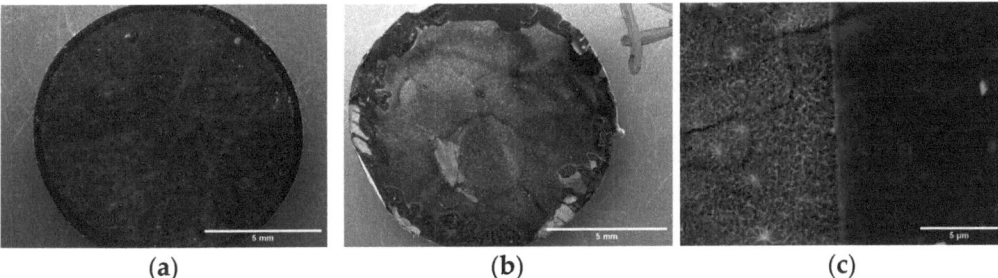

Figure 11. SEM images of TTNT + MNZ + 1PVA group, (a) before and (b,c) after "in vitro" MNZ release assay.

Although the thickness of the film affects its water uptake, a parallel between PVA cast film and the PVA layer of TTNT + MNZ + 1PVA can be drawn. In order to estimate the water absorption capacity of the PVA layer on the Ti surface, a PVA hydrogel was produced by the casting technique with 0.2 mm in thickness and irradiated with a dose of 25 KGy of gamma rays. This film showed a maximum absorption of 135% after 1 h of immersion in PBS pH 7.4 and reached an equilibrium swollen degree (the stage in which the hydration forces are in equilibrium with crosslinking elastic forces) of 120% after approximately 24 h. Based on this, the release of metronidazole from the TTNT + MNZ + 1PVA system may be related not only to the degradation of the coating, but also to the swelling of the PVA layer due to fluid absorption (a swelling-induced mechanism), since the period of the achievement of MNZ constant release (Figure 6, Table 2) was coincident with the point of the maximum absorption of the PVA film.

The biological fluid uptake by systems coated with PVA provides a hydrated environment that could facilitate the distribution of the antibiotic throughout the wound surgery site and contribute to wound healing at an early stage.

3.6. "In Vitro" Cytotoxicity

Considering the methodology for preparing the samples, the most critical step that could bring any damage to human cells is the hydrothermal surface treatment due to the alkaline solution used for this having the possibility of residual sodium. Moreover, although titanium implants are considered safe, with a high success rate in medical and dental applications, there are some reported cases of titanium toxicity related to corrosion, wear particle or ion release, and allergic reaction [40]. On the other hand, it can be inferred that the amount of MNZ used in our study would be safe to cells, since the exposure of human gingival fibroblasts to a dosage less than 50 µg/mL of MNZ up to 96 h did not induce the cytotoxicity effect [41]. In regard to PVA film, a previous study of the group using the same grade of PVA and employing the same methodology to produce hydrogels [17] showed that the samples were non-toxic to fibroblast cells. The irradiation method used to produce the PVA hydrogel layers leaves no residue or toxic materials in it. Furthermore, it uses only water as solvent, with no acid or toxic solvents.

In this context, the cytotoxicity of Ti and Ti + TTNT discs was assessed by evaluating human osteosarcoma MG63 cells' response to samples after being cultured for 24 h with the extracts of the discs. The MTT colorimetric assay was employed for this proposal. This assay measures the ability of viable cells to reduce a tetrazolium salt (MTT) to formazan, a process that produces a purple color that can be measured spectrophotometrically. If the cells are healthy and viable, they will be able to reduce the MTT and produce a strong purple color. However, if the cells are damaged or dying, they will not be able to reduce the MTT and the color will be weaker or absent.

According to Figure 12, cells cultured in extracts of the Ti and Ti + TTNT discs showed viability near the negative control (polystyrene), with no significant difference between them. These results indicate that there was no significant alteration in mitochondrial metabolic activity of cell population in the presence of the Ti and Ti + TTNT extracts, i.e., pure Ti and titanate nanostructured coating do not deliver toxic residues to the supernatant, even after 24 h soaking in a medium culture. This data is important for evaluating the safety of the biomaterial and for making decisions about its potential use in medical and dental applications.

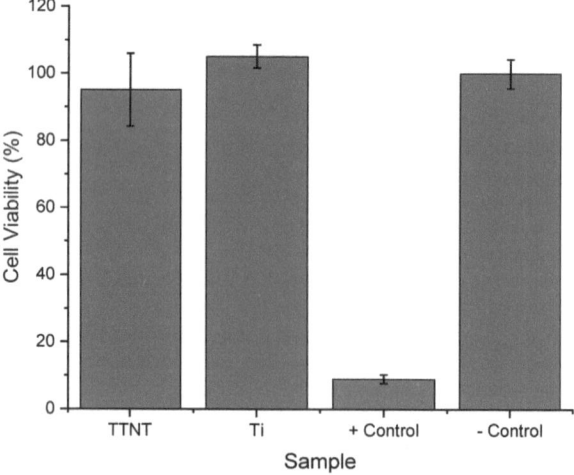

Figure 12. Cytotoxicity of Ti and TTNT discs extracts measured by MTT assay. + control (latex): indicates toxicity and—control (polystyrene): indicates the absence of toxicity. The results are expressed as mean ± standard deviation (SD) of six measurements for each group (n = 6).

4. Conclusions

In summary, alkaline hydrothermal treatment successfully produced intertwined nanostructures like a web on the titanium surface, in addition to good wettability and high bioactivity. With the aim of creating a local drug release device, the proposed surface modification strategy is simple, economical, and promising, since:

(1) It did not change the surface treatment and consequently the properties of the material;
(2) All groups reached the minimum inhibitory concentration described in the literature to help fight anaerobic bacteria with probably no cytoxicity effect;
(3) All groups allowed the immediate delivery of metronidazole, which could reduce implant complications during the early wound healing processes;
(4) Although TTNT + MNZ showed a higher percentage of antibiotic release within the studied groups, the PVA coating may absorb body fluids and water that provide

distribution of MNZ throughout the wound surgery site, besides contributing to the hydration of the implant site, facilitating wound healing;

(5) The design with one layer of PVA (TTNT + MNZ + 1PVA) was shown to be the best option, since it can combine the water absorption capacity of the PVA-coated regions with the higher bioactivity of the titanate nanostructure exposed in the degraded regions of the coating. Nevertheless, the effect of the crosslinking degree of PVA on the kinetic release of metronidazole should be better investigated.

The present study serves as proof that this method of surface modification can be a new alternative to the administration of systemic drugs, combining local antibiotic therapy with a surface treatment with proven efficacy. This delivery device could become a powerful approach to improve the integration of the titanium implant with the bone in dental applications, preventing early infections and bone failure. These results encourage further studies to evaluate the biological effectiveness of the proposed surface modification methodology.

Author Contributions: Conceptualization, P.M.J., I.R.S. and R.M.S.M.T.; methodology, I.R.S., R.S.S., A.T.S.B. and J.N.L.; data curation, A.T.S.B., I.R.S., R.S.S., J.N.L. and P.N.G.P.; writing—preparation of original draft, I.R.S., R.S.S. and A.T.S.B.; writing—proofreading and editing, I.R.S., A.T.S.B., P.N.G.P., P.M.J. and R.M.S.M.T.; project management, I.R.S., P.M.J. and R.M.S.M.T.; financing acquisition, P.M.J. and R.M.S.M.T. All authors have read and agreed to the published version of the manuscript.

Funding: The authors are grateful to the following Brazilian agencies: Coordenação de Aperfeiçoamento de Pessoal de Nível Superior—CAPES, National Council for Scientific and Technological Development-CNPq (Grant: 308789/2020-2), Fundação Carlos Chagas Filho de Amparo à Pesquisa do Estado do Rio de Janeiro-FAPERJ (Grant: Rede NanoSaúde—E-26/210.139/2019) for financial support.

Institutional Review Board Statement: Not applicable.

Informed Consent Statement: Not applicable.

Data Availability Statement: The data presented in this study are available on request from the corresponding authors.

Acknowledgments: We acknowledge the Center of Nanotechnology Characterization at INT /SISNANO (CNPq-SisNANO 442604/2019–0)), the Multiuser Nucleus of Microscopy and the Multiuser Laboratory of Materials Characterization (LMCM), both at PEMM/COPPE/Federal University of Rio de Janeiro (UFRJ) for their support with the use of equipments. The authors also acknowledge B. N. Teixeira (PEMM/COPPE/UFRJ) for the cytotoxicity analysis.

Conflicts of Interest: The authors declare no conflict of interest. The funders had no role in the design of the study; in the collection, analyses, or interpretation of data; in the writing of the manuscript; or in the decision to publish the results.

References

1. Rupp, F.; Liang, L.; Geis-Gerstorfer, J.; Scheideler, L.; Hüttig, F. Surface characteristics of dental implants: A review. *Dent. Mater.* **2018**, *34*, 40–57. [CrossRef]
2. Lin, L.; Wang, H.; Ni, M.; Rui, Y.; Cheng, T.-Y.; Cheng, C.-K.; Pan, X.; Li, G.; Lin, C. Enhanced osteointegration of medical titanium implant with surface modifications in micro/nanoscale structures. *J. Orthop. Transl.* **2014**, *2*, 35–42. [CrossRef]
3. Wang, Q.; Zhou, P.; Liu, S.; Attarilar, S.; Ma, R.L.-W.; Zhong, Y.; Wang, L. Multi-Scale Surface Treatments of Titanium Implants for Rapid Osseointegration: A Review. *Nanomaterials* **2020**, *10*, 1244. [CrossRef] [PubMed]
4. Oliveira, D.P.; Palmieri, A.; Carinci, F.; Bolfarini, C. Osteoblasts behavior on chemically treated commercially pure titanium surfaces. *J. Biomed. Mater. Res. Part A* **2013**, *102*, 1816–1822. [CrossRef] [PubMed]
5. Kang, B.; Lan, D.; Liu, L.; Dang, R.; Yao, C.; Liu, P.; Ma, F.; Qi, S.; Chen, X. Antibacterial Activity and Bioactivity of Zn-Doped TiO_2 Coating for Implants. *Coatings* **2022**, *12*, 1264. [CrossRef]
6. Eggert, F.; Levin, L. Biology of teeth and implants: The external environment, biology of structures, and clinical aspects. *Quintessence Int.* **2018**, *49*, 301–312. [CrossRef]
7. Kunrath, M.F.; Leal, B.F.; Hübler, R.; de Oliveira, S.D.; Teixeira, E.R. Antibacterial potential associated with drug-delivery built TiO_2 nanotubes in biomedical implants. *AMB Express* **2019**, *9*, 51. [CrossRef]
8. Pecoraro, C.; Carbone, D.; Deng, D.; Cascioferro, S.M.; Diana, P.; Giovannetti, E. Biofilm formation as valuable target to fight against severe chronic infections. *Curr. Med. Chem.* **2022**, *29*, 4307–4310. [CrossRef]

9. Chouirfa, H.; Bouloussa, H.; Migonney, V.; Falentin-Daudré, C. Review of titanium surface modification techniques and coatings for antibacterial applications. *Acta Biomater.* **2018**, *83*, 37–54. [CrossRef]
10. Li, Z.; Xu, W.; Wang, X.; Jiang, W.; Ma, X.; Wang, F.; Zhang, C.; Ren, C. Fabrication of PVA/PAAm IPN hydrogel with high adhesion and enhanced mechanical properties for body sensors and antibacterial activity. *Eur. Polym. J.* **2021**, *146*, 110253. [CrossRef]
11. Ebhodaghe, O.S. Hydrogel—Based biopolymers for regenerative medicine applications: A critical review. *Int. J. Polym. Mater. Polym. Biomater.* **2022**, *71*, 155–172. [CrossRef]
12. Rivera-Hernández, G.; Antunes-Ricardo, M.; Martínez-Morales, P.; Sánchez, M.L. Polyvinyl alcohol based-drug delivery systems for cancer treatment. *Int. J. Pharm.* **2021**, *600*, 120478. [CrossRef] [PubMed]
13. Gajra, B.; Pandya, S.S.; Vidyasagar, G.; Rabari, H.; Dedania, R.R.; Rao, S. Poly vinyl alcohol Hydrogel and its Pharmaceutical and Biomedical Applications: A Review. *Int. J. Pharm. Res.* **2012**, *4*, 20–26.
14. Kumar, A.; Han, S.S. PVA-based hydrogels for tissue engineering: A review. *Int. J. Polym. Mater. Polym. Biomater.* **2017**, *66*, 159–182. [CrossRef]
15. Dilley, M.; Geng, B. Immediate and Delayed Hypersensitivity Reactions to Antibiotics: Aminoglycosides, Clindamycin, Linezolid, and Metronidazole. *Clin. Rev. Allergy Immunol.* **2021**, *62*, 463–475. [CrossRef]
16. Muthuraj, M.S.A. Antimicrobial Susceptibility of Periodontopathogens. *Clin. Dent.* **2021**, *15*, 18–24. [CrossRef]
17. Oliveira, R.N.; Rouzé, R.; Quilty, B.; Alves, G.G.; Soares, G.D.A.; Thiré, R.M.S.M.; McGuinness, G.B. Mechanical properties and in vitro characterization of polyvinyl alcohol-nano-silver hydrogel wound dressings. *Interface Focus* **2013**, *4*, 20130049. [CrossRef]
18. ISO/FDIS 23317; Implants for Surgery—In Vitro Evaluation for Apatite-Forming Ability of Implant Materials. International Organization for Standardization: Geneva, Switzerland, 2007.
19. Da Silva, M.A.C.; Oliveira, R.N.; Mendonça, R.H.; Lourenço, T.G.B.; Colombo, A.P.V.; Tanaka, M.N.; Tude, E.M.O.; da Costa, M.F.; Thiré, R.M.S.M. Evaluation of metronidazole—Loaded poly(3-hydroxybutyrate) membranes to potential application in periodontist treatment. *J. Biomed. Mater. Res. Part B Appl. Biomater.* **2016**, *104B*, 106–115. [CrossRef]
20. Anitha, V.C.; Banerjee, A.N.; Joo, S.W.; Min, B.K. Morphology-dependent low macroscopic field emission properties of titania/titanate nanorods synthesized by alkali-controlled hydrothermal treatment of a metallic Ti surface. *Nanotechnology* **2015**, *26*, 355705. [CrossRef]
21. Manivasagam, V.K.; Popat, K.C. Hydrothermally treated titanium surfaces for enhanced osteogenic differentiation of adipose derived stem cells. *Mater. Sci. Eng. C* **2021**, *128*, 112315. [CrossRef]
22. Kokubo, T.; Matsushita, T.; Takadama, H.; Kizuki, T. Development of bioactive materials based on surface chemistry. *J. Eur. Ceram. Soc.* **2009**, *29*, 1267–1274. [CrossRef]
23. Huang, Y.-Z.; He, S.-K.; Guo, Z.-J.; Pi, J.-K.; Deng, L.; Dong, L.; Zhang, Y.; Su, B.; Da, L.-C.; Zhang, L.; et al. Nanostructured titanium surfaces fabricated by hydrothermal method: Influence of alkali conditions on the osteogenic performance of implants. *Mater. Sci. Eng. C* **2019**, *94*, 1–10. [CrossRef]
24. Bright, R.; Hayles, A.; Wood, J.; Ninan, N.; Palms, D.; Visalakshan, R.M.; Burzava, A.; Brown, T.; Barker, D.; Vasilev, K. Bio-Inspired Nanostructured Ti-6Al-4V Alloy: The Role of Two Alkaline Etchants and the Hydrothermal Processing Duration on Antibacterial Activity. *Nanomaterials* **2022**, *12*, 1140. [CrossRef] [PubMed]
25. Hosseini, S.H.; Kazemian, M.; Ghorbanzadeh, S. A brief overview of cellular and molecular mechanisms of osseointegration. *Int. J. Contemp. Med. Res.* **2015**, *12*, 13.
26. Morgado, E.; de Abreu, M.A.; Pravia, O.R.; Marinkovic, B.A.; Jardim, P.M.; Rizzo, F.C.; Araújo, A.S. A study on the structure and thermal stability of titanate nanotubes as a function of sodium content. *Solid State Sci.* **2006**, *8*, 888–900. [CrossRef]
27. Scarano, A.; Rexhep, S.T.; Leo, L.; Lorusso, F. Wettability of implant surfaces: Blood vs autologous platelet liquid (APL). *J. Mech. Behav. Biomed. Mater.* **2021**, *126*, 104773. [CrossRef]
28. Terheyden, H.; Lang, N.P.; Bierbaum, S.; Stadlinger, B. Osseointegration—Communication of cells. *Clin. Oral Implant. Res.* **2011**, *23*, 1127–1135. [CrossRef] [PubMed]
29. He, Y.; Gao, Y.; Ma, Q.; Zhang, X.; Zhang, Y.; Song, W. Nanotopographical cues for regulation of macrophages and osteoclasts: Emerging opportunities for osseointegration. *J. Nanobiotechnol.* **2022**, *20*, 1–22. [CrossRef]
30. Ferencík, M.; Rovensky, J.; Matha, V.; Herold, M. *Kompendium der Immunologie: Grundlagen und Klinik*; Springer: Berlin/Heidelberg, Germany, 2006.
31. Poulet, P.P.; Duffaut, D.; Lodter, J.P. Metronidazole susceptibility testing of anaerobic bacteria associated with periodontal disease. *J. Clin. Periodontol.* **1999**, *26*, 261–263. [CrossRef]
32. Yoshida, R.; Suzuki, Y.; Yoshikawa, S. Syntheses of TiO_2(B) nanowires and TiO_2 anatase nanowires by hydrothermal and post-heat treatments. *J. Solid State Chem.* **2005**, *178*, 2179–2185. [CrossRef]
33. Xie, J.; Wang, X.; Zhou, Y. Understanding Formation Mechanism of Titanate Nanowires through Hydrothermal Treatment of Various Ti-Containing Precursors in Basic Solutions. *J. Mater. Sci. Technol.* **2012**, *28*, 488–494. [CrossRef]
34. Mansur, H.; Sadahira, C.M.; Souza, A.N.; Mansur, A. FTIR spectroscopy characterization of poly (vinyl alcohol) hydrogel with different hydrolysis degree and chemically crosslinked with glutaraldehyde. *Mater. Sci. Eng. C* **2008**, *28*, 539–548. [CrossRef]
35. Oliveira, R.N.; McGuinness, G.; Ramos, M.E.T.; Kajiyama, C.E.; Thiré, R. Properties of PVA Hydrogel Wound-Care Dressings Containing UK Propolis. *Macromol. Symp.* **2016**, *368*, 122–127. [CrossRef]
36. Zainuddin, H.D.J.T.; Le, T.T. An ESR study on γ-irradiated poly(vinyl alcohol). *Radiat. Phys. Chem.* **2001**, *62*, 283–291. [CrossRef]

37. Herculano, R.D.; Guimarães, S.A.C.; Belmonte, G.C.; Duarte, M.A.H.; de Oliveira Júnior, O.N.; Kinoshita, A.; de Oliveira Graeff, C.F. Metronidazole release using natural rubber latex as matrix. *Mater. Res.* **2010**, *13*, 57–61. [CrossRef]
38. Brako, F.; Luo, C.; Matharu, R.K.; Ciric, L.; Harker, A.; Edirisinghe, M.; Craig, D.Q.M. A Portable Device for the Generation of Drug-Loaded Three-Compartmental Fibers Containing Metronidazole and Iodine for Topical Application. *Pharmaceutics* **2020**, *12*, 373. [CrossRef]
39. Pavia, D.L.; Lampman, G.M.; Kriz, G.S.; Vyvyan, J.A. *Introduction to Spectroscopy*; Cengage Learning: Boston, MA, USA, 2014.
40. Kim, K.T.; Eo, M.Y.; Nguyen, T.T.H.; Kim, S.M. General review of titanium toxicity. *Int. J. Implant. Dent.* **2019**, *5*, 10. [CrossRef]
41. Ferreira, M.B.; Myiagi, S.; Nogales, C.G.; Campos, M.S.; Lage-Marques, J.L. Time- and concentration-dependent cytotoxicity of antibiotics used in endodontic therapy. *J. Appl. Oral Sci.* **2010**, *18*, 259–263. [CrossRef]

Disclaimer/Publisher's Note: The statements, opinions and data contained in all publications are solely those of the individual author(s) and contributor(s) and not of MDPI and/or the editor(s). MDPI and/or the editor(s) disclaim responsibility for any injury to people or property resulting from any ideas, methods, instructions or products referred to in the content.

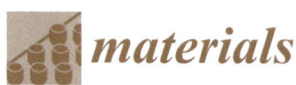 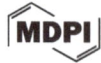

Review

Zirconia Dental Implant Designs and Surface Modifications: A Narrative Review

Michał Ciszyński [1], Bartosz Chwaliszewski [1], Wojciech Simka [2], Marzena Dominiak [1], Tomasz Gedrange [1,3] and Jakub Hadzik [1,*]

1. Department of Dental Surgery, Faculty of Medicine and Dentistry, Medical University of Wroclaw, 50-425 Wroclaw, Poland; michal.ciszynski@umw.edu.pl (M.C.); marzena.dominiak@umw.edu.pl (M.D.); tomasz.gedrange1@tu-dresden.de (T.G.)
2. Faculty of Chemistry, Silesian University of Technology, 44-100 Gliwice, Poland; wojciech.simka@polsl.pl
3. Department of Orthodontics, Technische Universität Dresden, 01069 Dresden, Germany
* Correspondence: jakub.hadzik@umw.edu.pl

Abstract: Titanium currently has a well-established position as the gold standard for manufacturing dental implants; however, it is not free of flaws. Mentions of possible soft-tissue discoloration, corrosion, and possible allergic reactions have led to the development of zirconia dental implants. Various techniques for the surface modification of titanium have been applied to increase titanium implants' ability to osseointegrate. Similarly, to achieve the best possible results, zirconia dental implants have also had their surface modified to promote proper healing and satisfactory long-term results. Despite zirconium oxide being a ceramic material, not simply a metal, there have been mentions of it being susceptible to corrosion too. In this article, we aim to review the literature available on zirconia implants, the available techniques for the surface modification of zirconia, and the effects of these techniques on zirconia's biological properties. Zirconia's biocompatibility and ability to osseointegrate appears unquestionably good. Despite some of its mechanical properties being, factually, inferior to those of titanium, the benefits seem to outweigh the drawbacks. Zirconia implants show very good success rates in clinical research. This is partially due to available methods of surface treatment, including nanotopography alterations, which allow for improved wettability, bone-to-implant contact, and osseointegration in general.

Keywords: dental; implants; zirconia; surface; modifications; corrosion

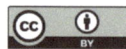

1. Introduction

In the past few decades, the extensive use of and extensive research on titanium implants has resulted in them being perceived as the gold standard in oral implantology. Currently, it can be agreed that their overall osseointegration rate is very high, above 95% [1].

Despite the obvious advantages, titanium and its alloys as dental implant materials have some drawbacks, which include possible discolorations of peri-implant soft tissues, leading to esthetic problems; possible hypersensitivity; and/or allergic reactions [1]. Following titanium corrosion, titanium compounds and ions have been found in the peri-implant tissues of patients who developed peri-implantitis [2]. It is argued that such compounds may contribute to osseointegration failure. Some authors even report an accumulation of titanium compounds in regional lymph nodes, lungs, and bones after the placement of titanium plasma-sprayed implants [3]. In the case of implants made not of pure titanium but of alloys like Grade 5 titanium (Ti6Al4V), corrosion could potentially result in vanadium compounds migrating to the peri-implant tissues as well as titanium. A meta-analysis by Chun-Teh Lee et al. has shown that even 30.7% implants develop peri-implant mucositis after placement [3,4].

Those drawbacks have prompted researchers to develop a new material. The first ceramic dental implants date back to as early as 1968, when alumina (Al_2O_3) implants were developed [5]. Several implant systems were developed later, in the seventies and eighties, including the Cerasand, Pfeilstift, Bonit, and Tubingen implants. However, their poor biomechanical properties often led to fractures when loaded extra-axially [6]. At the beginning of the 1990s, a new ceramic material, yttrium oxide–partially stabilized zirconia (YPSZ), was introduced to dentistry [7]. Zirconia is a crystalline oxide of zirconium [8]. Zirconia as a mineral was discovered in 1892. Stabilized zirconia was developed in 1929 [9]. It holds good mechanical, optical, and biological properties [10]. Zirconia's fracture resistance and bending strength are significantly higher than those of Al_2O_3, allowing zirconia implants to withstand occlusal forces [11]. This makes zirconia the material of choice for the fabrication of ceramic dental implants.

While reviewing the available literature, one can find information concerning zirconia implants' properties (often in comparison to conventional titanium dental implants), different methods of obtaining zirconia implants, and possible surface modifications, as well as the effects of these variables on an implant's clinical effects. In this article, we authors aim to summarize the available information and present the current trends concerning zirconia dental implants, focusing in particular on the possible effects of surface treatment of zirconia on the performance of zirconia dental implants.

2. Properties of Zirconia as an Implant Material

As was mentioned in the introduction, one of the main concerns regarding titanium as a dental implant material is the possible discoloration following gingival recessions around dental implants. As authors of this review, we believe that in most cases, such esthetic problems can be avoided or solved through the careful choice of surgical techniques in each particular clinical case. For example, proper 3D implant position and soft-tissue thickness can prevent titanium from causing visible discolorations [12,13]. Moreover, anodization, a process often applied to modify titanium implants' surface characteristics, can also be used to change an implant's color, which can also be helpful for avoiding grayish discoloration visible in peri-implant soft tissues [14].

Nonetheless, as zirconia (ZrO_2), introduced to dental implantology in 2005, is a tooth-colored material, it can significantly enhance the patient's esthetic outcome, which could, in case of complications, reduce the need for additional surgical procedures. Zirconia tends not to be visible as much as titanium through thin soft tissues [15,16].

Similarly to titanium, zirconium oxide shows high biocompatibility and osteoconductivity. The bone-to-implant contact values and osseointegration rates are similar for zirconia and titanium dental implants. While titanium has been criticized for the possible corrosion and release of titanium particles and ions into the peri-implant tissues, this does not seem to be a problem in the case of zirconia implants, which show excellent resistance to corrosion and thus cause less irritation. Titanium compounds can promote local inflammatory reactions and possibly account for the lack of osseointegration [3,17].

The polymorphic zirconia structure is present in three different crystal forms: monoclinic, tetragonal, and cubic. At room temperature, zirconia acquires a monoclinic structure, which changes into tetragonal at 1170 °C and into cubic at 2370 °C. The tetragonal structure has superior fracture toughness and flexural strength thanks to the martensitic toughening mechanism [6]. The tetragonal and cubic phases are unstable at room temperature and disintegrate while cooling. It is, nonetheless, possible to stabilize zirconia in its cubic phase by adding CaO, MgO, and Y_2O_3 (yttria), resulting in a material called partially stabilized zirconia (PSZ). This combines all three phases. Tetragonal zirconia polycrystals (TZP) can be obtained by adding Y_2O_3 at room temperature. Yttria-stabilized TZP (Y-TZP) have low porosity, high density, significant bending and compression strengths, high fracture toughness, and high fatigue resistance, and their form is suitable for medical applications. On top of their favorable mechanical properties, they also promote the proliferation of osteogenic cells during osseointegration. The mechanical characteristics that are measured to assess an implant's strength are, for example, tensile strength, bending strength, Young's modulus, Vickers hardness, and fracture toughness. A review by Takao Hanawa states that the bending strength is 1100 MPa for Y-TZP, 400 MPa for commercially pure (Grade 2) titanium, and 950 MPa for a Ti-6Al-4V alloy. The Young's modulus values are 210, 100 and 110 GPa, respectively. Vickers Hardness measures 1200, 150–170 and 270–320 HV, respectively. The fracture toughness of Y-TZP is 6–8 MPa/m^2. This is significantly lower than that of Grade 2 titanium (66 MPa/m^2) and Ti-6Al-4V alloy material (50 MPa/m^2). Tensile strength cannot be measured for naturally brittle materials like ceramics. Bending strength is satisfactory for all of the aforementioned materials. The fracture toughness of Y-TZP is significantly lower than that of titanium. As zirconia abutments are usually screwed in with titanium retentive screws, this leads to zirconia abutments fracturing before the abutment screw. It is, however, worth noting that Y-TZP' fracture toughness is still significantly higher than that of Al_2O_3 (3.1–5.5 MPa/m$^{2)}$. Young's modulus is important, as there is no periodontal ligament between the implant and bone. High values of Young's modulus make it impossible for a material to absorb occlusal forces, which are then conducted directly to alveolar bone. A large Young's modulus makes it difficult to fasten prosthetic abutment screws. Therefore, a problem with fixation can be encountered when employing Y-TZP by screwing [9,18,19].

Mechanical characteristics are important as they correlate directly to implant failures caused by possible fractures. Zirconia implants are often considered inferior to titanium ones for fear of them fracturing and requiring removal. A systematic review and meta-analysis by Bethke et al. concluded that despite some studies showing very promising results for two-piece zirconia implants, one-piece implants are in general more fracture-resistant. Moreover, implants made of alumina-toughened zirconia have been shown to be more fracture-resistant than implants made from Y-TZP [20].

Regarding osteoconductivity, it has been suggested that zirconia implants might display favorable properties compared to titanium implants. Various studies have been conducted and it has been, in fact, confirmed that zirconia as a material is osteoconductive. No clear advantage has, however, been documented over titanium surfaces [3,11].

Zirconia can however be associated with less biofilm formation than titanium, which might further decrease the risk of peri-implantitis [21]. This fact is associated with the lower surface energy and surface wettability of zirconia [22]. It has also been proven that early-formed (3-day-old) biofilms show greater accumulation on titanium rather than zirconia implants, while 14-day-old biofilms were comparable [21]. Rough or hydrophobic surfaces can, in general, increase bacterial adhesion, which suggests that different surface treatments (described in further parts of this article) of dental implants can influence biofilm formation. This appears to be true regardless of the material used. The same applies for the implant's design—its macrostructure also affects bacterial colonization [21,23,24].

3. Manufacturing Zirconia Dental Implants

The vast majority of zirconia-based dental implants are produced utilizing subtractive manufacturing methods, such as machining and milling; however, progressive processes like additive manufacturing are more promising for the future, alongside the development of digital dentistry, which gives a green light to the further progression of perfecting and polishing CAD/CAM individual zirconia implant solutions [25].

Regarding traditional subtractive manufacturing methods for zirconia implants, one can list the following techniques: dry pressing (uniaxial compaction), cold isostatic pressing, and hot isostatic pressing.

The predominant goal of these techniques is to decrease the volumetric percentage of void spaces in the block of material to the lowest possible amount during the compaction process. These empty fragments, called pores, tend to act in contradiction to the desirable physical properties of zirconia ceramics, decreasing its hardness and stiffness [26].

The first technique—uniaxial compaction—is based on hydraulic compression of the zirconia powder into a semi-finished product, which is called a blank. A lack of consistency and homogeneity leads to variable and unpredictable mechanical properties. Uniaxially pressed 3Y-TZP blanks, because of their properties, can be used successfully in manufacturing single-point prosthetic solutions, like dental crowns; however, their usage in manufacturing bridges has its limitations. The greatest asset of dry pressing is the low costs of its machinery and operation in comparison to other methods. Considering the previously mentioned characteristics, dry pressing is widely used as a preliminary stage, prior to introducing isostatic pressing as a final stage of manufacturing the product, hence eliminating the heterogeneities in the material [26].

In the cold isostatic pressing (CIP) method, a high-pressure liquid container is utilized to compress ceramic powder that is embodied inside a pliable form. CIP produces more homogenic and higher-density zirconia blanks compared to uniaxial compaction, which leads to the production of mechanically more durable blanks and enables a simplified and additionally efficient sintering process of the zirconia [27]. On the other hand, final products of the CIP method lack precision; thus, extra milling is required afterwards in order to produce more refined shapes, which causes material wastage [28].

The general idea of hot isostatic pressing (HIP) is quite akin to the concept of the cold isostatic pressing method; however, a main difference between these two processes is that HIP makes use of hot gasses (with temperatures ranging from 1300 °C to 1600 °C), like argon, compressed under high pressure, instead of the liquid utilized in CIP. Final products of the HIP method tend to be sintered, and thus they do not need any additional, complementary procedures. While costly in use, the HIP method fabricates product of the highest toughness of all three methods; that is why milling is required to achieve a desired shape afterwards. In conclusion, the hot isostatic pressing method is said to be the most costly technique when it comes to producing zirconia blanks because of its high running costs and increased cycle times. Nevertheless, different approaches have been explored by manufacturers with the aim of simplifying the whole process and refining the cycle parameters and cycle times, thus reducing the overall cost and enabling it to be more accessible for an average patient [28,29].

A constantly growing novelty in the field of manufacturing processes for zirconia oxide implants is exploiting CAD/CAM (Computer-Aided Design/Computer-Aided Manufacturing) methods. This is seen as a prospective changing factor in the near future for dental ceramics. These procedures are classified as a subtractive manufacturing technology, which allows a dental technician to digitally prepare a virtual project using a computer and then transfer this information to a milling machine for producing an implant from a blank. This technology possesses numerous advantages over a classic, analog approach. It diminishes possible occurrences of human error throughout the process, thus making it more predictable. The final product is of superior quality and precision, and also takes less time to manufacture. CAD/CAM technology, relying on digitally computed predictions, takes into consideration material shrinkage while sintering, which allows for better marginal adaptation of zirconia suprastructures. On the other hand, one of the very few disadvantages to this technology is its high cost; however, with constant technological development, it will eventually become within the reach of technicians, doctors, and patents [26,30].

Recent studies and developments in the field of CAD/CAM production processes for zirconia implants have resulted in the appearance of root-analog implant systems. They allow for the immediate implantation of an implant, mimicking the shape of an extracted tooth. An alternative way of acquiring the desired shape is the copy milling process [31].

Another intriguing branch being developed and researched involves employing additive manufacturing methods for producing zirconia oxide (3Y-TZP and ATZ) implant solutions. Currently, two technologies can be used for this procedure—direct light processing and laser-based stereolithography. New ways and opportunities open for manufacturers with these methods since they let them create implants of complex surface topography, thus improving the implant's osteoinductive properties, while simultaneously eliminating the risk of impairing the implant's surface through post-processes like sandblasting or acid-etching. This, being one of potential benefits of additive manufacturing, improves the firmness and endurance of zirconia oxide implants, casting a bright light for future development and research in the field of additive-manufactured ceramic solutions [32].

4. Surface Modifications

Many different factors affecting the results of implantation have been extensively studied and described in the scientific literature. These may include patient-specific medical conditions, medication, and biological characteristics such as the width, height, and thickness of the peri-implant-attached gingiva, bone mineral density, and vitamin D levels [33–36].

Other factors influencing osseointegration can be related directly to implant design and surface treatment. These include topography, roughness, and wettability [37].

The implant's topography has been proven to affect the osseointegration process though the means of primary stability, sealing, and marginal bone level maintenance. These finding have led manufacturers to continuous changes over the years. Surface topography can be divided into three levels: macrotopography (on a scale ranging from 10 μm to mm), microtopography (1–10 μm), and nanotopography (1–100 nm). Macrotopography is known to affect implant stability, while microtopography can influence bone-to-implant contact, the pace of osseointegration, and the extent of adhesion between mineralized bone and the implant surface. Nanotopography is believed to affect protein adsorption and cell adhesion [37,38]. Different types of surface-modifying methods, such as UV light exposure, heat treatment, and reactive plasma treatment, can change the surface's wettability, thus promoting the process of cell migration along the implant's surface, and consequently shortening the osseointegration period to about a month [39].

Surface roughness has been shown to affect bone-to-implant contact, healing rates, and osteogenic responses. According to a classification created in 2009, one can distinguish smooth (machined) surfaces when the average roughness over a measurement area (Sa) is less than 0.5 μm, minimally rough surfaces when the Sa ranges from 0.5 to 1 μm, moderately rough surfaces when the Sa is 1–2 μm, and rough surfaces when the Sa is $\geq$2 μm [38]. Later, many studies aimed to discover the possible responses of bone and soft tissues to varying levels of implant roughness. It has been shown that fibroblasts displayed enhanced proliferation and spread on smooth surfaces [40,41]. Regarding bone cells' behavior, it is currently agreeable that a moderately rough surface (Sa 1–2 μm) is ideal for achieving the best osteogenic effect [42–45]. Some researchers have suggested that such surfaces may promote bacterial colonization and peri-implantitis [46]. Further studies have, however, shown no evidence of an increased risk of peri-implantitis for moderately rough surfaces [45].

Surface wettability is believed to affect the adhesion of macromolecules to surfaces, the interaction of hard and soft tissues with the surfaces, biofilm formation, and clinical osseointegration rates. Surfaces can be, in general, divided into two groups according to wettability: hydrophilic and hydrophobic. Wettability is assessed by measuring the contact angle (CA) between a solid surface and a liquid when they meet. The lower the CA, the higher the wettability of a surface. In general, surfaces characterized by CA values higher and lower than 90° are considered hydrophobic and hydrophilic, respectively. The existing literature concerning wettability is relatively scarce; nonetheless, it is believed that wettability may promote tissue healing and modulate cellular adhesion levels [37,47,48].

Many processes have been tested to make titanium and zirconia implants' surfaces promote osseointegration as much as possible. The surface modifications of titanium implants are more numerous, as they have been in use for a significantly longer time than zirconia implants. Surface treatment options only applicable to titanium include anodizing, hydroxylation, and plasma oxidation. Anodization results in a TiO_2 layer being deposited onto the implant's surface, which, in turn, enhances gingival fibroblast deposition, adhesion, and proliferation; improves osteoblast adhesion; and provides favorable bone-to-implant contact and success rates. Hydroxylation leads to an increase in hydrophilicity and osseointegration rates through the means of bone-to-implant contact, increased bone density, enhanced cell attachment, and osteoblast differentiation. Plasma oxidation has been shown to lead to an increase in removal torque and bone-to-implant contact. Some surface modification techniques, however, have also been applied to zirconia implants. These processes can be of a physical or chemical nature and include machining, acid-etching, sandblasting, laser modification, coating, and UV treatment [15].

Currently, a strong emphasis is put on improving and developing zirconia implant surfaces as well, especially making them additionally rough and operative. It is possible to successfully enhance cellular responses, and thus the cells' function and reaction to the implant surface, by utilizing chemical, physical, and thermomechanical means [39]. Machine treatment of zirconia surfaces results in an average roughness around 0.96 μm. Machined zirconia implants display similar values of bone-to-implant contact to those of titanium implants, at 33.74–84.17% and 31.8–87.95%, respectively. Machined zirconia surfaces have shown a significant decrease in biofilm thickness compared to machined titanium. The osteoblast proliferation on machined titanium, however, is significantly better than that on machined zirconia. The early generation of implants used before the 1990s mostly had machined surfaces. As was mentioned earlier, a more solid bone fixation can be achieved with higher levels of surface roughness, namely above 0.96 μm. For this reason, further surface modification methods have been developed to increase the roughness, bone-to implant contact, and osseointegration rates [15,49].

Sandblasting and acid-etching were originally used on titanium implants to increase the surface area for osseointegration, and the resulting surface was called an SLA (sandblasted, large-grit, acid-etched) titanium surface (Figure 1). Similar processes can be used in the case of zirconia implants [50,51]. One study by Aifang Han et al. compared the characteristics of zirconia surfaces treated with grit-blasting with 110 μm silica-coated alumina particles (group GB), zirconia surfaces etched with 40% hydrofluoric acid for 25 min at 100 °C (group HF), zirconia surfaces that were grit-blasted as well as etched (group GBHP), and untreated zirconia (group C). The results showed that etching zirconia results in a desirable roughness regardless of whether it has been grit-blasted ($R_a = 1.47 \pm 0.04$ μm for group HF and $R_a = 1.49 \pm 0.05$ μm for group GBHF). The surface roughness in group GB measured 0.56 ± 0.05 μm, which is not satisfactory for implant purposes. Acid-etching was also shown to increase wettability. Moreover, contrary to the SLA titanium surface, acid-etching the zirconia vastly prohibited *S. sanguis* and *P. gingivalis* biofilm maturation, regardless of whether the surface had been grit-blasted or not [15,52]. In a systematic review by Gul et al., one-piece zirconia dental implants were shown to have promising 5-year clinical outcomes (95–98, 4% survival rates) regardless of their varying lengths and diameters. In the same study, acid-etching showed significantly better clinical outcomes compared to other surface designs [6]. Another study has shown that blasting zirconia with larger-sized (250 μm) particles resulted in even further enhancement of osteoblast cell adhesion in vitro [15,52,53]. It has been argued that grit-blasting Y-TZP can induce compressive stress concentration, which can lead to improvements in the zirconia's mechanical properties. It has also been shown that grit-blasting Y-TZP causes an increase in flexural strength. Unfortunately, grit-blasting can cause deep micro-cracks, which worsen zirconia's strength to an extent that cannot be compensated by the compression. Real clinical conditions are resembled by high-static-load and fatigue tests, which cause zirconia with micro-cracks to fail. It has been described that the changes caused by grit-blasting may increase the risk of future implant fractures. Surface treatment is only one of the many reasons that may contribute to zirconia implant fractures. Nonetheless, the fear of fractures is undoubtedly one of the reasons for zirconia still being a less popular choice than titanium, which is characterized by a 20–30-times-higher fracture toughness for Grade 4 titanium. The formation of micro-cracks can be diminished by using soft and round particles for blasting. Regarding acid-etching, high concentrations of acids and a too-long process duration can damage the zirconia's structure and decrease its flexural strength [54–56].

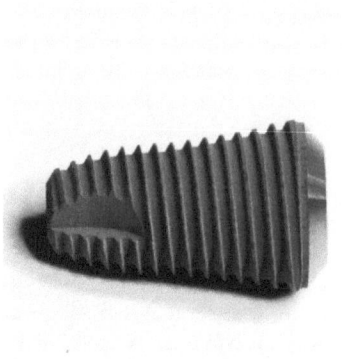
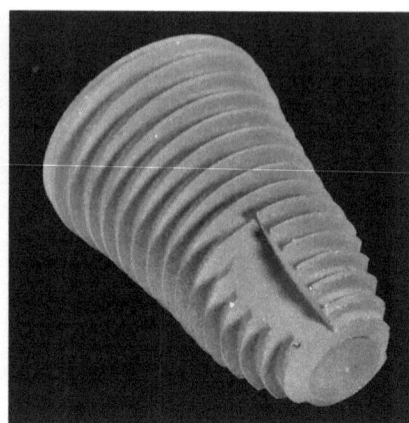

Figure 1. An example of an implant utilizing an SLA titanium surface [Dentium Superline 2, Dentium, Suwon, Republic of Korea].

Anodizing does play a role in modifying zirconia implant structures as well as titanium ones. In vitro studies have shown a significant increase in bone mineralization factors near anodized implants in comparison to control groups. A study conducted on rats by de la Hoz et al. showed that ZrO anodized at 60 Voltz is able to promote a significant increase in cancellous bone volume, trabecular thickness, and trabecular number, and a decrease in trabecular separation [39].

The next approach for modifying zirconia surfaces involves the use of lasers. Various types of lasers and various methods have been tested to improve zirconia surfaces for implantological needs. For example, fabricating micro-structures on zirconia with a wavelength of 1064 nm, a repetition rate of 20 kHz, an average power of 18 W, a pulse duration of 50 ns, and a fluence of 14.5 J/cm^2 leads to an increase in the surface free energy, which leads directly to an increase in wettability [48]. In vivo animal studies have concluded that modifying zirconia implants with pulses of a hundred femtoseconds, wavelengths of 795 nm, and 10 nJ energy with a repetition rate of 80 MHz could account for bone-to-implant contact and crestal resorption rates that are comparable to those of SLA titanium implants at one and three months [57]. Another animal study has shown that using fiber laser irradiation could increase the surface roughness and lead to greater bone-to-implant contact and removal torque in comparison to machined implants. Phosphatase activity, osteocalcin expression, cell proliferation, and calcification are among the processes that benefit from the laser modification of zirconia surfaces [58]. Most of the changes are, however, associated with the creation of microgrooves and surface structures, resulting in a change in roughness [15]. It is worth noting that aside from the above-mentioned surface modification methods, lasers can also be used in treating peri-implantitis. The parameters, however, need to be chosen carefully so as not to cause overheating of the peri-implant tissues [59].

The surface properties of zirconium oxide can also be, similarly to those of titanium, altered by applying various coatings. Regarding zirconia, these may include silica, magnesium, nitrogen, carbon, hydroxyapatite, calcium phosphate, and dopamine, all of which have been described as able to improve zirconia's biological properties [54]. More coating types are still being developed, not only for titanium and zirconia implants but also for prosthetic abutments. Among the researched possibilities, chitosan emerges as an interesting option due to its hemostatic and antimicrobial properties, and good biocompatibility [60]. Here, it is worth noting that some commercially available implants are made of a titanium core and coated with a thin ceramic layer. The idea behind this is to determine the mechanical properties of titanium and the benefits of zirconia, while also preventing titanium's corrosion. An example of such surface technology is the Cerid® ceramic coating on MyPlant Bio implants (Figure 2). In that particular case, the zirconium oxide coating is 4–7 µm thick. A comparison of different implant surfaces as visible under different magnifications through a scanning electron microscope can be seen in Figure 3.

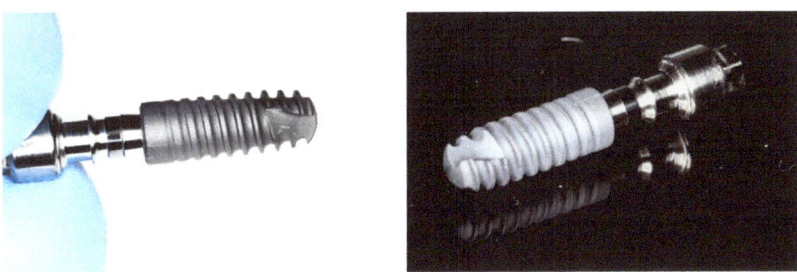

Figure 2. Myplant bio implant [MYPLANT GMBH, Neuss, Federal Republic of Germany] with Cerid® ceramic coating.

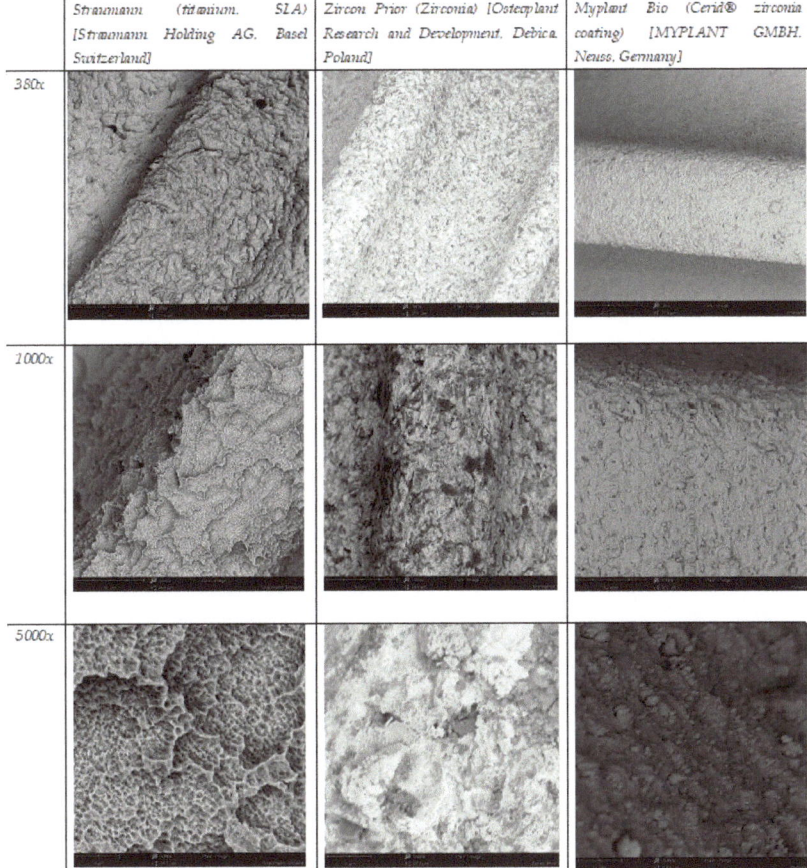

Figure 3. A comparison of different implant surfaces as visible through a scanning electron microscope under different magnifications.

Silica coatings can reduce bacterial adhesion to zirconia surfaces. Microstructured bioactive silica coatings can also assist in fibrin network formation and cell growth, and improve soft-tissue adherence. Magnesium can favor osteoblast proliferation, while the addition of nitrogen and carbon improves biological and mechanical properties of zirconia. A layer of nitrogen-doped hydrogenated amorphous carbon causes an increase in hydrophilicity and reduces bacterial adhesion. Some studies have tested coatings made of functionalized, multi-walled carbon nanotubes, which were shown to increase roughness, wettability, and cell adhesion. Hydroxyapatite, being of a similar mineral composition to bone, shows bioactive properties enhancing osseointegration, and leads to the formation of greater volumes of new bone. Calcium phosphate coating itself is too unstable to provide sufficient boding to the substrate. Because of this, studies have used tricalcium phosphate-reinforced hydroxyapatite coatings, which displayed bioresorbable and osteoconductive properties. Polydopamine as a coating has antimicrobial properties and facilitates protein adsorption and fibroblast adherence; therefore, it is very promising for improving soft-tissue integration around zirconia abutments. Graphene coatings have been shown to improve zirconia mechanical properties, leading to decreased wear and reduced occurrence of microfractures [54,61]. Nanoporous tantalum coatings can be fabricated by using tantalum nanotubes—recent studies have shown that they are able to improve osteoblasts' differentiation and proliferation processes, thus enhancing osseointegration. Moreover, ZrO_2/TaNS surfaces promote protein adsorption and hydrophilicity [62].

UV treatment of zirconia leads to electron excitation, which increases the surface free energy and hence also the wettability of zirconia. The available literature shows that treating zirconia with UV light for 12 or 15 min improves osteoblast attachment, proliferation, and differentiation. It also causes an increase in the osseointegration speed, bone volume, and bone-to-implant contact [15,54].

5. Discussion

We believe that the relatively scarce use of zirconia implants, when compared to titanium implants, can be associated with the early mentions of possible fractures. The majority of research papers focusing on zirconia implants' survival rates have been conducted on one-piece implants. Currently, one-piece implants are hardly used, regardless of the material they are made of. One-piece zirconia implants pioneered the way for zirconia implants overall and displayed rather good clinical results, but had some significant limitations. Two-piece implants allow for the use of screw-retained restorations, which allow reintervention if necessary and are not associated with the risk of cement residues remaining in the peri-implant tissues. Moreover, they allow for the use of different prosthetic abutment designs (angulations) and more predictable reconstructive surgeries, if necessary.

There are, however, some aspects that we authors find relevant when considering early two-piece zirconia implants too. First of all, the first two-piece zirconia implants were used together with titanium prosthetic abutments. As was mentioned earlier in this text, the differences in their material properties may have led to some of the technical complications occurring—screwing titanium into a zirconia implant would cause some tensions that titanium could withstand thanks to it being more plastic and able to adapt its shape, while the same forces could cause the zirconia to fracture. Currently, zirconia implants are usually paired with zirconia abutments, so the differences appear to be less relevant. Nonetheless, the abutment is still connected using a titanium screw—more research is needed to confirm whether such a solution is suitable for long-term restorations. The position of the European Association of Osseointegration on this matter is that there is evidence of similar results for one-piece zirconia implants compared to titanium implants for the fixed replacement of one to three missing teeth. In contrast, currently available clinical data evaluating two-piece zirconia implants with an adhesively bonded implant–abutment interface suggest an inferior outcome. Data evaluating the clinical applicability of screw-retained solutions, even if revealing sufficient fracture resistance in laboratory investigations, are still missing [63].

It is worth noting here that, to omit the problems emerging as results of the high Young's modulus of Y-TZP, a company named Patent has created a system of two-piece tissue-level zirconia implants with fiberglass abutments cemented adhesively into the implants. The abutments can be customized to any desired shape using a high-speed handpiece before a crown is fabricated and cemented onto the abutment. Such a solution aims to attenuate masticatory forces transferred from the crown to the implant and minimize the risk of implant fracture. Using a cemented restoration instead of a screw-retained one minimizes the occurrence of possible problems associated with the use of metal screws. Such implants restored with all-ceramic single crowns have demonstrated no fractures, stable soft-tissue levels, and a survival rate of 94.1% in a 9-year follow-up [64]. Studies show that this method can also be applied successfully to perform immediate implantations and immediate loading [65,66].

Regardless of all of the aspects mentioned above, recent research on two-piece zirconia implants' clinical performance shows very good results. A meta-analysis by Roehling et al. estimated that zirconia dental implants after 5 years of observation displayed a mean survival rate of 97.2%, marginal bone loss of 1.1 mm, and a probing depth of 3 mm. This is a strong evidence that zirconia implants are a reliable treatment option [67]. Similarly to titanium, zirconia shows better clinical results when proper surface treatment techniques are applied [64,65]. A systematic review and meta-analysis by Padhye et al. concluded that there was no statistically significant difference between zirconia and titanium implant survival at 12 months, while the pink esthetic score was higher for zirconia. Zirconia implants have shown to present a lower inflammation rate compared to titanium implants due to lower bacterial attachment [68]. It is, however, worth noting that longer observations are needed to confirm zirconia implants' good outcomes. Research papers comparing zirconia and titanium implants still appear to be limited.

The causes for peri-implantitis are similar for titanium and zirconia dental implants. The methods of treating peri-implantitis, however, differ. As zirconia has different mechanical properties, mechanical debridement cannot be applied to zirconia implants that develop peri-implantitis. Er:YAG laser therapy is the most promising option in these cases [69].

Research has shown that microbial corrosion is not more intensive for TiZr or zirconia in comparison to commercially pure titanium implants [70]. The effect of different mouthwash solutions, fluoride ions, or chlorhexidine on titanium aging and corrosion have been mentioned and it is a known fact that corroded titanium surfaces can promote bacterial colonization, reduce the ability of host cells to attach and proliferate, and impair regeneration procedures overall [71,72]. Oral bacteria are also known to play a crucial role in the corrosion of dental implants [73]. This corrosion appears important as it correlates with the occurrence of peri-implantitis. It has been shown that fluorides and toothpaste abrasives together can affect the topography and roughness of titanium, which further increases bacterial adhesion [74]. Moreover, the presence of fluoride ions damages the protective layer made of titanium oxide. This further promotes corrosion and enhances the release of titanium compounds [75]. High concentrations of fluoride ions in oral cavities lead to the formation of hydrofluoric acid (HF), which strongly promotes the corrosion of titanium [76]. Increased levels of dissolved titanium are associated with peri-implantitis [77]. Relatively low concentrations of titanium ions show cytotoxic effects on epithelial cells and cause increased monocyte migration and increased inflammation of peri-implant tissues [78,79]. Ti also stimulates osteoclastogenesis directly and indirectly through the release of inflammatory cytokines (Il-6, IL-1β, TNFα), and increases the activity of osteoclasts. The inflammatory reaction spreads into areas not in direct contact with the titanium [80,81]. Despite signs that zirconia implants can also corrode and that zirconium was in fact found in oral mucosa in gingival tissues, the literature discussing zirconia implants' corrosion is relatively scarce [82]. Similarly, the literature concerning different factors that could potentially affect zirconia's corrosion is almost non-existent. Some studies do, in fact, describe the mechanisms of zirconia's wear: stress corrosion and chemical degradation. Stress corrosion is the slow transformation of surface particles to the monoclinic phase over time, while chemical degradation is a chemisorption of OH$^-$ from water at the surface of zirconia grains to form Y(OH)$_3$. As was written in the aforementioned study by Thomas et al., the oral cavity is an aqueous, electrochemical environment susceptible to various changes in pH, which can promote the corrosion of zirconia [83].

Oral hygiene products can contain various chemicals, whose effects on the corrosion of zirconia are not yet known. Taking this and all of the above into consideration, we authors of this narrative review believe that further research needs to be conducted on zirconia corrosion, especially in response to different concentrations of substances applied in daily oral hygiene.

6. Conclusions

Zirconia implants in general seem to present satisfactory mechanical properties, undoubtedly sufficient for clinical use. While some of their properties may cause difficulties, available solutions allow clinicians to provide successful treatment. Their osseointegration ability and biocompatibility are equally good or even superior to those of titanium implants. Many research papers suggest that superior esthetic outcomes, especially in the anterior region, can be achieved by using zirconia implants rather than titanium. Nonetheless, the available observations on zirconia implants are relatively scarce and more research needs to be conducted.

Author Contributions: Conceptualization, M.C.; methodology, M.C.; validation, W.S., M.D., T.G. and J.H.; formal analysis, W.S., M.D., T.G. and J.H.; investigation, M.C. and B.C.; data curation, M.C. and B.C.; writing—original draft preparation, M.C. and B.C.; writing—review and editing, W.S., M.D., T.G. and J.H.; supervision, W.S., T.G. and J.H. All authors have read and agreed to the published version of the manuscript.

Funding: This research was funded and supported by the Wrocław University, grant no. SUBZ.B040.24.008.

Institutional Review Board Statement: Not applicable.

Informed Consent Statement: Not applicable.

Data Availability Statement: Data can be made available on request.

Conflicts of Interest: The authors declare no conflicts of interest.

References

1. Sales, P.H.d.H.; Barros, A.W.P.; de Oliveira-Neto, O.B.; de Lima, F.J.C.; Carvalho, A.d.A.T.; Leão, J.C. Do zirconia dental implants present better clinical results than titanium dental implants? A systematic review and meta-analysis. *J. Stomatol. Oral Maxillofac. Surg.* **2023**, *124*, 101324. [CrossRef] [PubMed]
2. Olmedo, D.G.; Nalli, G.; Verdú, S.; Paparella, M.L.; Cabrini, R.L. Exfoliative cytology and titanium dental implants: A pilot study. *J. Periodontol.* **2013**, *84*, 78–83. [CrossRef]
3. Sadowsky, S.J. Has zirconia made a material difference in implant prosthodontics? A review. *Dent. Mater.* **2020**, *36*, 1–8. [CrossRef]
4. Lee, C.-T.; Huang, Y.-W.; Zhu, L.; Weltman, R. Prevalences of peri-implantitis and peri-implant mucositis: Systematic review and meta-analysis. *J. Dent.* **2017**, *62*, 1–12. [CrossRef] [PubMed]
5. Roehling, S.; Schlegel, K.A.; Woelfler, H.; Gahlert, M. Performance and outcome of zirconia dental implants in clinical studies: A meta-analysis. *Clin. Oral Implant. Res.* **2018**, *29*, 135–153. [CrossRef]
6. Gul, A.; Papia, E.; Naimi-Akbar, A.; Ruud, A.; von Steyern, P.V. Zirconia dental implants; the relationship between design and clinical outcome: A systematic review. *J. Dent.* **2024**, *143*, 104903. [CrossRef]
7. Christel, P.; Meunier, A.; Heller, M.; Torre, J.P.; Peille, C.N. Mechanical properties and short-term in-vivo evaluation of yttrium-oxide-partially-stabilized zirconia. *J. Biomed. Mater. Res.* **1989**, *23*, 45–61. [CrossRef]
8. Kongkiatkamon, S.; Rokaya, D.; Kengtanyakich, S.; Peampring, C. Current classification of zirconia in dentistry: An updated review. *PeerJ* **2023**, *11*, e15669. [CrossRef]
9. Hanawa, T. Zirconia versus titanium in dentistry: A review. *Dent. Mater. J.* **2020**, *39*, 24–36. [CrossRef]
10. Bapat, R.A.; Yang, H.J.; Chaubal, T.V.; Dharmadhikari, S.; Abdulla, A.M.; Arora, S.; Rawal, S.; Kesharwani, P. Review on synthesis, properties and multifarious therapeutic applications of nanostructured zirconia in dentistry. *RSC Adv.* **2022**, *12*, 12773–12793. [CrossRef] [PubMed]
11. Andreiotelli, M.; Wenz, H.J.; Kohal, R. Are ceramic implants a viable alternative to titanium implants? A systematic literature review. *Clin. Oral Implant. Res.* **2009**, *20*, 32–47. [CrossRef] [PubMed]

12. Hadzik, J.; Błaszczyszyn, A.; Gedrange, T.; Dominiak, M. Soft-Tissue Augmentation around Dental Implants with a Connective Tissue Graft (CTG) and Xenogeneic Collagen Matrix (CMX)—5-Year Follow-Up. *J. Clin. Med.* **2023**, *12*, 924. [CrossRef] [PubMed]
13. Hadzik, J.; Kubasiewicz-Ross, P.; Nawrot-Hadzik, I.; Gedrange, T.; Pitułaj, A.; Dominiak, M. Short (6 mm) and Regular Dental Implants in the Posterior Maxilla—7-Years Follow-up Study. *J. Clin. Med.* **2021**, *10*, 940. [CrossRef] [PubMed]
14. Hadzik, J.; Kubasiewicz-Ross, P.; Gębarowski, T.; Waloszczyk, N.; Maciej, A.; Stolarczyk, A.; Gedrange, T.; Dominiak, M.; Szajna, E.; Simka, W. An Experimental Anodized Titanium Surface for Transgingival Dental Implant Elements-Preliminary Report. *J. Funct. Biomater.* **2023**, *14*, 34. [CrossRef]
15. Kligman, S.; Ren, Z.; Chung, C.-H.; Perillo, M.A.; Chang, Y.-C.; Koo, H.; Zheng, Z.; Li, C. The impact of dental implant surface modifications on osseointegration and biofilm formation. *J. Clin. Med.* **2021**, *10*, 1641. [CrossRef]
16. Saini, M.; Singh, Y.; Arora, P.; Arora, V.; Jain, K. Implant biomaterials: A comprehensive review. *World J. Clin. Cases* **2015**, *3*, 52–57. [CrossRef]
17. Sivaraman, K.; Chopra, A.; Narayan, A.I.; Balakrishnan, D. Is zirconia a viable alternative to titanium for oral implant? A critical review. *J. Prosthodont. Res.* **2018**, *62*, 121–133. [CrossRef]
18. Almas, K.; Smith, S.; Kutkut, A. What is the best micro and macro dental implant topography? *Dent. Clin. N. Am.* **2019**, *63*, 447–460. [CrossRef]
19. Kohal, R.J.; Wolkewitz, M.; Tsakona, A. The effects of cyclic loading and preparation on the fracture strength of zirconium-dioxide implants: An in vitro investigation. *Clin. Oral Implant. Res.* **2011**, *22*, 808–814. [CrossRef]
20. Bethke, A.; Pieralli, S.; Kohal, R.-J.; Burkhardt, F.; Von Stein-Lausnitz, M.; Vach, K.; Spies, B.C. Fracture Resistance of Zirconia Oral Implants in Vitro: A Systematic Review and Meta-Analysis. *Materials* **2020**, *13*, 562. [CrossRef]
21. Chiou, L.-L.; Panariello, B.H.D.; Hamada, Y.; Gregory, R.L.; Blanchard, S.; Duarte, S. Comparison of in vitro biofilm formation on titanium and zirconia implants. *BioMed Res. Int.* **2023**, *2023*, 8728499. [CrossRef]
22. Al-Radha, A.S.D.; Dymock, D.; Younes, C.; O'Sullivan, D. Surface properties of titanium and zirconia dental implant materials and their effect on bacterial adhesion. *J. Dent.* **2012**, *40*, 146–153. [CrossRef]
23. Bermejo, P.; Sánchez, M.C.; Llama-Palacios, A.; Figuero, E.; Herrera, D.; Sanz Alonso, M. Biofilm formation on dental implants with different surface micro-topography: An in vitro study. *Clin. Oral Implant. Res.* **2019**, *30*, 725–734. [CrossRef] [PubMed]
24. Bermejo, P.; Sánchez, M.C.; Llama-Palacios, A.; Figuero, E.; Herrera, D.; Sanz, M. Topographic characterization of multispecies biofilms growing on dental implant surfaces: An in vitro model. *Clin. Oral Implant. Res.* **2019**, *30*, 229–241. [CrossRef]
25. Aldesoki, M.; Keilig, L.; Dörsam, I.; Evers-Dietze, B.; Elshazly, T.M.; Bourauel, C. Trueness and precision of milled and 3D printed root-analogue implants: A comparative in vitro study. *J. Dent.* **2023**, *130*, 104425. [CrossRef] [PubMed]
26. Grech, J.; Antuneş, E. Zirconia in dental prosthetics: A literature review. *J. Mater. Res. Technol.* **2019**, *8*, 4956–4964. [CrossRef]
27. Arnaud, G. The truth about zirconia. *Dent. Technol.* 80, 59–72. Available online: https://www.bnddental.com/wp-content/uploads/2023/05/everythingyouveeverwantedtoknowaboutzirconia.pdf (accessed on 22 August 2024).
28. Muñoz-Saldaña, J.; Balmori-Ramírez, H.; Jaramillo-Vigueras, D.; Iga, T.; Schneider, G.A. Mechanical properties and low-temperature aging of tetragonal zirconia polycrystals processed by hot isostatic pressing. *J. Mater. Res.* **2003**, *18*, 2415–2426. [CrossRef]
29. Stawarczyk, B.; Ozcan, M.; Trottmann, A.; Hämmerle, C.H.F.; Roos, M. Evaluation of flexural strength of hipped and presintered zirconia using different estimation methods of Weibull statistics. *J. Mech. Behav. Biomed. Mater.* **2012**, *10*, 227–234. [CrossRef] [PubMed]
30. Davidowitz, G.; Kotick, P.G. The use of CAD/CAM in dentistry. *Dent. Clin. N. Am.* **2011**, *55*, 559–570. [CrossRef] [PubMed]
31. Regish, K.M.; Sharma, D.; Prithviraj, D.R. An overview of immediate root analogue zirconia implants. *J. Oral Implant.* **2013**, *39*, 225–233. [CrossRef]
32. Nakai, H.; Inokoshi, M.; Nozaki, K.; Komatsu, K.; Kamijo, S.; Liu, H.; Shimizubata, M.; Minakuchi, S.; Van Meerbeek, B.; Vleugels, J.; et al. Additively manufactured zirconia for dental applications. *Materials* **2021**, *14*, 3694. [CrossRef]
33. Jiang, X.; Zhu, Y.; Liu, Z.; Tian, Z.; Zhu, S. Association between diabetes and dental implant complications: A systematic review and meta-analysis. *Acta Odontol. Scand.* **2021**, *79*, 9–18. [CrossRef] [PubMed]
34. Fiorillo, L.; Cicciù, M.; Tözüm, T.F.; D'Amico, C.; Oteri, G.; Cervino, G. Impact of bisphosphonate drugs on dental implant healing and peri-implant hard and soft tissues: A systematic review. *BMC Oral Health* **2022**, *22*, 291. [CrossRef]
35. Monje, A.; González-Martín, O.; Ávila-Ortiz, G. Impact of peri-implant soft tissue characteristics on health and esthetics. *J. Esthet. Restor. Dent.* **2023**, *35*, 183–196. [CrossRef] [PubMed]
36. Werny, J.G.; Sagheb, K.; Diaz, L.; Kämmerer, P.W.; Al-Nawas, B.; Schiegnitz, E. Does vitamin D have an effect on osseointegration of dental implants? A systematic review. *Int. J. Implant. Dent.* **2022**, *8*, 16. [CrossRef]
37. Cruz, M.B.; Silva, N.; Marques, J.F.; Mata, A.; Silva, F.S.; Caramês, J. Biomimetic Implant Surfaces and Their Role in Biological Integration—A Concise Review. *Biomimetics* **2022**, *7*, 74. [CrossRef] [PubMed]
38. Wennerberg, A.; Albrektsson, T. Effects of titanium surface topography on bone integration: A systematic review. *Clin. Oral Implant. Res.* **2009**, *20* (Suppl. S4), 172–184. [CrossRef]
39. Gupta, S.; Noumbissi, S.; Kunrath, M.F. Nano modified zirconia dental implants: Advances and the frontiers for rapid osseointegration. *Med. Devices Sens.* **2020**, *3*, e10076. [CrossRef]
40. Yamano, S.; Ma, A.K.-Y.; Shanti, R.M.; Kim, S.-W.; Wada, K.; Sukotjo, C. The influence of different implant materials on human gingival fibroblast morphology, proliferation, and gene expression. *Int. J. Oral Maxillofac. Implant.* **2011**, *26*, 1247–1255.

41. Cionca, N.; Hashim, D.; Mombelli, A. Zirconia dental implants: Where are we now, and where are we heading? *Periodontology 2000* **2017**, *73*, 241–258. [CrossRef] [PubMed]
42. Matos, G.R.M. Surface roughness of dental implant and osseointegration. *J. Maxillofac. Oral Surg.* **2021**, *20*, 1–4. [CrossRef] [PubMed]
43. Pellegrini, G.; Francetti, L.; Barbaro, B.; Del Fabbro, M. Novel surfaces and osseointegration in implant dentistry. *J. Investig. Clin. Dent.* **2018**, *9*, e12349. [CrossRef] [PubMed]
44. Lee, J.W.Y.; Bance, M.L. Physiology of Osseointegration. *Otolaryngol. Clin. N. Am.* **2019**, *52*, 231–242. [CrossRef]
45. Zetterqvist, L.; Feldman, S.; Rotter, B.; Vincenzi, G.; Wennström, J.L.; Chierico, A.; Stach, R.M.; Kenealy, J.N. A prospective, multicenter, randomized-controlled 5-year study of hybrid and fully etched implants for the incidence of peri-implantitis. *J. Periodontol.* **2010**, *81*, 493–501. [CrossRef]
46. Albouy, J.-P.; Abrahamsson, I.; Persson, L.G.; Berglundh, T. Spontaneous progression of ligatured induced peri-implantitis at implants with different surface characteristics. An experimental study in dogs II: Histological observations. *Clin. Oral Implant. Res.* **2009**, *20*, 366–371. [CrossRef] [PubMed]
47. Harawaza, K.; Cousins, B.; Roach, P.; Fernandez, A. Modification of the surface nanotopography of implant devices: A translational perspective. *Mater. Today Bio* **2021**, *12*, 100152. [CrossRef]
48. Pu, Z.; Jing, X.; Yang, C.; Wang, F.; Ehmann, K.F. Wettability modification of zirconia by laser surface texturing and silanization. *Int. J. Appl. Ceram. Technol.* **2020**, *17*, 2182–2192. [CrossRef]
49. Kubasiewicz-Ross, P.; Dominiak, M.; Gedrange, T.; Botzenhart, U.U. Zirconium: The material of the future in modern implantology. *Adv. Clin. Exp. Med.* **2017**, *26*, 533–537. [CrossRef] [PubMed]
50. Kubasiewicz-Ross, P.; Hadzik, J.; Dominiak, M. Osseointegration of zirconia implants with 3 varying surface textures and a titanium implant: A histological and micro-CT study. *Adv. Clin. Exp. Med.* **2018**, *27*, 1173–1179. [CrossRef]
51. Gredes, T.; Kubasiewicz-Ross, P.; Gedrange, T.; Dominiak, M.; Kunert-Keil, C. Comparison of surface modified zirconia implants with commercially available zirconium and titanium implants: A histological study in pigs. *Implant Dent.* **2014**, *23*, 502–507. [CrossRef]
52. Han, A.; Tsoi, J.; Matinlinna, J.; Chen, Z. Influence of Grit-Blasting and Hydrofluoric Acid Etching Treatment on Surface Characteristics and Biofilm Formation on Zirconia. *Coatings* **2017**, *7*, 130. [CrossRef]
53. Al Qahtani, W.M.S.; Schille, C.; Spintzyk, S.; Al Qahtani, M.S.; Engel, E.; Geis-Gerstorfer, J.; Rupp, F.; Scheideler, L. Effect of surface modification of zirconia on cell adhesion, metabolic activity and proliferation of human osteoblasts. *BioMed. Tech.* **2017**, *62*, 75–87. [CrossRef]
54. Schünemann, F.H.; Galárraga-Vinueza, M.E.; Magini, R.; Fredel, M.; Silva, F.; Souza, J.C.; Zhang, Y.; Henriques, B. Zirconia surface modifications for implant dentistry. *Mater. Sci. Eng. C Mater. Biol. Appl.* **2019**, *98*, 1294–1305. [CrossRef] [PubMed]
55. Zhang, F.; Monzavi, M.; Li, M.; Čokić, S.; Manesh, A.; Nowzari, H.; Vleugels, J.; Van Meerbeek, B. Fracture analysis of one/two-piece clinically failed zirconia dental implants. *Dent. Mater.* **2022**, *38*, 1633–1647. [CrossRef]
56. Scherrer, S.S.; Mekki, M.; Crottaz, C.; Gahlert, M.; Romelli, E.; Marger, L.; Durual, S.; Vittecoq, E. Translational research on clinically failed zirconia implants. *Dent. Mater.* **2019**, *35*, 368–388. [CrossRef] [PubMed]
57. La Monaca, G.; Iezzi, G.; Cristalli, M.P.; Pranno, N.; Sfasciotti, G.L.; Vozza, I. Comparative Histological and Histomorphometric Results of Six Biomaterials Used in Two-Stage Maxillary Sinus Augmentation Model after 6-Month Healing. *Biomed Res. Int.* **2018**, *2018*, 9430989. [CrossRef]
58. Taniguchi, Y.; Kakura, K.; Yamamoto, K.; Kido, H.; Yamazaki, J. Accelerated Osteogenic Differentiation and Bone Formation on Zirconia with Surface Grooves Created with Fiber Laser Irradiation. *Clin. Implant Dent. Relat. Res.* **2016**, *18*, 883–894. [CrossRef]
59. Matys, J.; Botzenhart, U.; Gedrange, T.; Dominiak, M. Thermodynamic effects after Diode and Er:YAG laser irradiation of grade IV and V titanium implants placed in bone—An ex vivo study. Preliminary report. *Biomed. Tech.* **2016**, *61*, 499–507. [CrossRef]
60. Paradowska-Stolarz, A.; Mikulewicz, M.; Laskowska, J.; Karolewicz, B.; Owczarek, A. The importance of chitosan coatings in dentistry. *Mar. Drugs* **2023**, *21*, 613. [CrossRef]
61. Laranjeira, M.S.; Carvalho, A.; Pelaez-Vargas, A.; Hansford, D.; Ferraz, M.P.; Coimbra, S.; Costa, E.; Santos-Silva, A.; Fernandes, M.H.; Monteiro, F.J. Modulation of human dermal microvascular endothelial cell and human gingival fibroblast behavior by micropatterned silica coating surfaces for zirconia dental implant applications. *Sci. Technol. Adv. Mater.* **2014**, *15*, 025001. [CrossRef]
62. Wu, L.; Dong, Y.; Yao, L.; Liu, C.; Al-Bishari, A.M.; Yie, K.H.R.; Zhang, H.; Liu, J.; Wu, G. Nanoporous tantalum coated zirconia implant improves osseointegration. *Ceram. Int.* **2020**, *46*, 17437–17448. [CrossRef]
63. Balmer, M.; Payer, M.; Kohal, R.-J.; Spies, B.C. EAO position paper: Current level of evidence regarding zirconia implants in clinical trials. *Int. J. Prosthodont.* **2022**, *35*, 560–566. [CrossRef]
64. Brunello, G.; Rauch, N.; Becker, K.; Hakimi, A.R.; Schwarz, F.; Becker, J. Two-piece zirconia implants in the posterior mandible and maxilla: A cohort study with a follow-up period of 9 years. *Clin. Oral Implant. Res.* **2022**, *33*, 1233–1244. [CrossRef] [PubMed]
65. Karapataki, S.; Vegh, D.; Payer, M.; Fahrenholz, H.; Antonoglou, G.N. Clinical Performance of Two-Piece Zirconia Dental Implants After 5 and Up to 12 Years. *Int. J. Oral Maxillofac. Implant.* **2023**, *38*, 1105–1114. [CrossRef] [PubMed]
66. Brüll, F.; van Winkelhoff, A.J.; Cune, M.S. Zirconia dental implants: A clinical, radiographic, and microbiologic evaluation up to 3 years. *Int. J. Oral Maxillofac. Implant.* **2014**, *29*, 914–920. [CrossRef]

67. Roehling, S.; Gahlert, M.; Bacevic, M.; Woelfler, H.; Laleman, I. Clinical and radiographic outcomes of zirconia dental implants—A systematic review and meta-analysis. *Clin. Oral Implant. Res.* **2023**, *34*, 112–124. [CrossRef] [PubMed]
68. Padhye, N.M.; Calciolari, E.; Zuercher, A.N.; Tagliaferri, S.; Donos, N. Survival and success of zirconia compared with titanium implants: A systematic review and meta-analysis. *Clin. Oral Investig.* **2023**, *27*, 6279–6290. [CrossRef]
69. Schwarz, F.; John, G.; Hegewald, A.; Becker, J. Non-surgical treatment of peri-implant mucositis and peri-implantitis at zirconia implants: A prospective case series. *J. Clin. Periodontol.* **2015**, *42*, 783–788. [CrossRef]
70. Siddiqui, D.A.; Guida, L.; Sridhar, S.; Valderrama, P.; Wilson, T.G.; Rodrigues, D.C. Evaluation of oral microbial corrosion on the surface degradation of dental implant materials. *J. Periodontol.* **2019**, *90*, 72–81. [CrossRef]
71. Faverani, L.P.; Barao, V.A.R.; Pires, M.F.A.; Yuan, J.C.-C.; Sukotjo, C.; Mathew, M.T.; Assunção, W.G. Corrosion kinetics and topography analysis of Ti-6Al-4V alloy subjected to different mouthwash solutions. *Mater. Sci. Eng. C Mater. Biol. Appl.* **2014**, *43*, 1–10. [CrossRef]
72. Chen, W.-Q.; Zhang, S.-M.; Qiu, J. Surface analysis and corrosion behavior of pure titanium under fluoride exposure. *J. Prosthet. Dent.* **2020**, *124*, 239.e1–239.e8. [CrossRef] [PubMed]
73. Sridhar, S.; Wilson, T.G.; Palmer, K.L.; Valderrama, P.; Mathew, M.T.; Prasad, S.; Jacobs, M.; Gindri, I.M.; Rodrigues, D.C. In vitro investigation of the effect of oral bacteria in the surface oxidation of dental implants. *Clin. Implant Dent. Relat. Res.* **2015**, *17*, e562–e575. [CrossRef] [PubMed]
74. Fais, L.M.G.; Fernandes-Filho, R.B.; Pereira-da-Silva, M.A.; Vaz, L.G.; Adabo, G.L. Titanium surface topography after brushing with fluoride and fluoride-free toothpaste simulating 10 years of use. *J. Dent.* **2012**, *40*, 265–275. [CrossRef] [PubMed]
75. Insua, A.; Galindo-Moreno, P.; Miron, R.J.; Wang, H.-L.; Monje, A. Emerging factors affecting peri-implant bone metabolism. *Periodontology 2000* **2024**, *94*, 27–78. [CrossRef]
76. Noguti, J.; de Oliveira, F.; Peres, R.C.; Renno, A.C.M.; Ribeiro, D.A. The role of fluoride on the process of titanium corrosion in oral cavity. *Biometals* **2012**, *25*, 859–862. [CrossRef]
77. Safioti, L.M.; Kotsakis, G.A.; Pozhitkov, A.E.; Chung, W.O.; Daubert, D.M. Increased levels of dissolved titanium are associated with peri-implantitis—A cross-sectional study. *Br. Dent. J.* **2017**, *223*, 203. [CrossRef]
78. Noumbissi, S.; Scarano, A.; Gupta, S. A literature review study on atomic ions dissolution of titanium and its alloys in implant dentistry. *Materials* **2019**, *12*, 368. [CrossRef]
79. Makihira, S.; Mine, Y.; Nikawa, H.; Shuto, T.; Iwata, S.; Hosokawa, R.; Kamoi, K.; Okazaki, S.; Yamaguchi, Y. Titanium ion induces necrosis and sensitivity to lipopolysaccharide in gingival epithelial-like cells. *Toxicol. Vitr.* **2010**, *24*, 1905–1910. [CrossRef]
80. Eger, M.; Hiram-Bab, S.; Liron, T.; Sterer, N.; Carmi, Y.; Kohavi, D.; Gabet, Y. Mechanism and Prevention of Titanium Particle-Induced Inflammation and Osteolysis. *Front. Immunol.* **2018**, *9*, 2963. [CrossRef]
81. Revell, P.A. The combined role of wear particles, macrophages and lymphocytes in the loosening of total joint prostheses. *J. R. Soc. Interface* **2008**, *5*, 1263–1278. [CrossRef]
82. Cionca, N.; Meyer, J.; Michalet, S.; Varesio, E.; Hashim, D. Quantification of titanium and zirconium elements in oral mucosa around healthy dental implants: A case—Control pilot study. *Clin. Oral Investig.* **2023**, *27*, 4715–4726. [CrossRef] [PubMed]
83. Thomas, A.; Sridhar, S.; Aghyarian, S.; Watkins-Curry, P.; Chan, J.Y.; Pozzi, A.; Rodrigues, D.C. Corrosion behavior of zirconia in acidulated phosphate fluoride. *J. Appl. Oral Sci.* **2016**, *24*, 52–60. [CrossRef] [PubMed]

Disclaimer/Publisher's Note: The statements, opinions and data contained in all publications are solely those of the individual author(s) and contributor(s) and not of MDPI and/or the editor(s). MDPI and/or the editor(s) disclaim responsibility for any injury to people or property resulting from any ideas, methods, instructions or products referred to in the content.

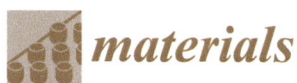

Review

From Tooth Adhesion to Bioadhesion: Development of Bioabsorbable Putty-like Artificial Bone with Adhesive to Bone Based on the New Material "Phosphorylated Pullulan"

Ko Nakanishi [1], Tsukasa Akasaka [1], Hiroshi Hayashi [2], Kumiko Yoshihara [3], Teppei Nakamura [4], Mariko Nakamura [5], Bart Van Meerbeek [6] and Yasuhiro Yoshida [1,*]

[1] Department of Biomaterials and Bioengineering, Faculty of Dental Medicine, Hokkaido University, Kita 13, Nishi 7, Kita-ku, Sapporo 060-8586, Hokkaido, Japan; nakanishi-ko@den.hokudai.ac.jp (K.N.); akasaka@den.hokudai.ac.jp (T.A.)

[2] Section for Dental Innovation, Faculty of Dental Medicine, Hokkaido University, Kita13, Nishi7, Kita-ku, Sapporo 060-8586, Hokkaido, Japan; h.hayashi@den.hokudai.ac.jp

[3] Health and Medical Research Institute, National Institute of Advanced Industrial Science and Technology, 2217-14 Hayashi-Cho, Takamaysu 761-0395, Kagawa, Japan; kumiko.yoshihara@aist.go.jp

[4] Department of Applied Veterinary Science, Faculty of Veterinary Medicine, Hokkaido University, Kita 18, Nishi 9, Kita-ku, Sapporo 060-0818, Hokkaido, Japan; nakamurate@vetmed.hokudai.ac.jp

[5] School of Clinical Psychology, Kyushu University of Medical Science, 1714-1 Yoshinocho, Nobeoka 882-8508, Miyazaki, Japan; marin@phoenix.ac.jp

[6] KU Leuven, Department of Oral Health Sciences, BIOMAT & UZ Leuven, Dentistry, 3000 Leuven, Belgium; bart.vanmeerbeek@kuleuven.be

* Correspondence: yasuhiro@den.hokudai.ac.jp; Tel.: +81-11-706-4249

Abstract: Bioabsorbable materials have a wide range of applications, such as scaffolds for regenerative medicine and cell transplantation therapy and carriers for drug delivery systems. Therefore, although many researchers are conducting their research and development, few of them have been used in clinical practice. In addition, existing bioabsorbable materials cannot bind to the body's tissues. If bioabsorbable materials with an adhesive ability to biological tissues can be made, they can ensure the mixture remains fixed to the affected area when mixed with artificial bone or other materials. In addition, if the filling material in the bone defect is soft and uncured, resorption is rapid, which is advantageous for bone regeneration. In this paper, the development and process of a new bioabsorbable material "Phosphorylated pullulan" and its capability as a bone replacement material were demonstrated. Phosphorylated pullulan, which was developed based on the tooth adhesion theory, is the only bioabsorbable material able to adhere to bone and teeth. The phosphorylated pullulan and β-TCP mixture is a non-hardening putty. It is useful as a new resorbable bone replacement material with an adhesive ability for bone defects around implants.

Keywords: phosphorylated pullulan; bioabsorbable polymers; artificial bone; bio-adhesion

Citation: Nakanishi, K.; Akasaka, T.; Hayashi, H.; Yoshihara, K.; Nakamura, T.; Nakamura, M.; Meerbeek, B.V.; Yoshida, Y. From Tooth Adhesion to Bioadhesion: Development of Bioabsorbable Putty-like Artificial Bone with Adhesive to Bone Based on the New Material "Phosphorylated Pullulan". *Materials* 2024, 17, 3671. https://doi.org/10.3390/ma17153671

Academic Editors: Ines Despotović and Bongju Kim

Received: 20 May 2024
Revised: 13 July 2024
Accepted: 17 July 2024
Published: 25 July 2024

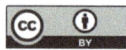

Copyright: © 2024 by the authors. Licensee MDPI, Basel, Switzerland. This article is an open access article distributed under the terms and conditions of the Creative Commons Attribution (CC BY) license (https://creativecommons.org/licenses/by/4.0/).

1. Introduction

Autogenous bone has the highest bone regenerative capacity among bone replacement materials for treating bone defects [1]. Autogenous bone contains many components important for bone formation, such as calcium phosphate, collagen, bone morphogenetic proteins (BMPs), and cells associated with bone formation. However, the amount of autogenous bone that can be harvested is limited, so artificial bone made of calcium phosphate is widely used as an alternative material because it has inorganic components and a crystal structure similar to natural bone [2,3]. However, the ability of this material to regenerate bone is inferior to that of autogenous bone. Also, in dental clinical practice, granule-type artificial bone with a particle diameter of several hundred μm is used. The resorption of artificial bone to replace natural bone occurs more rapidly with fine particles than with larger granules, resulting in the faster healing of bone defects. However, fine particles induce inflammation [4]. In addition, when they enter blood vessels, they may move into the bloodstream and accumulate in the body's organs. Thus, granular artificial bones currently on the market have a particle diameter of several hundred μm to several mm because they have been developed based on products that have obtained regulatory approval.

Nonetheless, new medical technology cannot advance by merely following predecessors. Different approaches from existing products are required to develop materials with novel functions. For this purpose, a collaboration with different fields is essential. Therefore, we used a strategy to develop bioabsorbable polymers that adhere to bone based on basic research on tooth adhesion. Here, we describe a novel bone replacement material with bone-adhesive properties and enhanced resorbability in the body.

2. Current Artificial Bone

There are various types of artificial bones made of calcium phosphate, such as granules, blocks, and hardened pastes. Granular artificial bones are the most common in dental clinical practice. Block-type artificial bone is intended to maintain its shape but could be slow to be absorbed in the body. Hardened pastes should be slightly resorbed because areas in contact with blood are insufficiently hardened, but the hardened body is basically nonabsorbable. Initially, non-absorbable hydroxyapatite was used for granular artificial bone. However, as the demand for resorption and bone replacement increased for artificial bone, β-tricalcium·phosphate (β-TCP) granules were introduced into clinical practice as an absorbable artificial bone. Subsequently, artificial bones that consisted mainly of apatite carbonate—the same inorganic component of natural bone [5]—and octacalcium phosphate (OCP), a precursor of apatite carbonate [6,7], were developed.

2.1. Hydroxyapatite

Hydroxyapatite ($Ca_{10}(PO_4)_6(OH)$) has a composition similar to that of bone. Therefore, it is highly biocompatible and can adhere directly to bone tissue during bone formation when used as a bone replacement material [8]. Nevertheless, simply synthesized hydroxyapatite does not contain trace elements such as Na^+ and Mg^{2+}, which are found in real bone. Over the past few decades, many researchers have demonstrated that adding various ionic substituents to synthetic hydroxyapatite can produce a mineral composition similar to that of natural bone tissue [9–12]. Furthermore, synthetic hydroxyapatite cannot reproduce the porosity that distinguishes it from natural bone. Synthesized hydroxyapatite is characterized by very slow or no absorption, due to a high Ca/P rate and crystallinity [13]. A limitation of using hydroxyapatite as a bone replacement material is its low mechanical strength and fragility. Nanotechnology is an important solution to this fragility. Reducing the size of the crystalline grain of hydroxyapatite to a smaller or nano-sized one can decrease internal pores and defects. Moreover, material plasticity can be improved by increasing the number of grain boundaries [14]. Zhao et al. successfully improved carbon nanofiber-reinforced hydroxyapatite by reducing the size of the hydroxyapatite grain using spark plasma sintering [15]. Zeng et al. also reduced the grain size of hydroxyapatite and improved its mechanical properties by creating hydroxyapatite using a two-step sintering process in the digital light processing of 3D printing technology [16].

2.2. β-Tricalcium Phosphate (β-TCP)

β-TCP (β-$Ca_3(PO_4)_2$) has been widely used as a bone replacement material for more than 30 years [17,18]. It has good osteoconductivity due to its porosity, which promotes vascular fiber growth and osteogenic cell adhesion [13,19]. β-TCP also has low immunogenicity in the body and high biosafety [13]. As described earlier, it possesses excellent properties as a bone replacement material. In their study of dog alveolar bone, Nakajima et al. found that the bone regenerative potential of β-TCP was comparable with that of freeze-dried heterologous bone, autogenous bone, demineralized freeze-dried bone, and inorganic bovine bone [20]. Galois et al. considered the use of β-TCP an optimal choice for moderate bone defects [18]. β-TCP is considered to be absorbed by osteoclasts, and its Ca/P rate is lower than that of hydroxyapatite, resulting in faster degradation and absorption in the body than hydroxyapatite [21]. However, its absorption rate is said to be unpredictable [22]. Furthermore, the interconnected porous structures of β-TCP can improve vascularization; however, the mechanical strength is reduced [23], thereby limiting applications and sites of use [17]. Recent studies have attempted to improve the mechanical strength of β-TCP using liquid phase sintering to increase the density of the material [24,25].

2.3. Carbonate Apatite

Carbonate apatite is the inorganic composition of bone, and the material was developed based on the idea that a material with a composition similar to that of bone would be best suited for use as a bone replacement material. Nevertheless, it was initially difficult to develop carbonate apatite because it pyrolyzes and therefore cannot be sintered. When calcium carbonate blocks are immersed in a phosphate solution, carbonate apatite precipitates on the block surface. This reaction progresses over time, transforming the entire block into carbonate apatite [5]. Using this technique, carbonate apatite can be produced in a clinically usable form. Carbonate apatite dissolves in the weak acid produced in the osteoclast Howship's lacuna, similar to bone, and is absorbed faster than hydroxyapatite [26]. Clinical trials have shown that carbonate apatite is an effective bone substitute in human sinus lifts [27]. Carbonate apatite also possesses an excellent bone-conducting ability. It has been reported that carbonate apatite has better bone formation around it in beagle dogs than hydroxyapatite and possesses a superior osteoconductive ability [28]. This superior osteoconductivity is due to intercellular signaling from osteoclasts. In other words, osteoclasts that absorb carbonate apatite release liquid factors known as clastokines that activate osteoblasts [29]. Hydroxyapatite is not absorbed or is absorbed slowly, causing this phenomenon to rarely occur. Moreover, osteoblasts are activated in carbonate apatite through information transfer between the material and the cells. When bone marrow cells are seeded on the surface of carbonate apatite and analyzed for differentiation markers to osteoblasts, they show higher values than those on the hydroxyapatite surface [30]. In recent years, carbonate apatite has been verified to be more porous in order to improve its osteogenic potential [31].

2.4. Octacalcium Phosphate (OCP)

OCP ($Ca_8H_2(PO_4)6-5H_2O$) was suggested as a precursor for hydroxyapatite formation from an aqueous solution [6] and for apatite crystal formation during mineralization [7]. OCP is composed of a repetitive apatite layer, similar to that in Ca-deficient hydroxyapatite, and a hydrated layer containing large amounts of water molecules, such as dicalcium phosphate dihydrate (DCPD) [7]. It was anticipated that OCP could be used as a bone replacement material because of its potential to function as a precursor phase, as observed in the formation of OCP before hydroxyapatite deposition in bone collagen matrices in natural bone [32]. When implanted in the mouse calvaria, OCP demonstrated earlier bone formation than hydroxyapatite and Ca-deficient hydroxyapatite. Furthermore, bone apatite crystals are bonded by OCP crystals during bone formation [33]. The degradation of OCP might be primarily caused by the phagocytosis of osteoclasts because OCP induces osteoclast formation in an in vitro coculture system of osteoblasts and osteoclast precursor cells [34]. The degradation rate of OCP is faster than that of hydroxyapatite and tricalcium phosphate [35]. Based on these characteristics of OCP, a human clinical trial was conducted using a mixture of OCP and collagen, which demonstrated effective results in cases of sinus floor elevation in the 1st and 2nd stages, socket preservation, cyst, and alveolar cleft procedures [36]. Various forms of OCP, including granules [37] and blocks [38], and various additives, such as biodegradable polymers [36,39,40] and ions [41,42], are now considered to improve the effectiveness of OCP.

3. Problems and Solutions of Existing Artificial Bone

These artificial bones made of calcium phosphate are osteoconductive [43], as mentioned above. Bone regeneration occurs around granules with a size of several μm before they are resorbed, and the artificial bone remains in the bone. Therefore, it is suggested that even β-TCP, carbonate apatite, and OCP also take a long time to be completely absorbed and replaced by natural bone in the human body. The larger the particle size of the resorbable artificial bone, the longer it takes for its resorption and replacement by natural bone in the human body. This may help reduce bone resorption but is a major problem for controlling infection because the implanted material that remains in the body increases the risk of infection (Figure 1). For example—as is evident in catheter infections—it is challenging to control infection when an implanted artificial material is exposed to the outside of the body and becomes infected. The same happens to artificial bones. When the infection on artificial bones cannot be controlled, they must be removed by curettage.

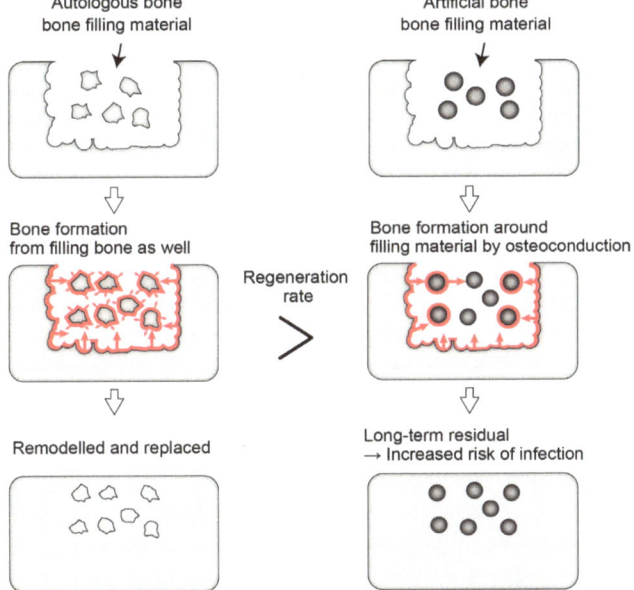

Figure 1. Differences between autogenous bone and artificial bone in terms of bone formation and resorption patterns. Red arrows show the direction of bone regeneration.

Furthermore, granular artificial bones are difficult to handle. Mixing with saline or blood improves handling but only slightly. The size of bone defects in dentistry is smaller than in orthopedics, and the particle size of the granular artificial bone used in dentistry is also smaller. Besides the oral cavity being a site of easy infection, osteogenesis of the alveolar ridge requires placing a granular artificial bone to fit the defect, which increases the procedure's difficulty. In addition, a smaller granular artificial bone results in greater risks of dispersal, migration, and leakage through the incision.

4. Necessity of Bioabsorbable Polymers that Adhere to Calcium Phosphate

A bioabsorbable material that can adhere to bone and artificial bone components is desirable because it would allow the artificial bone to be easily placed in a bone defect by mixing the artificial bone with it and making it patty-like. In addition to the improved handling due to enhanced formability and adhesion to the bone surface, the stronger sealing of the natural bone–artificial bone interface is expected to improve the treatment outcome. Furthermore, if the material that adheres to calcium phosphate can maintain its gel state in the body, and if fine powdered artificial bone can be used, it leads to the development of new artificial bone able to be quickly absorbed and replaced with natural bone. The rapid resorption of bone replacement materials and their substitution with natural bone is ideal for reducing the risk of infection.

5. Problems with Existing Bioabsorbable Polymers

For the above reasons, the development of absorbable polymers that can adhere to calcium phosphate, which is an inorganic component of bone and is used as artificial bone, has been long awaited. If such materials are available, innovative materials that contribute to implant therapy, such as putty-like artificial bones with short-term resorption and replacement by mixing a bioabsorbable polymer and calcium phosphate fine powder, are expected to be developed. However, materials that can be absorbed and replaced with tissue in the body are challenging to put to practical use. Collagen, hyaluronic acid, polyglycolic acid, and polylactic acid are still widely used as absorbable polymers that can be implanted in the body, but none of them can adhere to bone or tooth.

6. Development of Non-Animal-Derived Bioabsorbable Polymers

Phosphorylated pullulan was developed to solve problems with the above existing artificial bones. The raw material, pullulan, is a natural polysaccharide produced by fermentation with black yeast; it has water-soluble properties among polysaccharides and can be processed into powder and film. Pullulan has been used in the food industry for many years and was introduced as a non-gelatin capsule material in pharmaceuticals because its firm had excellent gas barrier properties when bovine spongiform encephalopathy became a major problem in Japan [44].

We hypothesized that introducing numerous phosphate groups into pullulan would yield a bioabsorbable material that adheres to bone (Table 1).

Table 1. Comparison of bioabsorbable polymers.

	Natural Bioabsorbable Polymer		Synthetic Bioabsorbable Polymer		New Bioabsorbable Polymer
	Collagen	Hyaluronic Acid	Polyglycolic Acid	Polylactic Acid	Phosphorylated Pullulan
Biocompatibility	Good	Good	Cause inflammation during degradation	Cause inflammation during degradation	Good
Adhesion	Poor	Adhesion to wet tissue	Poor	Poor	Good
Gamma sterilization	Poor	Poor	Poor	Poor	Good
Manufacturing Method	Animal-derived	Animal-derived	Synthesis	Synthesis	Non-animal-derived

7. Design Concept of Phosphorylated Pullulan

Mechanical mating between the adherend and the material and chemical bonding at the interface are important factors when considering adhesive materials. Mechanical mating is considered to affect the adhesive strength in tooth bonding, whereas chemical bonding contributes to bond durability [45]. It is also a concept agreed upon by all those involved in adhesive bonding that adhesive materials need to have adequate wettability to achieve a high adhesive strength. Pullulan is easily soluble in water, and the viscosity of a pullulan aqueous solution is very low among polysaccharides. Using pullulan as a backbone reduces viscosity, compared to other polysaccharides, leading to the creation of a bioabsorbable polymer with adequate wettability.

Phosphorylated pullulan was created based on the tooth adhesion theory, using pullulan as a backbone. In the dental field, the progress of tooth adhesion is particularly remarkable. It is well known that adhesive techniques and materials are applied to most current dental treatments, such as aesthetic restorations, including resin fillings, posts and cores, crown restorations, orthodontics, fixing mobile teeth, and bonding fractured teeth. Many dental adhesives have been developed and applied in clinical practice with repeated improvements and development. Nowadays, two types of adhesives (glass ionomer cement and resin cement) are commonly used in dental treatment.

Glass ionomer cement is cured by an acid-base reaction between polycarboxylic acid and the cations leached from aluminosilicate glass and can chemically bond well to untreated enamel and dentin. Thus, glass ionomer cements have the ability to chemically bond to the tooth [46]. Compared to resin-based tooth-bonding systems, glass ionomer cement can be used even in areas with insufficient moisture protection, which is thought to be largely due to the characteristics of polycarboxylic acid (the main component). Polycarboxylic acid has many carboxy groups that chemically bond to teeth. In addition, many of these carboxyl groups are considered to make glass ionomer cements somewhat hydrophilic and not as hydrophobic as resin-based tooth-bonding systems.

Furthermore, we previously compared three adhesive monomers: 4-methacryloxyethyl trimellitic acid (4-MET), 2-methacryloxyethyl phenyl hydrogen phosphate (phenyl-P), and 10-methacryloyloxydecyl dihydrogen phosphate (10-MDP) and found that 10-MDP had the best chemical bonding ability [47]. Since this report, the effectiveness of the divalent phosphate group has become clear, and 10-MDP has been used in various tooth-bonding systems. These results of basic research on tooth adhesion [48–52] allowed for the development of phosphorylated pullulan, based on the idea of "introducing a large number of phosphate groups into a polysaccharide with high water solubility" (Figure 2).

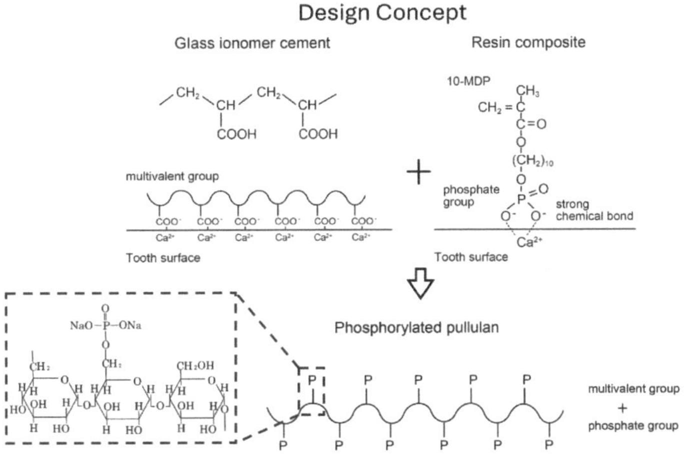

Figure 2. Design concept.

8. Efficacy of Phosphorylated Pullulan as a Bone Replacement Material

Phosphorylated pullulan has been applied in various ways, due to its characteristics, such as a coating agent for implants [53–56] and as a direct pulp-capping material [57–59]. Takahata et al. [60] and Morimoto et al. [61] reported the efficacy of phosphorylated pullulan as a bone replacement material (Table 2).

Takahata et al. [60] implanted a mixture of phosphorylated pullulan and β-TCP in the medullary cavity of a mouse femur, a rabbit ulnar, and a porcine vertebral body bone and evaluated bone formation. A histological evaluation of the medullary cavity of a mouse femur revealed that only phosphorylated pullulan remained 2 weeks after implantation. Five weeks after implantation, bone marrow replacement was observed in the group implanted with only phosphorylated pullulan, and bone formation was observed in the group implanted with a mixture of pullulan phosphate and β-TCP. After 8 weeks, additional new bone was observed in the group implanted with a mixture of phosphorylated pullulan and β-TCP, but no bone formation was observed in the group implanted with only phosphorylated pullulan. The effects of Biopex-R and a mixture of phosphorylated pullulan and β-TCP in the rabbit ulnar were compared. Eight weeks after implantation, a micro-CT showed that Biopex-R separated from the existing bone in the group implanted with only Biopex-R, but the bone defect was completely amended in the group implanted with a mixture of phosphorylated pullulan and β-TCP. Histologically, the type of this bone formation is classified as endochondral ossification. On the other hand, the formation of new bone in the porcine vertebral body bone in the group with no treatment for the defect and the group implanted with Biopex-R was not confirmed by micro-CT, even after 8 weeks. By contrast, a mixture of phosphorylated pullulan and β-TCP implanted in the bone defect of the porcine vertebral body bone resulted in new bone formation at 8 weeks. Histologically, only fibrotic changes were observed in the untreated group, even at 8 weeks. However, in the group implanted with a mixture of phosphorylated pullulan and β-TCP, the new bone began to form at 4 weeks, and trabecular bone formation began at 8 weeks. Based on this, Takahata et al. concluded that phosphorylated pullulan alone cannot induce bone formation, but when used together with β-TCP, it promotes bone remodeling.

Table 2. Application development of phosphorylated pullulan.

Clinical Application	Study	Materials and Methods	Note
Dental implant	Cardoso et al. (2014) [53]	Titanium plates treated with phosphorylated pullulan were implanted in the rabbit tibia.	The bone fraction in areas 100 μm remote from the implant surface was higher than in the water treatment.
	Cardoso et al. (2017) [54]	Phosphorylated pullulan-coated implants were implanted in the pig skull bone.	The titanium implant surface with phosphorylated pullulan could improve the mineralization of the implant–bone interface.
	Cardoso et al. (2017) [55]	Titanium implant treated with phosphorylated pullulan were implanted in the pig parietal bone.	The peri-implant bone formation and bone-to-implant contact were improved, compared to the water-treated group.
	Nagamoto et al. (2024) [56]	Cell culture on a titanium disk coated with phosphorylated pullulan.	Cell proliferation and calcification were improved by coating with phosphorylated pullulan.
Pulp-capping material	Pedano et al. (2018) [57]	Preparing the hydraulic calcium-silicate cement including phosphorylated pullulan and culturing human dental pulp cells using eluates from this cement.	The eluate of this cement stimulated the proliferation, migration, and odontogenic differentiation of human dental pulp cells.
	Pedano et al. (2020) [58]	An injectable phosphopullulan-based calcium-silicate cement was used for the pulp-capping material ex vivo and in vivo.	This cement stimulated the formation of fibrous tissue and mineralized foci ex vivo and promoted the inflammatory reaction and regeneration of the pulp–tissue interface.
	Islam et al. (2024) [59]	Calcium hydroxide including phosphorylate pullulan was applied to rat first molar cavities.	Calcium hydroxide including phosphorylate pullulan could have the potential to minimize pulpal inflammation and to promote mineralized tissue formation.
Bone replacement material	Takahata et al. (2015) [60]	A mixture of phosphorylated pullulan and β-TCP was implanted in the medullary cavity of a mouse femur, a rabbit ulnar, and porcine vertebral body bone.	Phosphorylated pullulan and β-TCP promoted bone remodeling when phosphorylated pullulan and β-TCP were used together.
	Morimoto et al. (2023) [61]	A mixture of phosphorylated pullulan and β-TCP was implanted in rats with a tibia bone defect.	Phosphorylated pullulan mixed with β-TCP exhibited osteoblast anchorage and osteoconductive ability as a scaffold material and might induce calcification by retaining calcium

Morimoto et al. [61] implanted a mixture of phosphorylated pullulan and β-TCP in rats with a tibia bone defect, analyzed the bone regeneration process histologically and microstructurally, and reported that phosphorylated pullulan may have osteoconductive and calcification retention properties. These authors created a cylindrical bone defect with a diameter of 2.0 mm in the tibia of 10-week-old rats, and two materials, namely β-TCP (mean granule diameter = 100–250 μm) and a mixture of pullulan phosphate and β-TCP (4:6, w/w), were implanted in the animals and compared. A group with the bone defect but without an implant was used as the control. In the control group, a large amount of new bone was observed in the bone defect after 1 week, but these new bones decreased 4 weeks after implantation. By contrast, in the β-TCP implantation group, β-TCP granules were surrounded by numerous fibroblast-like cells 1 week after implantation; then, new bone was formed at 2 to 4 weeks, using β-TCP as a scaffold. This new bone remained in the bone defect 4 weeks after implantation. In the group implanted with a mixture of phosphorylated pullulan and β-TCP, numerous fibroblast-like cells were observed around phosphorylated pullulan and β-TCP 1 week after implantation, and new bone was observed on the phosphorylated pullulan and β-TCP granules after 2 weeks (Figures 3 and 4).

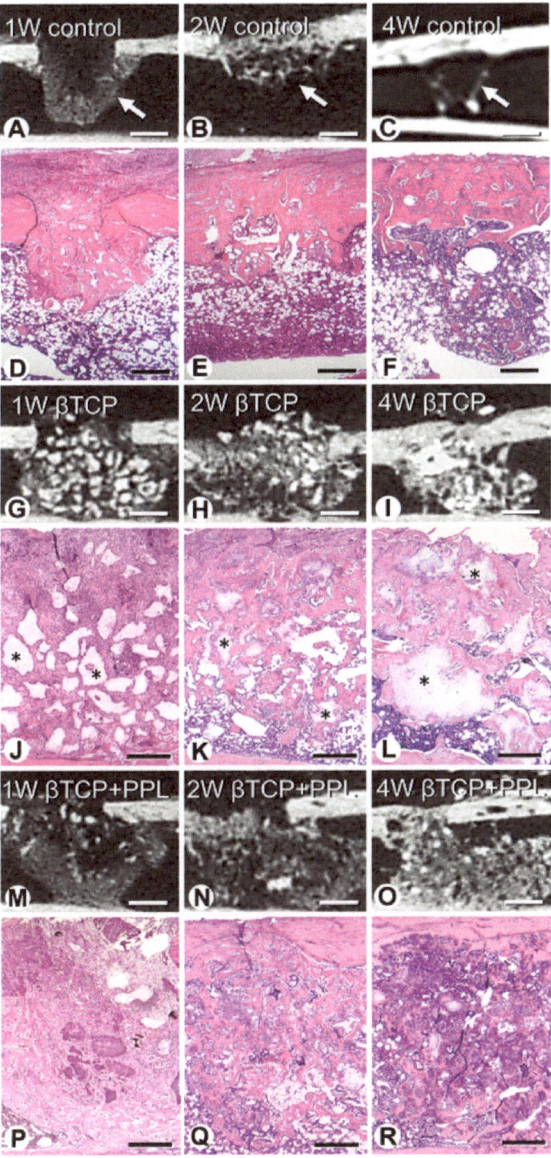

Figure 3. Micro-CT images and histological images after the implantation of β-TCP or β-TCP and phosphorylated pullulan in rats with a tibia bone defect. (**A–C**): Micro-CT images of the control group.

(**D–F**): Histological images of the control group. (**G–I**): Micro-CT images of the β-TCP implantation group. (**J–L**): Histological images of the β-TCP implantation group. (**M–O**): Micro-CT images of the group implanted with a mixture of phosphorylated pullulan and β-TCP. (**P–R**): Histological images of the group implanted with a mixture of phosphorylated pullulan and β-TCP. *: β-TCP. Bar, (**A–C,G–I,M–O**): 1 mm, (**D–F**): 400 μm, (**J–L,P–R**): 300 μm. (Morimoto et al. Frontiers in Bioengineering and Biotechnology, 2023, 11 [61]).

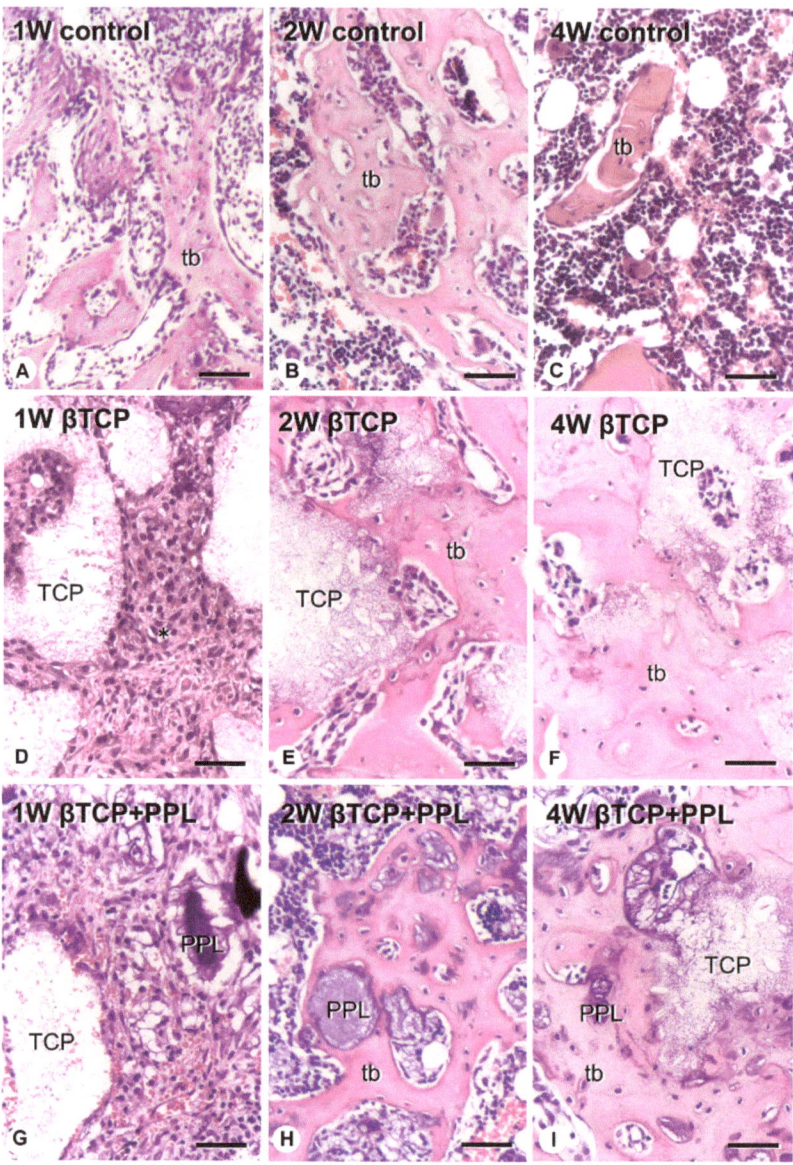

Figure 4. High-magnification histological images after the implantation of β-TCP or β-TCP and phosphorylated pullulan in rats with a tibia bone defect. (**A–C**): Control group. (**D–F**): β-TCP implantation group. (**G–I**): Group implanted with a mixture of phosphorylated pullulan and β-TCP. tb: trabecular bone, TCP: β-TCP, PPL: phosphorylated pullulan. Bar: 30 μm (Morimoto et al. Frontiers in Bioengineering and Biotechnology, 2023, 11 [61]).

Osteoblast lineage cells and bone formation at the bone regeneration site were evaluated by immunohistochemistry for alkaline phosphatase (ALP) (Figure 5A–F), PHOSPHO1 (Figure 5G–L), and osteopontin (Figure 5M–R). In the control group (without implantation), numerous ALP-positive osteoblast lineage cells (osteoblasts and preosteoblasts) were present on the surface of new bone during all postoperative periods. Moreover, PHOSPHO1-positive reactions—expressed on osteoblasts responsible for matrix vesicular calcification—were also observed on the bone surface. In the β-TCP implantation group, ALP-positive osteoblast lineage cells and PHOSPHO1-positive osteoblasts were found on the surface of new bone and on β-TCP granules. Thereafter, ALP-positive osteoblast lineage cells were more widespread on the surface of new bone than PHOSPHO1-positive osteoblasts. In the group implanted with a mixture of phosphorylated pullulan and β-TCP, ALP-positive osteoblast lineage cells and PHOSPHO1-positive osteoblasts were located not only on the surfaces of β-TCP and new bone but also on phosphorylated pullulan. Interestingly, osteopontin, a bone matrix protein able to bind to crystalline calcium, was found on the surfaces of β-TCP and phosphorylated pullulan, suggesting that phosphorylated pullulan may function as a scaffold material for osteoblast fixation. In addition, an analysis using strain-derived osteoblasts (MC3T3-E1 cells) suggested that phosphorylated pullulan did not have a direct effect on osteoblast differentiation or function.

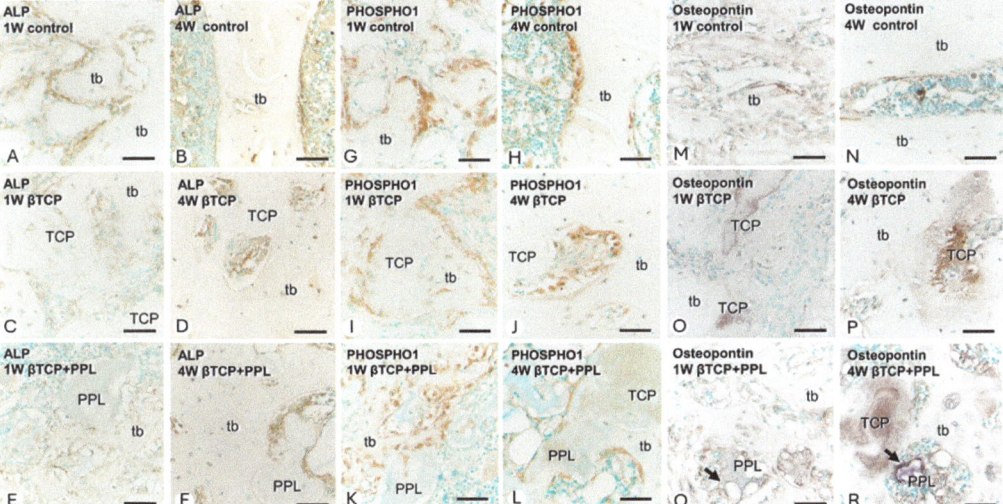

Figure 5. Immunohistochemical staining images of ALP, PHOSPHO1, and osteopontin. (**A–F**): ALP, (**G–L**): PHOSPHO1, (**M–R**): osteopontin. tb: trabecular bone, TCP: β-TCP, PPL: phosphorylated pullulan, Arrow: immunohistochemical reaction of PPL surface, Bar: 30 μm (Morimoto et al. Frontiers in Bioengineering and Biotechnology, 2023, 11, partially modified [61]).

On the other hand, bone resorption was evaluated by osteoclast distribution using tartrate-resistant acid phosphatase (TRAP) staining. Osteoclasts were most abundant 2 weeks after implantation in all groups and then decreased. In the control group, TRAP-positive osteoclasts were located on the surface of the new bone, whereas in the β-TCP implantation group, they were located not only on the new bone but also on β-TCP. In the group implanted with a mixture of phosphorylated pullulan and β-TCP, the TRAP-positive osteoclasts were mainly located on the surface of the new bone, but some osteoclasts were also localized on the surface of phosphorylated pullulan.

In addition, Morimoto et al. evaluated calcification related to phosphorylated pullulan using the elemental mapping of calcium and phosphorus using an electron probe microanalyzer. Calcium and phosphorus were not detected in the phosphorylated pullulan

1 week after implantation, but 2 to 4 weeks after implantation, calcium and phosphorus deposits were observed on the phosphorylated pullulan surface and the surrounding new bone. Although the X-ray fluorescence intensity of phosphorus on phosphorylated pullulan 2 and 4 weeks after implantation did not differ, the X-ray fluorescence intensity of calcium increased over time (Figure 6). These results suggested that calcium might accumulate in phosphorylated pullulan and the surrounding new bone over time. Microstructural analysis revealed the formation of numerous calcite spheres and needle-like calcified crystal masses on the surface of pullulan phosphate (Figure 7), suggesting that phosphorylated pullulan may have an affinity for crystalline calcium and may promote calcification.

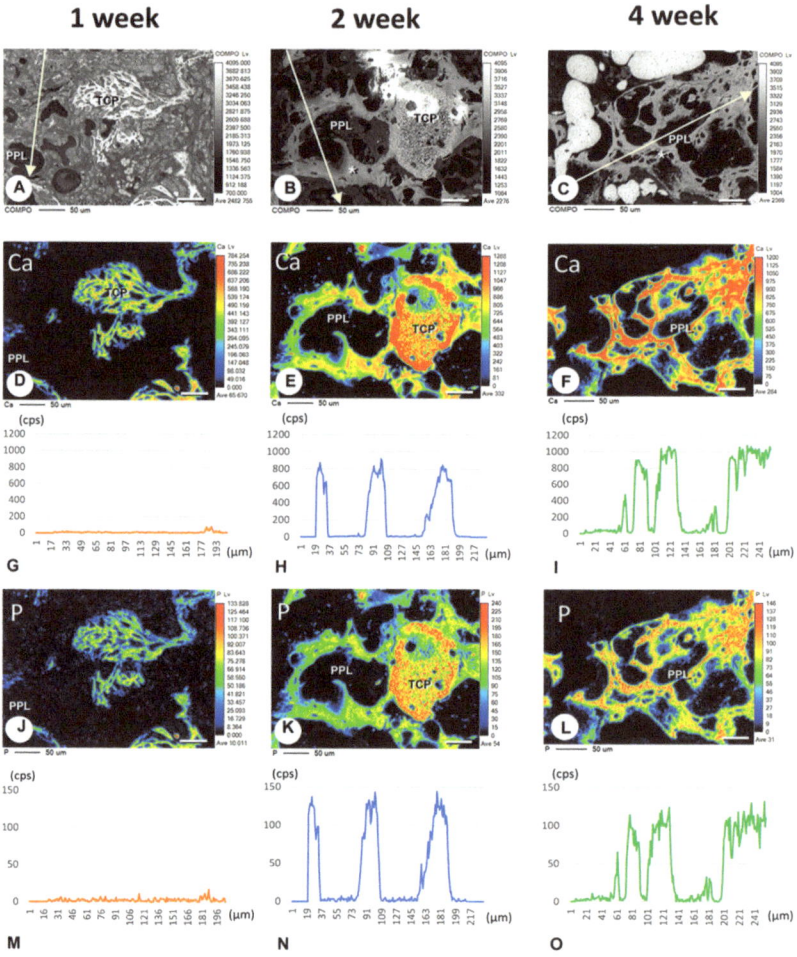

Figure 6. Results of the electron probe micro-analyzer measurement after the implantation of β-TCP and phosphorylated pullulan in rats with a tibia bone defect. The composition (COMPO) images of the bone defect region at 1, 2, and 4 weeks after the implantation of β-TCP and phosphorylated pullulan are illustrated. (A–C) The electron probe micro-analyzes images of Ca (D–F) and P (J–L) are shown in (D–F) and (J–L). The intensities of X-ray fluorescence from Ca (G–I) and P (M–O) on the arrow in (A–C) are displayed in (G–I) and (M–O). In 2 and 4 weeks after implantation, calcium and phosphorus deposits were observed on the phosphorylated pullulan surface and surrounding new bone (E,F,K,L). PPL: phosphorylated pullulan, TCP: β-TCP, *: trabecular bone Bar, (A–F,J–L): 50 μm (Morimoto et al. Frontiers in Bioengineering and Biotechnology, 2023, 11 [61]).

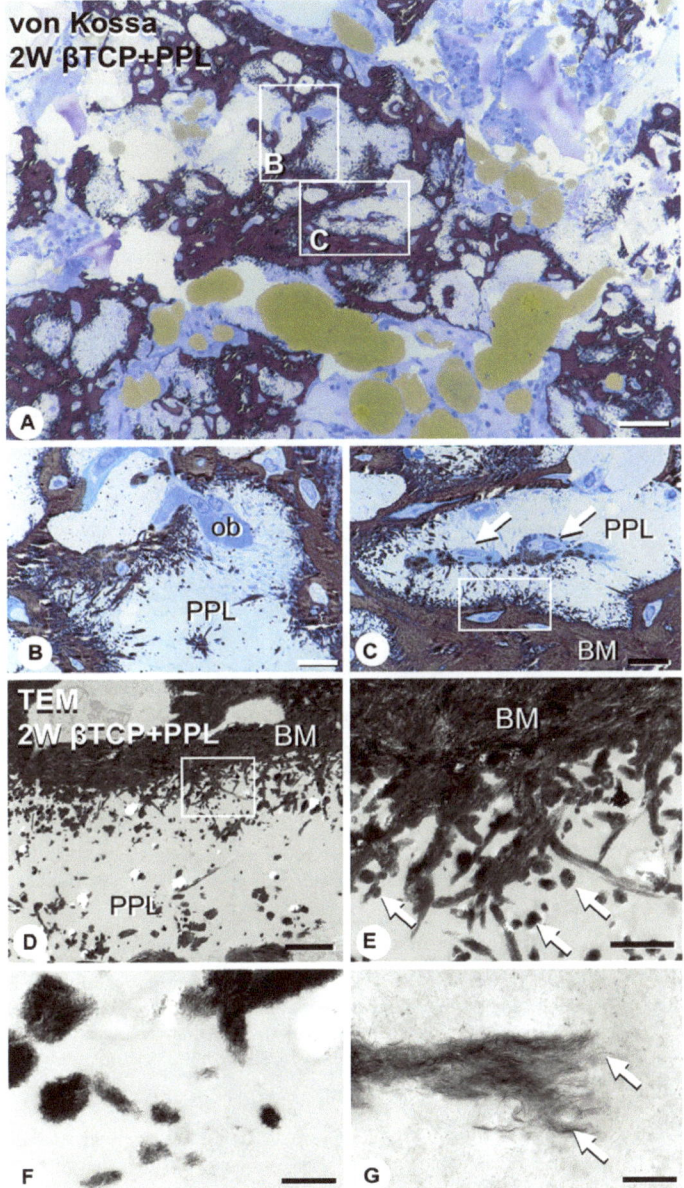

Figure 7. Von Kossa-stained images and transmission electron microscope images after the implantation of β-TCP and phosphorylated pullulan in rats with a tibia bone defect. (**A**): the low magnified image of von Cossa, (**B**,**C**): the high magnified image on the frame part in (**A**), arrow shows osteoblasts, (**D**): the low magnified TEM image, (**E**): the high magnified image on the frame part in (**D**), arrow shows calcified nodules, (**F**,**G**): the high magnified image from (**E**), arrow shows fine needle-like mineral crystals, PPL: phosphorylated pullulan, BM: bone matrix, ob: osteoblast Bar, (**A**): 50 μm, (**B**,**C**): 10 μm, (**D**): 3 μm, (**E**): 1 μm, (**F**): 0.3 μm, (**G**): 0.2 μm. (Morimoto et al. Frontiers in Bioengineering and Biotechnology, 2023, 11 [61]).

Based on these results, Morimoto et al. speculated that phosphorylated pullulan mixed with β-TCP exhibited osteoblast anchorage and osteoconductive ability as a scaffold material and might induce calcification by retaining calcium.

9. Application of Phosphorylated Pullulan to Areas Other than Hard Tissue

Phosphorylated pullulan is promoted for practical use in fields other than hard tissue. The submucosal injection material used for the endoscopic resection of gastric and other cancers is one of them. Satomi et al. confirmed that submucosal injection material-based phosphorylated pullulan could demonstrate a tissue elevation volume and duration comparable to existing submucosal injection materials using pigs and has high operability [62]. From these characteristics, the submucosal injection material containing phosphorylated pullulan as a key component has been approved under the Pharmaceutical Affairs Law in Japan and is marketed as "enRise".

10. Conclusions

Phosphorylated pullulan is an unprecedented bioabsorbable material with bone adhesion properties developed based on experience in basic research on dental adhesive materials. It also can assist with bone formation. From these characteristics, phosphorylated pullulan is expected to be a novel bone replacement material. Currently, clinical trials of this material will begin in 2024 as a Class IV medical device, which is defined by the Japanese Act on Securing Quality, Efficacy, and Safety of Products Including Pharmaceuticals and Medical Devices. In addition to bone, phosphorylated pullulan is also expected to be used as a scaffold for the regeneration of various organs, as a carrier for drug delivery systems, and in a wide range of applications as a bioabsorbable material able to replace collagen and hyaluronic acid.

Author Contributions: Conceptualization, K.N. and Y.Y.; methodology, K.N. and Y.Y.; formal analysis, K.N., T.A. and Y.Y.; investigation, K.N., H.H., K.Y., T.N. and M.N.; data curation, K.N.; writing—original draft preparation, K.N., T.A. and Y.Y.; writing—review and editing, K.N., H.H., B.V.M. and Y.Y.; visualization, K.N. and T.A.; supervision, B.V.M. and Y.Y.; project administration, Y.Y.; funding acquisition, Y.Y. All authors have read and agreed to the published version of the manuscript.

Funding: Parts of these researches were supported by AMED under Grant Numbers JP18hk0102055 and JP22hk0102087 and by the Suzuken Memorial Foundation.

Data Availability Statement: The raw data supporting the conclusions of this article will be made available by the authors on request.

Conflicts of Interest: The corresponding author, Yasuhiro Yoshida, owns shares in Japan MDB Solutions Co., Inc., the manufacturer and distributor of the endoscopic submucosal injection material "enRize". The remaining authors declare that the research was conducted in the absence of any commercial or financial relationships that could be construed as a potential conflict of interest.

References

1. Noelken, R.; Pausch, T.; Wagner, W.; Al-Nawas, B. Peri-implant defect grafting with autogenous bone or bone graft material in immediate implant placement in molar extraction sites—1- to 3-year results of a prospective randomized study. *Clin. Oral Implant. Res.* **2020**, *31*, 1138–1148. [CrossRef] [PubMed]
2. Cheng, L.; Lin, T.; Khalaf, A.T.; Zhang, Y.; He, H.; Yang, L.; Zhu, J.; Shi, Z. The preparation and application of calcium phosphate biomedical composites in filling of weight-bearing bone defects. *Sci. Rep.* **2021**, *11*, 4283. [CrossRef]
3. Graham, S.M.; Leonidou, A.; Aslam-Pervez, N.; Hamza, A.; Panteliadis, P.; Heliotis, M.; Mantalaris, A.; Tsiridis, E. Biological therapy of bone defects: The immunology of bone allo-transplantation. *Expert Opin. Biol. Ther.* **2010**, *10*, 885–901. [CrossRef] [PubMed]
4. Yang, C.; Wang, W.; Zhu, K.; Liu, W.; Luo, Y.; Yuan, X.; Wang, J.; Cheng, T.; Zhang, X. Lithium chloride with immunomodulatory function for regulating titanium nanoparticle-stimulated inflammatory response and accelerating osteogenesis through suppression of MAPK signaling pathway. *Int. J. Nanomed.* **2019**, *14*, 7475–748823. [CrossRef]
5. Ishikawa, K. Bone Substitute Fabrication Based on Dissolution-Precipitation Reactions. *Materials* **2010**, *3*, 1138–1155. [CrossRef]
6. Brown, W.E.; Smith, J.P.; Lehr, J.R.; Frazier, A.W. Octacalcium Phosphate and Hydroxyapatite: Crystallographic and Chemical Relations between Octacalcium Phosphate and Hydroxyapatite. *Nature* **1962**, *196*, 1050–1055. [CrossRef]

7. Suzuki, O.; Hamai, R.; Sakai, S. The material design of octacalcium phosphate bone substitute: Increased dissolution and osteogenecity. *Acta Biomater.* **2023**, *158*, 1–11. [CrossRef]
8. Kattimani, V.S.; Kondaka, S.; Lingamaneni, K.P. Hydroxyapatite—Past, Present, and Future in Bone Regeneration. *Bone Tissue Regen. Insights* **2016**, *7*. [CrossRef]
9. Ratnayake, J.T.B.; Mucalo, M.; Dias, G.J. Substituted hydroxyapatites for bone regeneration: A review of current trends. *J. Biomed. Mater. Res. B Appl. Biomater.* **2017**, *105*, 1285–1299. [CrossRef]
10. Shepherd, J.H.; Shepherd, D.V.; Best, S.M. Substituted hydroxyapatites for bone repair. *J. Mater. Sci. Mater. Med.* **2012**, *23*, 2335–2347. [CrossRef]
11. Bracci, B.; Torricelli, P.; Panzavolta, S.; Boanini, E.; Giardino, R.; Bigi, A. Effect of Mg^{2+}, Sr^{2+}, and Mn^{2+} on the chemico-physical and in vitro biological properties of calcium phosphate biomimetic coatings. *J. Inorg. Biochem.* **2009**, *103*, 1666–1674. [CrossRef] [PubMed]
12. Landi, E.; Logroscino, G.; Proietti, L.; Tampieri, A.; Sandri, M.; Sprio, S. Biomimetic Mg-substituted hydroxyapatite: From synthesis to in vivo behaviour. *J. Mater. Sci. Mater. Med.* **2008**, *19*, 239–247. [CrossRef] [PubMed]
13. Zhao, R.; Yang, R.; Cooper, P.R.; Khurshid, Z.; Shavandi, A.; Ratnayake, J. Bone Grafts and Substitutes in Dentistry: A Review of Current Trends and Developments. *Molecules* **2021**, *26*, 3007. [CrossRef] [PubMed]
14. Feng, P.; Zhao, R.; Tang, W.; Yang, F.; Tian, H.; Peng, S.; Pan, H.; Shuai, C. Structural and Functional Adaptive Artificial Bone: Materials, Fabrications, and Properties. *Adv. Funct. Mater.* **2023**, *33*, 2214726. [CrossRef]
15. Zhao, X.; Chen, X.; Gui, Z.; Zheng, J.; Yang, P.; Liu, A.; Wei, S.; Yang, Z. Carbon fiber reinforced hydroxyapatite composites with excellent mechanical properties and biological activities prepared by spark plasma sintering. *Ceram. Int.* **2020**, *46*, 27446–27456. [CrossRef]
16. Zeng, Y.; Yan, Y.; Yan, H.; Liu, C.; Li, P.; Dong, P.; Zhao, Y.; Chen, J. 3D printing of hydroxyapatite scaffolds with good mechanical and biocompatible properties by digital light processing. *J. Mater. Sci.* **2018**, *53*, 6291–6301. [CrossRef]
17. Fernandez de Grado, G.; Keller, L.; Idoux-Gillet, Y.; Wagner, Q.; Musset, A.M.; Benkirane-Jessel, N.; Bornert, F.; Offner, D. Bone substitutes: A review of their characteristics, clinical use, and perspectives for large bone defects management. *J. Tissue Eng.* **2018**, *9*, 2041731418776819. [CrossRef] [PubMed]
18. Galois, L.; Mainard, D.; Delagoutte, J.P. Beta-tricalcium phosphate ceramic as a bone substitute in orthopaedic surgery. *Int. Orthop.* **2002**, *26*, 109. [PubMed]
19. Frayssinet, P.; Mathon, D.; Lerch, A.; Autefage, A.; Collard, P.; Rouquet, N. Osseointegration of composite calcium phosphate bioceramics. *J. Biomed. Mater. Res.* **2000**, *50*, 125–130. [CrossRef]
20. Nakajima, Y.; Fiorellini, J.; Kim, D.; Weber, H. Regeneration of standardized mandibular bone defects using expanded polytetrafluoroethylene membrane and various bone fillers. *Int. J. Periodontics Restor. Dent.* **2007**, *27*, 151–159.
21. Wang, W.; Yeung, K.W.K. Bone grafts and biomaterials substitutes for bone defect repair: A review. *Bioact. Mater.* **2017**, *2*, 224. [CrossRef]
22. Nery, E.B.; LeGeros, R.Z.; Lynch, K.L.; Lee, K. Tissue response to biphasic calcium phosphate ceramic with different ratios of HA/beta TCP in periodontal osseous defects. *J. Periodontol.* **1992**, *63*, 729–735. [CrossRef] [PubMed]
23. Bhatt, R.A.; Rozental, T.D. Bone Graft Substitutes. *Hand Clin.* **2012**, *28*, 457–468. [CrossRef]
24. Zhang, H.; Xiong, Y.; Dong, L.; Shen, Y.; Hu, H.; Gao, H.; Zhao, S.; Li, X. Microstructural, mechanical properties and strengthening mechanism of DLP produced β-tricalcium phosphate scaffolds by incorporation of MgO/ZnO/58S bioglass. *Ceram. Int.* **2021**, *47*, 25863–25874. [CrossRef]
25. Bose, S.; Bhattacharjee, A.; Banerjee, D.; Boccaccini, A.R.; Bandyopadhyay, A. Influence of random and designed porosities on 3D printed tricalcium phosphate-bioactive glass scaffolds. *Addit. Manuf.* **2021**, *40*, 101895. [CrossRef]
26. Ishikawa, K.; Hayashi, K. Carbonate apatite artificial bone. *Sci. Technol. Adv. Mater.* **2021**, *22*, 683–694. [CrossRef] [PubMed]
27. Kudoh, K.; Fukuda, N.; Kasugai, S.; Tachikawa, N.; Koyano, K.; Matsushita, Y.; Ogino, Y.; Ishikawa, K.; Miyamoto, Y. Maxillary Sinus Floor Augmentation Using Low-Crystalline Carbonate Apatite Granules With Simultaneous Implant Installation: First-in-Human Clinical Trial. *J. Oral Maxillofac. Surg.* **2019**, *77*, e1–e985. [CrossRef]
28. Ishikawa, K. Carbonate apatite bone replacement: Learn from the bone. *J. Ceram. Soc. Jpn.* **2019**, *127*, 595–601. [CrossRef]
29. Ishikawa, K.; Miyamoto, Y.; Tsuchiya, A.; Hayashi, K.; Tsuru, K.; Ohe, G. Physical and Histological Comparison of Hydroxyapatite, Carbonate Apatite, and β-Tricalcium Phosphate Bone Substitutes. *Materials* **2018**, *11*, 1993. [CrossRef]
30. Nagai, H.; Kobayashi-Fujioka, M.; Fujisawa, K.; Ohe, G.; Takamaru, N.; Hara, K.; Uchida, D.; Tamatani, T.; Ishikawa, K.; Miyamoto, Y. Effects of low crystalline carbonate apatite on proliferation and osteoblastic differentiation of human bone marrow cells. *J. Mater. Sci. Mater. Med.* **2015**, *26*, 99. [CrossRef]
31. Elsheikh, M.; Kishida, R.; Hayashi, K.; Tsuchiya, A.; Shimabukuro, M.; Ishikawa, K. Effects of pore interconnectivity on bone regeneration in carbonate apatite blocks. *Regen. Biomater.* **2022**, *9*, rbac010. [CrossRef]
32. Suzuki, O.; Miyasaka, Y.; Sakurai, M.; Nakamura, M.; Kagayama, M. Bone Formation on Synthetic Precursors of Hydroxyapatite. *Tohoku J. Exp. Med.* **1991**, *164*, 37–50. [CrossRef] [PubMed]
33. Davies, E.; Müller, K.H.; Wong, W.C.; Pickard, C.J.; Reid, D.G.; Skepper, J.N.; Duer, M.J. Citrate bridges between mineral platelets in bone. *Proc. Natl. Acad. Sci. USA* **2014**, *111*, E1354–E1363. [CrossRef] [PubMed]

34. Takami, M.; Mochizuki, A.; Yamada, A.; Tachi, K.; Zhao, B.; Miyamoto, Y.; Anada, T.; Honda, Y.; Inoue, T.; Nakamura, M.; et al. Osteoclast differentiation induced by synthetic octacalcium phosphate through receptor activator of NF-kappaB ligand expression in osteoblasts. *Tissue Eng. Part A* **2009**, *15*, 3991–4000. [CrossRef]
35. Chow, L.C. Next generation calcium phosphate-based biomaterials. *Dent. Mater. J.* **2009**, *28*, 1–10. [CrossRef] [PubMed]
36. Kawai, T.; Kamakura, S.; Matsui, K.; Fukuda, M.; Takano, H.; Iino, M.; Ishikawa, S.; Kawana, H.; Soma, T.; Imamura, E.; et al. Clinical study of octacalcium phosphate and collagen composite in oral and maxillofacial surgery. *J. Tissue Eng.* **2020**, *11*, 2041731419896449. [CrossRef]
37. Komlev, V.S.; Barinov, S.M.; Bozo, I.I.; Deev, R.V.; Eremin, I.I.; Fedotov, A.Y.; Gurin, A.N.; Khromova, N.V.; Kopnin, P.B.; Kuvshinova, E.A.; et al. Bioceramics composed of octacalcium phosphate demonstrate enhanced biological behavior. *ACS Appl. Mater. Interfaces* **2014**, *6*, 16610–16620. [CrossRef] [PubMed]
38. Sugiura, Y.; Ishikawa, K. Fabrication of pure octacalcium phosphate blocks from dicalcium hydrogen phosphate dihydrate blocks via a dissolution–precipitation reaction in a basic solution. *Mater. Lett.* **2019**, *239*, 143–146. [CrossRef]
39. Hamada, S.; Mori, Y.; Shiwaku, Y.; Hamai, R.; Tsuchiya, K.; Baba, K.; Oizumi, I.; Kanabuchi, R.; Miyatake, N.; Aizawa, T.; et al. Octacalcium Phosphate/Gelatin Composite (OCP/Gel) Enhances Bone Repair in a Critical-sized Transcortical Femoral Defect Rat Model. *Clin. Orthop. Relat. Res.* **2022**, *480*, 2043–2055. [CrossRef]
40. Oizumi, I.; Hamai, R.; Shiwaku, Y.; Mori, Y.; Anada, T.; Baba, K.; Miyatake, N.; Hamada, S.; Tsuchiya, K.; Nishimura, S.; et al. Impact of simultaneous hydrolysis of OCP and PLGA on bone induction of a PLGA-OCP composite scaffold in a rat femoral defect. *Acta Biomater.* **2021**, *124*, 358–373. [CrossRef]
41. Shi, H.; Ye, X.; Wu, T.; Zhang, J.; Ye, J. Regulating the physicochemical and biological properties in vitro of octacalcium phosphate by substitution with strontium in a large doping range. *Mater. Today Chem.* **2017**, *5*, 81–91. [CrossRef]
42. Inoue, S.; Koshiro, K.; Yoshida, Y.; De Munck, J.; Nagakane, K.; Suzuki, K.; Sano, H.; Van Meerbeek, B. Hydrolytic stability of self-etch adhesives bonded to dentin. *J. Dent. Res.* **2005**, *84*, 1160–1164. [CrossRef] [PubMed]
43. Koyama, S.; Hamai, R.; Shiwaku, Y.; Kurobane, T.; Tsuchiya, K.; Takahashi, T.; Suzuki, O. Angio-osteogenic capacity of octacalcium phosphate co-precipitated with copper gluconate in rat calvaria critical-sized defect. *Sci. Technol. Adv. Mater.* **2022**, *23*, 120–139. [CrossRef] [PubMed]
44. LeGeros, R.Z. Calcium phosphate-based osteoinductive materials. *Chem. Rev.* **2008**, *108*, 4742–4753. [CrossRef] [PubMed]
45. Singh, R.S.; Jayr, N.; Singh, D.; Purewal, S.S.; Kennedy, J.F. Pullulan in pharmaceutical and cosmeceutical formulations: A review. *Int. J. Biol. Macromol.* **2023**, *231*, 123353. [CrossRef] [PubMed]
46. Yoshida, Y.; Van Meerbeek, B.; Nakayama, Y.; Snauwaert, J.; Hellemans, L.; Lambrechts, P.; Vanherle, G.; Wakasa, K. Evidence of chemical bonding at biomaterial-hard tissue interfaces. *J. Dent. Res.* **2000**, *79*, 709–714. [CrossRef] [PubMed]
47. Yoshida, Y.; Nagakane, K.; Fukuda, R.; Nakayama, Y.; Okazaki, M.; Shintani, H.; Inoue, S.; Tagawa, Y.; Suzuki, K.; De Munck, J.; et al. Comparative study on adhesive performance of functional monomers. *J. Dent. Res.* **2004**, *83*, 454–458. [CrossRef] [PubMed]
48. Yoshihara, K.; Yoshida, Y.; Nagaoka, N.; Fukegawa, D.; Hayakawa, S.; Mine, A.; Nakamura, M.; Minagi, S.; Osaka, A.; Suzuki, K.; et al. Nano-controlled molecular interaction at adhesive interfaces for hard tissue reconstruction. *Acta Biomater.* **2010**, *6*, 3573–3582. [CrossRef] [PubMed]
49. Yoshihara, K.; Yoshida, Y.; Hayakawa, S.; Nagaoka, N.; Irie, M.; Ogawa, T.; Van Landuyt, K.; Osaka, A.; Suzuki, K.; Minagi, S.; et al. Nanolayering of phosphoric acd ester monomer on enamel and dentin. *Acta Biomater.* **2011**, *7*, 3187–3195. [CrossRef]
50. Yoshida, Y.; Inoue, S. Chemical analyses in dental adhesive technology. *Jpn. Dent. Sci. Rev.* **2012**, *48*, 141–152. [CrossRef]
51. Yoshida, Y.; Yoshihara, K.; Nagaoka, N.; Hayakawa, S.; Torii, Y.; Ogawa, T.; Osaka, A.; Van Meerbeek, B. Self-assembled nano-layering at the adhesive interface. *J. Dent. Res.* **2012**, *91*, 376–381. [CrossRef] [PubMed]
52. Yoshihara, K.; Nagaoka, N.; Yoshida, Y.; Van Meerbeek, B.; Hayakawa, S. Atomic level observation and structural analysis of phosphoric-acid ester interaction at dentin. *Acta Biomater.* **2019**, *97*, 544–556. [CrossRef] [PubMed]
53. Cardoso, M.V.; Chaudhari, A.; Yoshida, Y.; Van Meerbeek, B.; Naert, I.; Duyck, J. Bone tissue response to implant surfaces functionalized with phosphate-containing polymers. *Clin. Oral Implants Res.* **2014**, *25*, 91–100. [CrossRef] [PubMed]
54. Cardoso, M.V.; Chaudhari, A.; Yoshihara, K.; Mesquita, M.F.; Yoshida, Y.; Van Meerbeek, B.; Vandamme, K.; Duyck, J. Phosphorylated Pullulan Coating Enhances Titanium Implant Osseointegration in a Pig Model. *Int. J. Oral Maxillofac. Implants* **2017**, *32*, 282–290. [CrossRef] [PubMed]
55. Cardoso, M.V.; de Rycker, J.; Chaudhari, A.; Coutinho, E.; Yoshida, Y.; Van Meerbeek, B.; Mesquita, M.F.; da Silva, W.J.; Yoshihara, K.; Vandamme, K.; et al. Titanium implant functionalization with phosphate-containing polymers may favour in vivo osseointegration. *J. Clin. Periodontol.* **2017**, *44*, 950–960. [CrossRef] [PubMed]
56. Nagamoto, K.; Nakanishi, K.; Akasaka, T.; Abe, S.; Yoshihara, K.; Nakamura, M.; Hayashi, H.; Takemoto, S.; Tamura, M.; Kitagawa, Y.; et al. Investigation of a new implant surface modification using phosphorylated pullulan. *Front. Bioeng. Biotechnol.* **2024**, *12*, 1378039. [CrossRef] [PubMed]
57. Pedano, M.S.; Li, X.; Li, S.; Sun, Z.; Cokic, S.M.; Putzeys, E.; Yoshihara, K.; Yoshida, Y.; Chen, Z.; Van Landuyt, K.; et al. Freshly-mixed and setting calcium-silicate cements stimulate human dental pulp cells. *Dent. Mater.* **2018**, *34*, 797–808. [CrossRef] [PubMed]
58. Pedano, M.S.; Li, X.; Camargo, B.; Hauben, E.; De Vleeschauwer, S.; Yoshihara, K.; Van Landuyt, K.; Yoshida, Y.; Van Meerbeek, B. Injectable phosphopullulan-functionalized calcium-silicate cement for pulp-tissue engineering: An in-vivo and ex-vivo study. *Dent. Mater.* **2020**, *36*, 512–526. [CrossRef] [PubMed]

59. Islam, M.R.R.; Islam, R.; Liu, Y.; Toida, Y.; Yoshida, Y.; Sano, H.; Ahmed, H.M.A.; Tomokiyo, A. Biological evaluation of novel phosphorylated pullulan-based calcium hydroxide formulations as direct pulp capping materials: An in-vivo study on rat molars. *Int. Endod. J.* 2024. in printing.
60. Takahata, T.; Okihara, T.; Yoshida, Y.; Yoshihara, K.; Shiozaki, Y.; Yoshida, A.; Yamane, K.; Watanabe, N.; Yoshimura, M.; Nakamura, M.; et al. Bone engineering by phosphorylated-pullulan and β-TCP composite. *Biomed. Mater.* **2015**, *10*, 065009. [CrossRef]
61. Morimoto, Y.; Hasegawa, T.; Hongo, H.; Yamamoto, T.; Maruoka, H.; Haraguchi-Kitakamae, M.; Nakanishi, K.; Yamamoto, T.; Ishizu, H.; Shimizu, T.; et al. Phosphorylated pullulan promotes calcification during bone regeneration in the bone defects of rat tibiae. *Front. Bioeng. Biotechnol.* **2023**, *11*, 1243951. [CrossRef]
62. Satomi, T.; Ochi, Y.; Okihara, T.; Fujii, H.; Yoshida, Y.; Mominoki, K.; Hirayama, H.; Toyosawa, J.; Yamasaki, Y.; Kawano, S.; et al. Innovative submucosal injection solution for endoscopic resection with phosphorylated pullulan: A preclinical study. *Gastrointest. Endosc.* **2024**, *99*, 1039–1047. [CrossRef] [PubMed]

Disclaimer/Publisher's Note: The statements, opinions and data contained in all publications are solely those of the individual author(s) and contributor(s) and not of MDPI and/or the editor(s). MDPI and/or the editor(s) disclaim responsibility for any injury to people or property resulting from any ideas, methods, instructions or products referred to in the content.

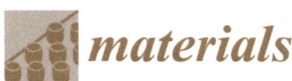 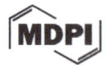

Systematic Review

Immediate Implant Placement with Soft Tissue Augmentation Using Acellular Dermal Matrix Versus Connective Tissue Graft: A Systematic Review and Meta-Analysis

Andrea Galve-Huertas *, Louis Decadt, Susana García-González, Federico Hernández-Alfaro and Samir Aboul-Hosn Centenero

Department of Oral and Maxillofacial Surgery, Universitat Internacional de Catalunya, 08195 Sant Cugat del Vallès, Spain; louis_decadt@uic.es (L.D.); susanagarcia@uic.es (S.G.-G.); samir@uic.es (S.A.-H.C.)
* Correspondence: andreagalve@uic.es

Abstract: This systematic review investigates the efficacy of using connective tissue grafting (CTG) versus an acellular dermal matrix (ADM) for soft tissue management in immediate implant placement (IIP). The study focuses on comparing the soft tissue thickness (STT) and keratinized tissue width (KTW) changes post-implantation. Adhering to the PRISMA guidelines, a comprehensive literature search was conducted, targeting randomized clinical trials and cohort studies involving soft tissue grafting in conjunction with IIP. Data extraction and analysis focused on STT and KTW measurements from baseline to follow-up intervals of at least 6 months. The statistical analyses included the weighted mean differences and heterogeneity assessments among the studies. The meta-analysis revealed no significant difference in the STT gain between CTG and ADM at 12 months, with the weighted mean differences favoring the control group but lacking statistical significance (CTG: 0.46 ± 0.53 mm, $p = 0.338$; ADM: 0.33 ± 0.44 mm, $p = 0.459$). The heterogeneity was high among the studies, with discrepancies notably influenced by individual study variations. Similarly, the changes in KTW were not significantly different between the two grafting materials. Conclusions: Both CTG and ADM are viable options for soft tissue management in IIP, with no significant difference in efficacy regarding the soft tissue thickness and keratinized tissue width outcomes. Future research should aim to minimize the heterogeneity and explore the long-term effects to better inform clinical decisions.

Keywords: immediate implant; soft tissue augmentation; acellular dermal matrix; connective tissue; single tooth; soft tissue thickness

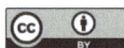

1. Introduction

Achieving optimal aesthetic outcomes in implant dentistry, particularly in the anterior region, remains a paramount goal for both clinicians and patients. Immediate implant placement (IIP) following tooth extraction has gained considerable attention due to its potential advantages in reducing the treatment time and preserving the peri-implant tissue [1–4].

Obtaining successful outcomes in the aesthetic zone demands meticulous planning, precise execution by clinicians with clinical experience and expertise, and the strategic management of soft tissue contours and biotypes. The restoration of missing teeth in the anterior maxilla demands not only osseointegration, but also the establishment of harmonious gingival contours that mimic natural dentition. Achieving and maintaining a stable soft tissue architecture around the implant is pivotal in creating a lifelike appearance and ensuring long-term aesthetic success [1–4].

A tooth extraction results in a series of changes occurring in the alveolar bone, which includes a bone remodeling phase. In the initial phase, due to the loss of the periodontal ligament and loss of the bundle bone, the lingual and buccal plate post-extraction undergo a series of changes that includes horizontal and vertical changes. In the anterior sector, this can compromise the aesthetics of the patient, especially if the extraction procedure was not atraumatic [5,6].

As a result of the volumetric changes, management to avoid unfavorable results has to be carried out [6].

Funato et al. describes and classifies the four scenarios in which immediate implants can be considered. However, he explains that extraction sockets with four walls show better aesthetic predictability [7]. On the other hand, Buser et al. describes protocols according to the time of placement, with the type 1 protocol involving immediate implant placement (IIP) directly into the alveolar socket via flapless implant placement with osseous augmentation and a connective tissue graft (CTG) or allograft, being a predictable approach [8].

Following the work of Chu et al., the classification of the different types of sockets has been used as a tool to aid clinicians in carrying out surgical interventions with several protocols known to fill the gap [9].

It is not only the management of hard tissue that must be considered in immediate implant therapy, but also that of soft tissue. This is due to the risk of deterioration in the soft tissue in the follow-up period; horizontal ridge deficiency, which results in the loss of the mid-facial contour; soft tissue recessions; and shine-through discoloration, leading to aesthetic compromises [10–12].

Considering the series of changes following a tooth extraction when placing an immediate implant, the patient characteristics also need to be evaluated, including the buccal position of the implant, the hard tissue status according to the classification of Chu et al., and the patient's phenotype [9,11].

Soft tissue was previously left untreated. Various studies have described results favoring the use of an autologous connective tissue graft (aCTG) when compared with the use of no soft tissue grafting on the peri-implant tissue's health and stability, due to decreasing the risk and prevalence of peri-implant mucositis and peri-implantitis by reducing the horizontal changes in the alveolar ridge. Moreover, it allows the maintenance of the tissue contour due to an increase in the soft tissue thickness, leading to a better aesthetic result from both the patient and clinician's point of view [13,14].

Soft tissue augmentation is recommended and has been established as part of the gold-standard protocol for immediate implant therapy, particularly for patients with a thin periodontal phenotype [15]. This phenotype is typically associated with a thin buccal bone, which undergoes greater bone resorption and soft tissue contraction in the postoperative phase [9,11]. However, autologous CTG sources are associated with disadvantages, such as postoperative pain and increased medication use, which can negatively affect patient-reported outcome measures (PROMs) [16,17].

Tavelli et al. found that various soft tissue grafting techniques, including free gingival grafts and connective tissue grafts, significantly increase the mucosal thickness around dental implants compared to sites without grafts, leading to improved peri-implant health and stability [18].

The use of an acellular dermal matrix (ADM) as an alternative method for soft tissue grafting has become more favorable, with the benefits not only favoring the clinician but also improving the PROMs in the postoperative stage following the surgical intervention [16,17]. In the case of a lack of sufficient donor material, the ADM has been developed as a substitute for the aCTG and has presented a potential alternative to thicken the peri-implant soft tissue. An ADM is a type of biomaterial derived from human or animal tissue that has been processed to remove cells, leaving behind the extracellular matrix (ECM). The ECM is composed of proteins such as collagen, elastin, and glycosaminoglycans, which provide structural support and signaling cues for tissue regeneration.

Following a study conducted by Stefanini et al. on soft tissue augmentation around implants, it was concluded that surgical sites undergoing soft tissue augmentation typically retain their soft tissue margins and marginal bone levels over time, whereas implants without augmentation may experience the recession of the soft tissue margin [19]. This study found that the clinical parameters remained stable over time for both CTG and ADM grafts. These findings are consistent with the results of Tommasato et al., who also reported increased an mucosal thickness postoperatively with ADM grafts [20].

One of the key advantages of an ADM is its ability to be integrated with the patient's own tissue, promoting natural healing and minimizing the risk of rejection [16–20].

For these reasons, the aim of this article is to investigate the critical aspects of IIP, focusing on the challenges that clinicians face in the management of soft tissue volumetric changes during immediate implant therapy, as well as looking for any changes in keratinized tissue when the two soft tissue substitutes are compared. Therefore, the objective of the present systematic review is to compare the effectiveness of CTG versus ADM for soft tissue management in IIP.

2. Materials and Methods

2.1. Clinical Question and Search Strategy

This systematic review was designed in accordance with the Preferred Reporting Items for Systematic Review and Meta-Analyses (PRISMA) 2020 statement (Table S1) [18], using the following population, intervention, comparison, outcome, study design (PICOS) model.

- Population (P): Healthy patients receiving an immediate implant due to the tooth being unrestorable with a simultaneous soft tissue graft in all sites of the mouth.
- Intervention (I): Soft tissue grafting with an ADM in conjunction with IIP.
- Comparison (C): Soft tissue grafting with an aCTG in conjunction with IIP; differences in soft tissue thickness and keratinized tissue changes under IIP with either an ADM or an aCTG.
- Outcome (O): The soft tissue thickness and keratinized tissue changes when comparing the different soft tissue graft materials from baseline, during the surgical act of placing the immediate implant, to the follow-up interval of a minimum of 6 months, using an analog or digital volumetric analysis.
- Study Design (S): To evaluate human randomized clinical trials (RCTs), with prospective/retrospective cohorts, that evaluate the peri-implant tissue following soft tissue augmentation with the different grafts.

The main question was, "In systemically healthy patients, being treated by means of single IIP with a simultaneous soft tissue augmentation procedure, is the soft tissue thickness and the keratinized tissue width affected by the type of soft tissue graft used when comparing an acellular dermal matrix graft to aCTG?"

Electronic and manual literature searches were conducted by two independent reviewers (LD and AG) in the National Library of Medicine (Medline via PubMed) [USA] for articles published up until March 2024.

The following search terms were used: ((("immediate"[All Fields] OR "immediately"[All Fields]) AND ("dental implants"[MeSH Terms] OR ("dental"[All Fields] AND "implants"[All Fields]) OR "dental implants"[All Fields]) AND ("soft"[All Fields] AND ("tissue s"[All Fields] OR "tissues"[MeSH Terms] OR "tissues"[All Fields] OR "tissue"[All Fields]) AND ("augment"[All Fields] OR "augmentation"[All Fields] OR "augmentations"[All Fields] OR "augmented"[All Fields] OR "augmenting"[All Fields] OR "augments"[All Fields]))) NOT ("embryo s"[All Fields] OR "embryoes"[All Fields] OR "embryonic structures"[MeSH Terms] OR ("embryonic"[All Fields] AND "structures"[All Fields]) OR "embryonic structures"[All Fields] OR "embryo"[All Fields] OR "embryos"[All Fields]).

The study was prospectively registered in the International Prospective Register of Systematic Reviews (PROSPERO) database (ID: CRD42024571855). Moreover, a flowchart illustrating the search strategy and selection process was created (Figure 1).

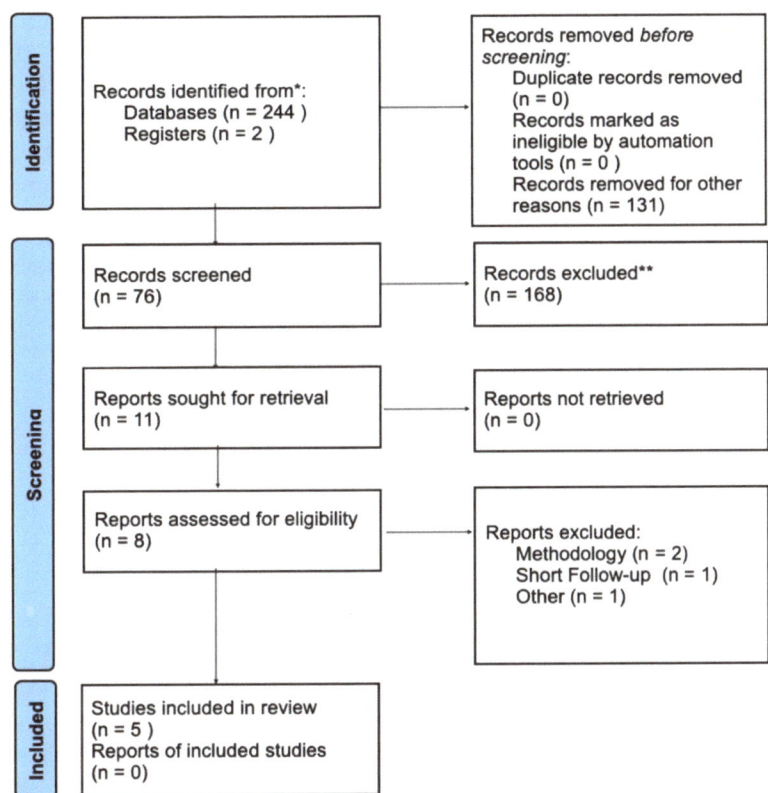

Figure 1. PRISMA flowchart of the search strategy. * Total amount of record identified. ** From the total amount of records identified, 168 Records were excluded after reviewing the abstacts of the studies found in the identification step.

2.2. Eligibility Criteria

The inclusion criteria were as follows: (1) publications in English; (2) human studies; (3) RCTs and prospective and retrospective cohort or case series studies where there were two groups to allow comparison; (4) the variables in the studies compared at least two groups of IIP + ADM versus IIP with aCTG; (5) healthy patients received an immediate implant with a soft tissue graft (CTG or ADM); (6) the studies had a minimum follow-up period of 6 months; (7) the reported outcome variables of the studies included the soft tissue thickness, the keratinized tissue width, and its standard deviation from the baseline to the follow-up interval.

Exclusion criteria: (1) studies that did not describe the outcome variables of the soft tissue thickness or keratinized tissue width; (2) studies that did not compare human ADMs versus aCTG as soft tissue substitutes in soft tissue augmentation in an immediate implant protocol; (3) publications in languages other than English, case reports, educational statements, expert opinions, animal studies, in vitro studies, narrative reviews on the subject of soft tissue grafting on immediate implants, or studies without a control group; (4) studies that did not provide any information concerning the research question.

2.3. Selection Process

In the first phase of the study selection, two reviewers (LD and AG) screened all identified titles and abstracts independently to assess their eligibility for the systematic review based on the predetermined inclusion and exclusion criteria.

In the second phase of study selection, the full-text articles of all studies identified in the first phase were retrieved and evaluated by the authors (LD and AG) on an independent basis. Any disagreements between the authors were resolved by discussion with two additional reviewers (SG and SAH).

2.4. Data Analysis

Full-text data extraction was performed independently for each eligible article by two reviewers (LD and AG).

The following variables were extracted from each study: (1) author(s); (2) year of publication; (3) type of study; (4) follow-up (FU); (5) study outcomes (soft tissue thickness, keratinized mucosa width, VAS, gingival biotype, pocket depth, peri-implant mucosal level, marginal bone level, bleeding index scores, perceived pain, VAS, and PES) (Table 1).

Additionally, the surgical protocol of each study was summarized and they were divided into a test group (ADM group) and control group (CTG): (1) author and year; (2) follow-up (FU); (3) number of implants; (4) methodology; (5) area of graft (palate or tuberosity); (6) flap or flawless design; (7) use of biomaterial or not; (8) gingival phenotype reported.

2.5. Risk of Bias and Quality of the Studies

Two reviewers (LD and AG) designed and assessed the proposal for the present project to ensure that the [21] guidelines were followed (Found in Supplementary Documents), as well as the use of the Strengthening the Reporting of Observational Studies in Epidemiology (STROBE) [22] statement. The STROBE statement is an international collaborative initiative for epidemiologists, methodologists, statisticians, researchers, and journal editors involved in the conduction and dissemination of observational studies and consists of a 22-item checklist to be fulfilled in a systematic review.

The quality of the included RCTs was established from the RCT checklist of the Cochrane Center and the Consolidated Standards of Reporting Trials (CONSORT) statement, which provided guidelines for the following parameters [23,24]: sequence generation; allocation concealment method; masking the examiner; addressing incomplete outcome data; free of selective outcome reporting.

2.6. Outcome Analysis

The primary outcome of the systematic review was the change in soft tissue thickness (STT) determined at the baseline and at the final follow-up, evaluated by comparing the volume through either an analogical method using manual calipers or K-files or by comparing digital STL files following an impression at both the baseline and follow-up periods.

The secondary outcome was the change in the keratinized mucosal width, evaluated using a periodontal probe, measured from the mucogingival junction towards the free gingival margin.

Table 1. Characteristics of included studies and methodologies used to obtain STT and KTW outcomes.

	Study Design	N° of Patients	N° of Implants	Tooth Replacement	Groups	Immediate Provisionalization	Follow-Up	Method of Measurement of Outcomes for STT and KTW
Panwar et al., 2021 [25]	Randomized Controlled Trial	20	20	Superior anterior zone (from second premolar to second premolar)	Group 1: IIP + ADM Group 2: IIP + CTG	None	6 m	1. Soft tissue thickness: use of Vernier calipers. 2. Keratinized mucosa width changes: use of a periodontal probe (measured from muco-gingival junction to mid-buccal gingival or per-implant mucosal level).
Happe et al., 2021 [26]	Randomized Controlled Trial	20	20	Superior anterior zone (from second premolar to second premolar)	Group 1: IIP + ADM Group 2: IIP + CTG	Not reported	12 m	1. Soft tissue thickness: superimposition of Standard Tessellation Language (STL) files in a digital imaging program.
Lee et al., 2023 [27]	Randomized Controlled Trial	30	30	Superior anterior zone (from second premolar to second premolar)	Group 1: IIP + ADM Group 2: IIP + CTG Group 3: IIP without graft	Healing abutment	12 m	1. Soft tissue thickness: use of endodontic files and use of digital impressions. 2. Keratinized mucosa width changes: use of a periodontal probe (measured from muco-gingival junction to mid-buccal gingival or per-implant mucosal level).
Abbas et al., 2020 [28]	Randomized Controlled Trial	14	14	Superior and inferior zone	Group 1: IIP + ADM Group 2: IIP + CTG	Temporary prothesis	12 m	1. KTW: use of a periodontal probe (measured from muco-gingival junction to mid-buccal gingival or per-implant mucosal level).
De Angelis et al., 2023 [29]	Prospective Clinical Trial	48	48	Superior anterior zone (from second premolar to second premolar)	Group 1: IIP + ADM Group 2: IIP + CTG	Depending on stability; 1 or 2 stages followed by a provisional.	12 m	1. Soft tissue thickness: use of endodontic files and use of digital impressions.

IIP: Immediate Implant Placement, CTG: Connective Tissue Graft, ADM: Acellular Dermal Matrix.

2.7. Statistical Analysis

A meta-analysis was carried out to estimate the global effect size (ΔSTT Baseline-12mo) in each of the groups. This was followed by a comparative intra-study meta-analysis between the two types of material, with the ADM being compared directly to CTG. Weighted mean differences (WMD) and 95% confidence intervals were calculated from random effects models with the DerSimonian and Laird estimator.

The results of the estimates, global effect measures, and confidence intervals are represented in the different forest graphs.

The heterogeneity index I^2 (percentage of variability in the estimated effect that could be attributed to heterogeneity of the true effects) and the corresponding statistical test of nullity of Q were applied. A threshold of $I^2 < 50\%$ was considered as an acceptable level of between-study heterogeneity. A forest plot was produced for each outcome to represent the difference graphically.

Publication bias was explored through funnel plots and the Egger test.

The level of significance used in the analyses was 5% ($\alpha = 0.05$).

The software used to carry out the meta-analysis was R 4.3.1 (R Core Team (2023), R: A language and environment for statistical computing, R Foundation for Statistical Computing, Vienna, Austria.

3. Results

3.1. Study Selection

The electronic search rendered 244 titles in total (Figure 1). One potentially eligible article was identified on the basis of a manual search. The gray literature did not result in any additional articles. Eleven articles of the remaining 76 were excluded after full-text analysis. The remaining eight articles were assessed for eligibility. Ultimately, five articles fully met the selection criteria for a qualitative analysis [25–29], as described in Table 1.

Exclusion was due to either the methodology or the primary outcome investigated. The articles of Guglielmi et al. [13] and Zuiderveld et al. [30] were excluded due to comparisons of soft tissue augmentation with an aCTG compared to no graft. Additionally, articles [31,32] were excluded due to the outcome variable not reflecting the outcome variable of this systematic review.

3.2. Intervention Types and Sample Characteristics

Table 1 illustrates the studies included. Four were RCT studies and one was a prospective study. All five studies were two-arm types comparing a test group (ADM) and control group (CTG) with IIP. The study of Lee et al. had three groups: test groups of IIP + CTG and IIP + ADM with a control of IIP placed with no graft (NG). Regarding the NG group, the data were excluded from this systematic review [27].

The total number of implants involved in the studies was 132: 66 in ADMs and 66 in CTG.

The main outcomes of the studies were the variations in the STT and KTW in both groups, with follow-up periods of a minimum of 6 months. Only some studies reported the mean variation with the SD, which was included in the meta-analysis [25,27,29]. For the meta-analysis, only three had 12-month information for the STT [25,27,29] and only one for the KTW [27]. Therefore, the statistical analysis was restricted to the variation in the STT at a follow-up period of 12 months, between the ADM group and the aCTG control group.

All surgeries were performed under local anesthesia, with the majority carrying out the surgery with a flapless approach, apart from Panwar et al. [25], where a non-traumatic extraction was carried out, followed by the debridement of the alveolar socket. All studies that were included in the systematic review used bone-level implants, leaving a buccal gap from the bone wall. Panwar et al. did not fill the gap with a biomaterial [25]. Three studies reported filling the gap with a xenograft [26,27,29]. Following this, the studies reported the division of two groups where an ADM graft was used and compared these to an aCTG obtained from the palate. Both grafts in all studies were sutured with sling sutures.

All studies had different rehabilitation procedures, with two studies not reporting provisional restoration rehabilitation [26,27]; however, all implants were reported as restored at 3 to 6 months postoperatively.

3.3. Soft Tissue Thickness Changes for CTG Group at 12 Months

The appropriate and valid studies for this analysis are described in Table 2.

Table 2. Studies involved in statistical analysis for soft tissue thickness in CTG at 12 months.

	n	Mean	SD
Happe et al., 2021 [26]	10	−0.6	0.49
Lee et al., 2023 [27]	15	0.8	0.26
De Angelis et al., 2023 [29]	24	1.16	0.41

Number (n); standard deviation (SD).

The STT gain estimate is 0.46 ± 0.53 mm, which not considered significant ($p = 0.388$) (Table 3).

Table 3. Meta-analysis results for STT in ADM group.

WM	SE	95% CI		Z (p-Value)	I^2	Q_H (p-Value)	Egger Test (p-Value)
0.46	0.53	−0.58	1.51	0.388	98.9%	<0.001 ***	0.013 *

WM: weighted mean; SE: standard error; CI: confidence interval; Z: Z-Test; QH: Cochrane's Q of heterogeneity. * $p < 0.05$; *** $p < 0.001$.

The forest plot also provides the relative weight of each study in the meta-analysis estimates. This illustrates that the three studies contributed to the calculations in a similar proportion (Figure 2).

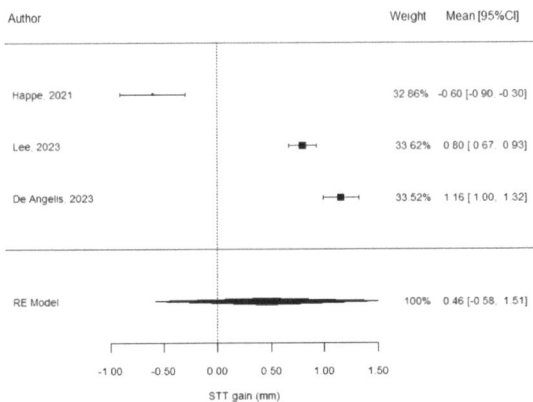

Figure 2. Forest plot for STT in the CTG group; Happe et al. [26], Lee et al. [27], De Angelis et al. [29].

The heterogeneity of the meta-analysis was found to be significant ($I^2 = 98.9\%$). The explanation for this lies in the great discrepancy between the results of Happe et al. [26] and those of the other two studies [31,33], whose confidence intervals did not intersect each other and hence the inter-study variability was, in general, much higher than the intra-study variability.

On the other hand, publication bias was detected ($p = 0.013$). This result was not conclusive due to the small number of articles, but the funnel graph shows asymmetry (Figure 3).

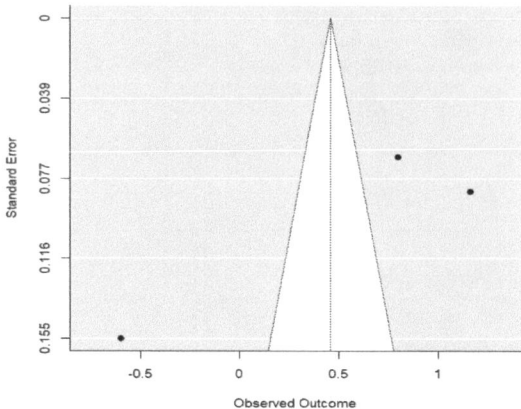

Figure 3. Funnel graph for the STT in the CTG group.

Due to the small number of implants and higher level of variability, Happe et al.'s study demonstrated a higher standard of error. When compared to the other two articles, the results appear more precise and exhibit the opposite correlation, reporting the true value of the soft tissue thickness.

3.4. Soft Tissue Thickness for ADM Group at 12 Months

Table 4 shows the appropriate and valid studies for this analysis.

Table 4. Studies involved in statistical analysis for soft tissue thickness in ADM at 12 months.

	n	Mean	SD
Happe et al., 2021 [26]	10	−0.55	0.33
Lee et al., 2023 [27]	15	0.86	0.36
De Angelis et al., 2023 [29]	24	0.66	0.31

Number (n); standard deviation (SD).

The forest plot (Figure 4) demonstrates an estimation of the results of the meta-analysis conducted for the soft tissue thickness in the ADM group at 12 months.

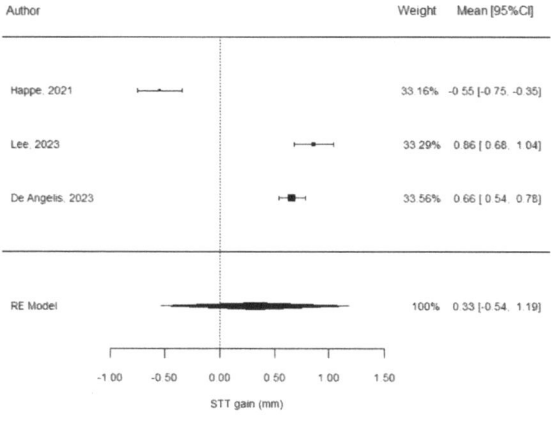

Figure 4. Forest plot for STT in the ADM group; Happe et al. [26], Lee et al. [27], De Angelis et al. [29].

The STT gain estimate for the ADM group was 0.33 ± 0.44 mm, and this value was also found not to be significant (p = 0.459) (Table 5).

Table 5. Meta-analysis results for STT in CTG group.

WM	SE	95% CI		Z (p-Value)	I^2	Q_H (p-Value)	Egger Test (p-Value)
0.33	0.44	−0.54	1.19	0.459	98.7%	<0.001 ***	0.434

WM: weighted mean; SE: standard error; CI: confidence interval; Z: Z-Test; QH: Cochrane's Q of heterogeneity. *** p < 0.001.

From the forest plot, it can be seen that each article contributed in a similar proportion (Figure 4).

There was a high level of heterogeneity among the values (I^2 = 98.7%). Following the trend in the other analysis, there was no correlation regarding the results between Happe et al. [26] and the other studies. In this part of the analysis, publication bias could not be detected. This was due to the three studies having a similar level of precision in regard to their analyses (Figure 5).

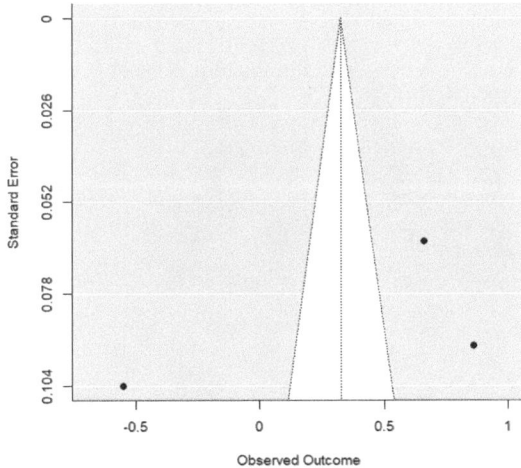

Figure 5. Funnel graph for the STT in the ADM group.

3.5. Soft Tissue Thickness Changes: ADM + IIP vs. CTG + IIP Intra-Study Comparison at 12 Months

The meta-analysis yielded a weighted mean difference (WMD) of −0.14 mm, favoring the control aCTG group, but with no significant statistical difference between the two groups (p = 0.490) (Table 6).

Table 6. Meta-analysis results for the mean differences in the STT gain according to the groups (ADM vs. CTG).

WM	SE	95% CI		Z (p-Value)	I^2	Q_H (p-Value)	Egger Test (p-Value)
−0.14	0.21	−0.55	0.26	0.493	86.8%	<0.001 ***	0.490

WM: weighted mean; SE: standard error; CI: confidence interval; Z: Z-Test; QH: Cochrane's Q of heterogeneity. *** p < 0.001.

The heterogeneity among the results was found to be high, as Happe et al. and Lee et al. obtained similar results when comparing both the CTG and ADM groups. However, this was not the case for De Angelis et al., who reported a greater gain in the soft tissue thickness with CTG (Figure 6).

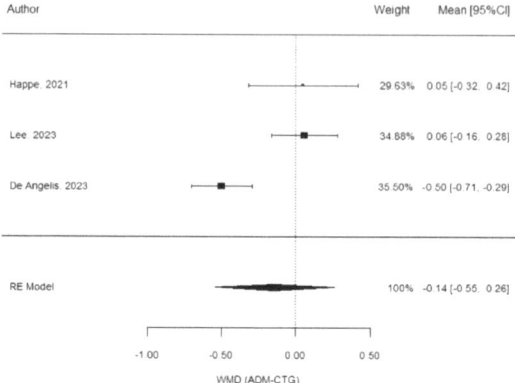

Figure 6. Forest plot for soft tissue thickness changes in ADM + IIP vs. CTG + IIP intra-study comparison at 12 months; Happe et al. [26], Lee et al. [27], De Angelis et al. [29].

There was also a small amount of publication bias found among the studies included (p = 0.490) (Figure 7).

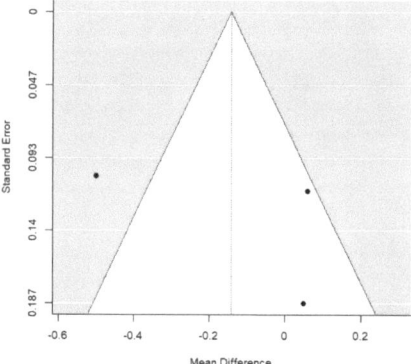

Figure 7. Funnel graph for the soft tissue thickness changes in the ADM + IIP vs. CTG + IIP intra-study comparison at 12 months.

For this reason, when comparing the use of the ADM and CTG when augmenting the soft tissue around the IIP, the soft tissue changes at 12 months showed similar average gains and no statistical difference.

3.6. Keratinized Tissue Width Changes

The results regarding the keratinized width changes reported in the selected studies are shown in Table 7.

The main findings were found in three of the five studies selected in the systematic review, with the results showing heterogeneity regarding when the keratinized tissue changes were reported [25,27,28].

Panwar et al. reported that the CTG group showed a statistically significant increase of 0.65 ± 0.0411 mm in the KTW; however, the gain was smaller than that found in the present literature. The reason for the reported decrease in the KTW in the ADM group was the use of a buccal flap advancement. The reason for this was to avoid the necrosis of the ADM graft due to having avascular properties compared to an aCTG [25].

Table 7. Selected studies evaluating keratinized tissue width changes.

		KMW Baseline (Mean ± SD)	KMW 6 m (Mean ± SD)	KMW 12 m (Mean ± SD)	KMW Difference at FU 6 m (Mean ± SD)	KMW Difference at FU 12 m (Mean ± SD)
Test	Panwar et al., 2021 [25]	3.200 ± 0.4216	2.950 ± 0.2838	NR	−0.250 ± 0.2635	NR
Control	Panwar et al., 2021 [25]	2.8 ± 0.788	3.400 ± 0.864	NR	0.65 ± 0.411	NR
Test	Lee et al., 2023 [27]	4.83 ± 1.32	NR	NR	NR	−0.80 ± 1.11
Control	Lee et al., 2023 [27]	4.70 ± 1.16	NR	NR	NR	−0.18 ± 1.07
Test	Abbas et al., 2020 [28]	4.786 ± 1.286	NR	4.429 ± 1.058	NR	NR
Control	Abbas et al., 2020 [28]	4.429 ± 1.397	NR	3.571 ± 1.397	NR	NR

KMW: keratinized tissue width; SD: standard deviation; NR: not reported; FU: follow-up; m: months.

Lee et al. [27] reported that, at the 12-month visit, the mean keratinized tissue widths were slightly decreased in the groups compared to the baseline. It was reported that the changes in the keratinized tissue width were not significantly different among the groups.

Abbas et al. [28] reported that there was no statistically significant difference found in the keratinized mucosa (KM) between the baseline, 4-month, and 12-month follow-up intervals in either Group 1 (ADM) or Group 2 (aCTG), with p-values of 0.338 and 0.156, respectively. Group 1 experienced a loss of 0.858 ± 1.199 mm in the KM, while Group 2 lost an average of 0.357 ± 1.488 mm. At the baseline, 4-month, and 12-month follow-up intervals, there was no statistically significant difference between the two groups, with p-values of 0.628, 0.598, and 0.220, respectively.

4. Discussion

Based on the literature analysis, there is limited published evidence comparing soft tissue augmentation between ADMs and aCTG in IIP. While there is abundant literature comparing the use of aCTG and ADMs independently or comparatively, especially around natural teeth, studies exploring techniques to enhance the gingival thickness around immediate implants are currently lacking.

The few clinical studies that do compare the two soft tissue graft options primarily evaluate the soft tissue thickness and keratinized tissue changes, while very few assess the PROMs or the PES score [25–29]. The studies by De Angelis et al., Aldhohrah et al., and Seyssens et al. demonstrate that using aCTG in IIP is more advantageous than not using a graft, improving the outcomes in terms of peri-implant marginal recession and marginal bone loss and increasing the soft tissue thickness [18,33,34]. To date, no systematic reviews have been published that solely assess the two soft tissue grafting options in the context of soft tissue augmentation during immediate implant therapy.

In this systematic review, five articles met the final inclusion criteria and were analyzed. Although there were limited data comparing the same primary outcomes, the studies chosen for the meta-analysis had a homogeneous methodology regarding their outcome variables, allowing for a quantitative analysis to be carried out evaluating the soft tissue thickness after 12 months [26,27,29]. A favorable aspect is that the studies involved had similar intervals and methodologies for the evaluation of the outcome variables, resulting in great homogeneity, which made the results highly comparable.

Regarding the soft tissue thickness, all studies investigated this outcome except for one [28]. The results of the meta-analysis showed that the STT for CTG + IIP was 0.46 ± 0.53 mm, and it was 0.33 ± 0.44 mm for ADM + IIP, indicating no statistical differences between the two groups reported across the meta-analysis [26,27,29]. The results of the meta-analysis demonstrated strong heterogeneity. Firstly, Happe et al. [26] reported results for each group that were significantly different from those of the other two articles. On the other hand, De Angelis et al. [29] were the only authors who reported the clear superiority of CTG compared to the other articles, which indicated greater homogeneity.

Concerning this outcome variable, great heterogeneity was observed between the studies, and the risk of bias was higher. This could be associated with the different follow-up intervals among the studies, as well as the varying methodological approaches to evaluating the soft tissue thickness and changes in keratinized tissue. Although all studies used either a manual caliper, endodontic files, or the superimposition of STLs using different types of digital software (Table 1), the heterogeneity in the methodologies regarding the outcome variable means that the results of each study should be interpreted with caution.

Additionally, the changes in the keratinized tissue width were evaluated in three studies. This outcome was considered as the secondary outcome [25,27,29].

Panwar et al. reported that there were no significant differences in the results when comparing thin and thick phenotype groups regarding keratinized mucosal changes. In the surgical protocol, a flap was raised to avoid exposing the ADM graft, which consequently led to a decrease in the amount of keratinized mucosa in the ADM + IIP group. Lee et al. reported that, in a flapless intervention, both groups resulted in a decrease in keratinized mucosa. It was noted that the ADM grafts were exposed during the healing phase or due to the submerged implant position. In contrast, Abbas et al. concluded that, when the phenotype was divided into thin and thick groups, the analysis of the two different grafts showed that they did not influence the width of the peri-implant keratinized tissue. No significant differences from the baseline to the 4- and 12-month follow-up intervals were reported. It was suggested that the patient's phenotype could affect the final amount of keratinized tissue, as well as raising the question of whether a larger graft size could influence the final result.

It has been reported that the use of a flapless technique shows a positive correlation with the keratinized gingiva thickness [35]; however, the act of raising a flap allows for more accurate implant placement [36]. Nevertheless, Grassi et al. reported that flap elevation does not seem to enhance the risk of increased bone levels, and there is a trend towards better results when using a flapless approach for peri-implant soft tissue [37].

Similarly, Park et al. [38] indicated that ADM grafts around implants in a delayed approach are a good alternative to increase the keratinized mucosa around dental implants. However, due to the lack of vascularity around dental implants, it is crucial for the ADM graft not to be exposed to allow for the integration of the graft within the peri-implant soft tissue following IIP [25]. Both Panwar et al. and Lee et al. experienced the exposure of the ADM grafts; Panwar et al. performed a flap to prevent the exposure and the consequent loss of keratinized tissue, while Lee et al. reported exposure during follow-ups, leading to necrosis and the loss of the grafts.

The results of this systematic review regarding changes in the keratinized width should be interpreted with caution due to the heterogeneity of the surgical protocols in each study, which has been shown to influence the results.

The overall success rate of the implants in this review was reported to be 100%, with minor complications noted in one of the studies [27]. The exposure of the grafts was also a common issue reported in these studies, which affected the final keratinized mucosa results.

The limitations of the present systematic review include the small number of studies that met the eligibility criteria, as well as the limited number of studies comparing the acellular dermal matrix as a substitute directly to an aCTG when performing soft tissue augmentation. Another limitation is the lack of a homogeneous methodology in the clinical studies when evaluating the outcome variables. Nevertheless, it was possible to conduct a thorough analysis of the most important outcomes of these five studies.

5. Conclusions

This review found that soft tissue augmentation using ADM with immediate implant placement (IIP) provides comparable results to connective tissue grafts (CTG) from the palate regarding soft tissue thickness and keratinized tissue changes.

1. Soft Tissue Thickness: ADM with IIP yields outcomes similar to CTG.
2. Keratinized Tissue: Comparable changes observed with ADM and CTG.
3. Research Needs: Additional RCTs and extended follow-ups are required to confirm long-term stability.

ADM appears viable as an alternative, though further studies are recommended.

Supplementary Materials: The following supporting information can be downloaded at: https://www.mdpi.com/article/10.3390/ma17215285/s1, Table S1: Prisma Main Checklist 2020, providing guidance for the systematic review [21].

Author Contributions: L.D. made substantial contributions to the study conception and design, data acquisition and analysis, and interpretation of the data. A.G.-H. made substantial contributions to the study conception and design, data acquisition and analysis, and interpretation of the data. S.G.-G. provided the final approval of the version for publication. S.A.-H.C. provided the final approval of the version for publication. F.H.-A. contributed to the critical review of the articles. All authors have read and agreed to the published version of the manuscript.

Funding: This research received no external funding.

Acknowledgments: The authors would like to thank Juan-Luis Gómez from Halley Statistics of Valencia Spain for his valuable contribution to the statistical work.

Conflicts of Interest: The authors declare no conflicts of interest.

References

1. Slagter, K.W.; Raghoebar, G.M.; Hentenaar, D.F.; Vissink, A.; Meijer, H.J. Immediate placement of single implants with or without immediate provisionalization in the maxillary aesthetic region: A 5-year comparative study. *J. Clin. Periodontol.* **2021**, *48*, 272–283. [CrossRef]
2. Tonetti, M.S.; Jung, R.E.; Avila-Ortiz, G.; Blanco, J.; Cosyn, J.; Fickl, S.; Figuero, E.; Goldstein, M.; Graziani, F.; Madianos, P.; et al. Management of the extraction socket and timing of implant placement: Consensus report and clinical recommendations of group 3 of the XV European Workshop in Periodontology. *J. Clin. Periodontol.* **2019**, *46* (Suppl. S21), 183–194. [CrossRef]
3. Slagter, K.W.; Meijer, H.J.A.; Bakker, N.A.; Vissink, A.; Raghoebar, G.M. Feasibility of immediate placement of single-tooth implants in the aesthetic zone: A 1-year randomized controlled trial. *J. Clin. Periodontol.* **2015**, *42*, 773–782. [CrossRef]
4. Slagter, K.W.; Raghoebar, G.M.; Bakker, N.A.; Vissink, A.; Meijer, H.J.A. Buccal bone thickness at dental implants in the aesthetic zone: A 1-year follow-up cone beam computed tomography study. *J. Cranio-Maxillofac. Surg.* **2017**, *45*, 13–19. [CrossRef]
5. Araújo, M.G.; Lindhe, J. Dimensional ridge alterations following tooth extraction. An experimental study in the dog. *J. Clin. Periodontol.* **2005**, *32*, 212–218. [CrossRef]
6. Tan, W.L.; Wong, T.L.T.; Wong, M.C.M.; Lang, N.P. A systematic review of post-extractional alveolar hard and soft tissue dimensional changes in humans. *Clin. Oral Implant. Res.* **2012**, *23* (Suppl. S5), 1–21. [CrossRef]
7. Funato, A.; Salama, M.A.; Ishikawa, T.; Garber, D.A.; Salama, H. Timing, Positioning, and Sequential Staging in Esthetic Implant Therapy: A Four-Dimensional Perspective. *Int. J. Periodontics Restor. Dent.* **2007**, *27*, 313–323.
8. Buser, D.; Chappuis, V.; Belser, U.C.; Chen, S. Implant placement post extraction in esthetic single tooth sites: When immediate, when early, when late? *Periodontology 2000* **2016**, *73*, 84–102. [CrossRef]
9. Chu, S.J.; Sarnachiaro, G.O.; Hochman, M.N.; Tarnow, D.P. Subclassification and Clinical Management of Extraction Sockets with Labial Dentoalveolar Dehiscence Defects. *Compend. Contin. Educ. Dent.* **2015**, *36*, 516, 518–520, 522.
10. Chen, S.T.; Buser, D. Clinical and esthetic outcomes of implants placed in postextraction sites. *Int. J. Oral Maxillofac. Implant.* **2009**, *24*, 186–217.
11. Chen, S.T.; Wilson, T.G., Jr.; Hämmerle, C.H.F. Immediate or early placement of implants following tooth extraction: Review of biologic basis, clinical procedures, and outcomes. *Int. J. Oral Maxillofac. Implant.* **2004**, *19*, 12–25.
12. Cosyn, J.; Eghbali, A.; Hermans, A.; Vervaeke, S.; De Bruyn, H.; Cleymaet, R. A 5-year prospective study on single immediate implants in the aesthetic zone. *J. Clin. Periodontol.* **2016**, *43*, 702–709. [CrossRef]

13. Guglielmi, D.; Di Domenico, G.L.; Aroca, S.; Vignoletti, F.; Ciaravino, V.; Donghia, R.; de Sanctis, M. Soft and hard tissue changes after immediate implant placement with or without a sub-epithelial connective tissue graft: Results from a 6-month pilot randomized controlled clinical trial. *J. Clin. Periodontol.* **2022**, *49*, 999–1011. [CrossRef]
14. Obreja, K.; Ramanauskaite, A.; Begic, A.; Galarraga-Vinueza, M.E.; Parvini, P.; Schwarz, F. The influence of soft-tissue volume grafting on the maintenance of peri-implant tissue health and stability. *Int. J. Implant. Dent.* **2021**, *7*, 15. [CrossRef]
15. Seyssens, L.; Eeckhout, C.; Cosyn, J. Immediate implant placement with or without socket grafting: A systematic review and meta-analysis. *Clin. Implant. Dent. Relat. Res.* **2022**, *24*, 339–351. [CrossRef]
16. Gargallo-Albiol, J.; Barootchi, S.; Tavelli, L.; Wang, H.-L. Efficacy of Xenogeneic Collagen Matrix to Augment Peri-implant Soft Tissue Thickness Compared with Autogenous Connective Tissue Graft: A Systematic Review and Meta-Analysis. *Int. J. Oral Maxillofac. Implant.* **2019**, *34*, 1059–1069. [CrossRef]
17. Thoma, D.S.; Zeltner, M.; Hilbe, M.; Hämmerle, C.H.F.; Hüsler, J.; Jung, R.E. Randomized controlled clinical study evaluating effectiveness and safety of a volume-stable collagen matrix compared to autogenous connective tissue grafts for soft tissue augmentation at implant sites. *J. Clin. Periodontol.* **2016**, *43*, 874–885. [CrossRef]
18. Tavelli, L.; Barootchi, S.; Di Gianfilippo, R.; Modarressi, M.; Cairo, F.; Wang, H.L. Peri-implant soft tissue phenotype modification and its impact on peri-implant health: A systematic review and network meta-analysis. *J. Periodontol.* **2023**, *94*, 12–25. [CrossRef]
19. Stefanini, M.; Felice, P.; Mazzotti, C.; Mounssif, I.; Pisa, C.; Wang, H.L.; Zucchelli, G. Do soft tissue augmentation techniques provide stable and favorable peri-implant conditions in the medium and long term? A systematic review. *Clin. Oral Implant. Res.* **2016**, *27*, 1293–1307. [CrossRef]
20. Tommasato, G.; Cavallucci, C.; Trullenque-Eriksson, A.; Baldini, N.; Felice, P. Autogenous graft versus collagen matrices for peri-implant soft tissue augmentation: A systematic review and network meta-analysis. *Clin. Oral Implant. Res.* **2023**, *34*, 388–402. [CrossRef]
21. Page, M.J.; McKenzie, J.E.; Bossuyt, P.M.; Boutron, I.; Hoffmann, T.C.; Mulrow, C.D.; Shamseer, L.; Tetzlaff, J.M.; Akl, E.A.; Brennan, S.E.; et al. The PRISMA 2020 statement: An updated guideline for reporting systematic reviews. *J. Clin. Epidemiol.* **2021**, *134*, 178–189. [CrossRef]
22. von Elm, E.; Altman, D.G.; Egger, M.; Pocock, S.J.; Gøtzsche, P.C.; Vandenbroucke, J.P.; STROBE Initiative. The Strengthening the Reporting of 447 Observational Studies in Epidemiology (STROBE) Statement: Guidelines for reporting observational studies. *Int. J. Surg.* **2014**, *12*, 1495–1499. [CrossRef]
23. Moher, D.; Hopewell, S.; Schulz, K.F.; Montori, V.; Gøtzsche, P.C.; Devereaux, P.J.; Elbourne, D.; Egger, M.; Altman, D.G. CONSORT 2010 explanation and elaboration: Updated guidelines for reporting parallel group randomised trials. *BMJ* **2010**, *340*, c869. [CrossRef]
24. Schulz, K.F.; Altman, D.G.; Moher, D.; CONSORT Group. CONSORT 2010 statement: Updated guidelines for reporting parallel group randomised trials. *BMJ* **2010**, *340*, c332. [CrossRef]
25. Panwar, M.; Kosala, M.; Malik, D.; Sharma, D. Comparison of acellular dermal matrix allografts and connective tissue autografts in soft-tissue augmentation around immediate implants: A pilot study. *Med. J. Armed Forces India* **2021**, *78*, S251–S257. [CrossRef]
26. Happe, A.; Debring, L.; Schmidt, A.; Fehmer, V.; Neugebauer, J. Immediate Implant Placement in Conjunction with Acellular Dermal Matrix or Connective Tissue Graft: A Randomized Controlled Clinical Volumetric Study. *Int. J. Periodontics Restor. Dent.* **2022**, *42*, 381–390. [CrossRef]
27. Lee, C.-T.; Tran, D.; Tsukiboshi, Y.; Min, S.; Kim, S.K.; Ayilavarapu, S.; Weltman, R. Clinical efficacy of soft-tissue augmentation on tissue preservation at immediate implant sites: A randomized controlled trial. *J. Clin. Periodontol.* **2023**, *50*, 1010–1020. [CrossRef]
28. Abbas, W.M.; Ali, F.M.; Elmahdi, F.M. Comparative Randomized Clinical Study of Acellular Dermal Matrix Allograft and Subepithelial Connective Tissue Graft Around Immediate Dental Implants: 12-Months Clinical and Esthetic Outcomes. *Egypt. Dent. J.* **2020**, *66*, 313–325. [CrossRef]
29. De Angelis, P.; Rella, E.; Manicone, P.F.; Liguori, M.G.; De Rosa, G.; Cavalcanti, C.; Galeazzi, N.; D'Addona, A. Xenogeneic collagen matrix versus connective tissue graft for soft tissue augmentation at immediately placed implants: A prospective clinical trial. *Int. J. Oral Maxillofac. Surg.* **2023**, *52*, 1097–1105. [CrossRef]
30. Zuiderveld, E.G.; van Nimwegen, W.G.; Meijer, H.J.A.; Jung, R.E.; Mühlemann, S.; Vissink, A.; Raghoebar, G.M. Effect of connective tissue grafting on buccal bone changes based on cone beam computed tomography scans in the esthetic zone of single immediate implants: A 1-year randomized controlled trial. *J. Periodontol.* **2021**, *92*, 553–561. [CrossRef]
31. Happe, A.; Schmidt, A.; Neugebauer, J. Peri-implant soft-tissue esthetic outcome after immediate implant placement in conjunction with xenogeneic acellular dermal matrix or connective tissue graft: A randomized controlled clinical study. *J. Esthet. Restor. Dent.* **2022**, *34*, 215–225. [CrossRef]
32. Puisys, A.; Deikuviene, J.; Vindasiute-Narbute, E.; Razukevicus, D.; Zvirblis, T.; Linkevicius, T. Connective tissue graft vs. porcine collagen matrix after immediate implant placement in esthetic area: A randomized clinical trial. *Clin. Implant. Dent. Relat. Res.* **2022**, *24*, 141–150. [CrossRef]
33. De Angelis, P.; Manicone, P.F.; Rella, E.; Liguori, M.G.; De Angelis, S.; Tancredi, S.; D'Addona, A. The effect of soft tissue augmentation on the clinical and radiographical outcomes following immediate implant placement and provisionalization: A systematic review and meta-analysis. *Int. J. Implant. Dent.* **2021**, *7*, 48. [CrossRef]
34. Aldhohrah, T.; Qin, G.; Liang, D.; Song, W.; Ge, L.; Mashrah, M.A.; Wang, L. Does simultaneous soft tissue augmentation around immediate or delayed dental implant placement using sub-epithelial connective tissue graft provide better outcomes compared

35. Puisys, A.; Linkevicius, T. The influence of mucosal tissue thickening on crestal bone stability around bone-level implants. A prospective controlled clinical trial. *Clin. Oral Implant. Res.* **2015**, *26*, 123–129. [CrossRef]
36. Barone, A.; Toti, P.; Piattelli, A.; Iezzi, G.; Derchi, G.; Covani, U. Extraction socket healing in humans after ridge preservation techniques: Comparison between flapless and flapped procedures in a randomized clinical trial. *J. Periodontol.* **2014**, *85*, 14–23. [CrossRef]
37. Grassi, F.R.; Grassi, R.; Rapone, B.; Alemanno, G.; Balena, A.; Kalemaj, Z. Dimensional changes of buccal bone plate in immediate implants inserted through open flap, open flap and bone grafting and flapless techniques: A cone-beam computed tomography randomized controlled clinical trial. *Clin. Oral Implant. Res.* **2019**, *30*, 1155–1164. [CrossRef]
38. Park, J.B. Increasing the width of keratinized mucosa around endosseous implant using acellular dermal matrix allograft. *Implant. Dent.* **2006**, *15*, 275–281. [CrossRef]

Disclaimer/Publisher's Note: The statements, opinions and data contained in all publications are solely those of the individual author(s) and contributor(s) and not of MDPI and/or the editor(s). MDPI and/or the editor(s) disclaim responsibility for any injury to people or property resulting from any ideas, methods, instructions or products referred to in the content.

MDPI AG
Grosspeteranlage 5
4052 Basel
Switzerland
Tel.: +41 61 683 77 34

Materials Editorial Office
E-mail: materials@mdpi.com
www.mdpi.com/journal/materials

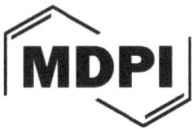

Disclaimer/Publisher's Note: The title and front matter of this reprint are at the discretion of the Guest Editor. The publisher is not responsible for their content or any associated concerns. The statements, opinions and data contained in all individual articles are solely those of the individual Editor and contributors and not of MDPI. MDPI disclaims responsibility for any injury to people or property resulting from any ideas, methods, instructions or products referred to in the content.

www.ingramcontent.com/pod-product-compliance
Lightning Source LLC
LaVergne TN
LVHW072358090526
838202LV00019B/2570